For Vera, with warm regards

David 1/90

Clinical Implications of ABNORMAL DIGESTIVE TRACT RADIOGRAPHS

DAVID A. MOROWITZ, M.D.

Clinical Professor of Medicine
Georgetown University Hospital and
Medical School
Senior Attending Physician
The Washington Hospital Center
Washington, D.C.

Clinical Implications of ABNORMAL DIGESTIVE TRACT RADIOGRAPHS

Lea & Febiger
Philadelphia • London
1990

Lea & Febiger
200 Chesterfield Parkway
Malvern, Pennsylvania 19355
U.S.A.
1-800-444-1785

Lea & Febiger (UK) Ltd.
145a Croydon Road
Beckenham, Kent BR3 3RB
U.K.

Library of Congress Cataloging in Publication Data

Morowitz, David A.
Clinical implications of abnormal digestive tract radiographs / David A. Morowitz.
p. cm.
ISBN 0-8121-1268-7
1. Digestive organs—Radiography. 2. Digestive organs—Diseases—Diagnosis. I. Title.
[DNLM: 1. Digestive System—pathology. 2. Digestive System—radiography. WI 141 M869c]
RC804.R6M67 1990
616.3'07572—dc20
DNLM/DLC
for Library of Congress 89-12982
CIP

PRINTED IN THE UNITED STATES OF AMERICA

Print number: 5 4 3 2 1

For Joel, Nancy, and Barbara

FOREWORD

"Of all treasures, knowledge is the most precious, for it can neither be stolen, given away, or consumed."

—Hitopadesa, *Good Advice* (12th-century India)

Perhaps more than any other profession, medicine is a lifelong learning process for physicians of all disciplines and all ages. And certainly as much as any professional activity, medicine has endeavored to teach and to instruct its students in newer knowledge and improved diagnostic and therapeutic methodology. Yet despite this dedication to the educational process, the challenge of effective medical education has not been met completely, and medicine continues to seek additional ways of imparting information useful in the care of the sick. This commitment is reflected in the numerous educational programs and in the many journals and ever-enlarging textbooks characterizing today's medical scene.

Here, Dr. Morowitz has developed a concise and informative approach to the recognition of important digestive problems. In this book he combines his extensive clinical and teaching experience with the visual quality of the x ray, certainly utilizing, in addition, his own unique skills in photography.

Some may quibble with this emphasis upon x rays and barium studies of the digestive tract in the 1980s and 1990s as "old fashioned" and perhaps less revealing than ultrasonography, computerized abdominal tomography, or magnetic resonance imaging. But these newer techniques notwithstanding, plain and barium x rays of the gastrointestinal tract, like the complete, careful history and examination of the patient, will remain with us for many years to come, and rightfully so. Furthermore, physicians do indeed have difficulty in correctly interpreting such potentially useful diagnostic material. Here then is an opportunity to learn a great deal, clinically and "roentgenologically," about many important diagnostic problems in gastroenterology, privately and painlessly. Physicians already experienced in this methodology will welcome the renewed sense of confidence provided by this well-organized material. Those readers who are in the process of developing their diagnostic and clinical skills will especially appreciate this opportunity to upgrade their contributions during rounds or at the patient's bedside.

Overall, Dr. Morowitz has produced a practical and highly informative overview of clinical gastroenterology, useful not only to the medical student, resident, and family doctor, but also to the gastrointestinal internist and his radiologist colleagues. *Clinical Implications of Abnormal Digestive Tract Radiographs* is a worthy addition to our current literature.

Joseph B. Kirsner, M.D., Ph.D., M.A.C.P.
Louis Block Distinguished Service
Professor of Medicine
The University of Chicago
Chicago, IL

PREFACE

This attempt to link the visual and factual in one area of medical practice was nourished by two closely held convictions. First, despite the availability of ever more complex imaging techniques, plain and barium x rays remain the safest, most economic, and in some ways, best method for examining the gastrointestinal tract. And second, while most physicians recognize their continuing need for the information necessary to practice good medicine, "the real world" presents its obstacles, among which are crowded waiting rooms, the issues of one's own personal life, phone messages awaiting response, the spectre of malpractice, and a desk heaped with charts, junk mail, and uncompleted insurance forms.

It is not surprising then that practitioners will choose to seek their science where it is made concentrated, clear, and pragmatic. However, in conventional texts, these worthy informational nuggets are typically buried amidst less usable data that reflect their author's intellectual pride and understandable wish for thoroughness. Also, most chapters are appended with dozens, sometimes even hundreds, of references. Their conspicuous exclusion here satisfies another personal prejudice: to the usual reader, such citations are valueless, like an extravagant display of unearned medals on a military tunic. Thus, while purchased dutifully and replaced by thicker, costlier descendants, most medical books fill more shelves than minds.

This is a concise collection of related x rays and essays in medical and surgical gastroenterology. The films are from a personal practice; the discussions, a synthesis of experience, reading, and intuition. Only common digestive tract disorders are presented, but certain rarer ones, with important diagnostic or pathophysiologic implications, are included. Some are omitted. The remarks on each illness are limited to around 300 words, the length of most written hospital or office consultations. The language strives to be colloquial and personalized, like an informal conversation between colleagues.

One issue does receive some extra attention. Today, every x ray omitted, lost, improperly read, or inadequately performed exposes the doctor to costly, heartbreaking, and often unjustified litigation for "failure to diagnose" and his patient to unimaginable harm of another kind. The poorly prepared large intestine, thickened gastric mucosa, or overlapping bowel loops may each conceal a hidden, perhaps curable cancer. Thus, if comments about obligatory skepticism, or what to worry about, or how to better utilize our diagnostic opportunities seem repetitive or overemphasized, to me they are justified.

In sum, this is not an exhaustive text, nor does it contain all that a responsible doctor should want to know about a patient's disease. I hope it will serve its reader as a kind of "tell me now what I need to know" survival kit, to be read quickly and comfortably and, like a series of letters between friends, to be easily understood and remembered.

Washington, D.C. David A. Morowitz

CONTENTS

CHAPTER 1

THE ESOPHAGUS

SLIDING HIATAL HERNIA, ESOPHAGITIS AND BENIGN STRICTURE

Esophagitis is the anatomic equivalent of "heartburn," and its typical etiology is a hypotensive gastroesophageal sphincter, allowing gastric acid to migrate into and burn an unprotected esophageal epithelium. A sliding hiatal hernia, ineffective peristalsis, impaired gastric emptying, or hypersecretion also may play a role. The hernia aside, uncomplicated esophagitis is usually radiologically subtle, but instead of a usually smooth barium outline, careful inspection of the distal esophageal mucosa may demonstrate patches of tiny, saw-tooth irregularities, correlating endoscopically with exudate, free bleeding, luminal narrowing, or occasional ulcerations.

Management of peptic esophagitis is anything but complex, utilizing an understanding of the simplest physicochemical principles: acid irritates unprotected tissue, alkali neutralizes acid, fluids obey the law of gravity and flow from areas of high pressure (intra-abdominal stomach) to low (intrathoracic esophagus). Patients therefore first need protracted antacid and H_2-receptor-blocker therapy. Minimizing gastroesophageal reflux requires a patient to lose weight if obese, to avoid large meals and restrictive abdominal garments, and to stay upright for several hours after eating; the head of the patient's bed should be elevated by several inches (a thick telephone directory?) and he or she should be counseled to sleep *left* side down, to retain gastric juice in the dependent greater curvature reservoir. The long-term value of promotility agents (metoclopramide, and eventually domperidone) must be balanced against their potential extrapyramidal toxicity. The major clinical issue in esophagitis is not bleeding or perforation but stricture formation, resulting from recurrent healing with fibrosis. On barium-swallow examinations, most benign stenoses are smoothly tapered, lacking the shelf, ridge, or shoulder of malignant tumors. Therapeutic bougie dilation in the presence of an active inflammation or ulcer seems to risk perforation, but this occurs rarely when the physician is experienced and uses dilators of gradually increasing diameter.

A link between chronic peptic esophagitis and esophageal cancer is not established, except where a biopsy adjacent to the stricture or ulceration shows columnar mucosa (Barrett's esophagus), which is another matter entirely. Any antireflux surgery should be reserved for the most accomplished surgeons and only the severely symptomatic, intractably sick patient.

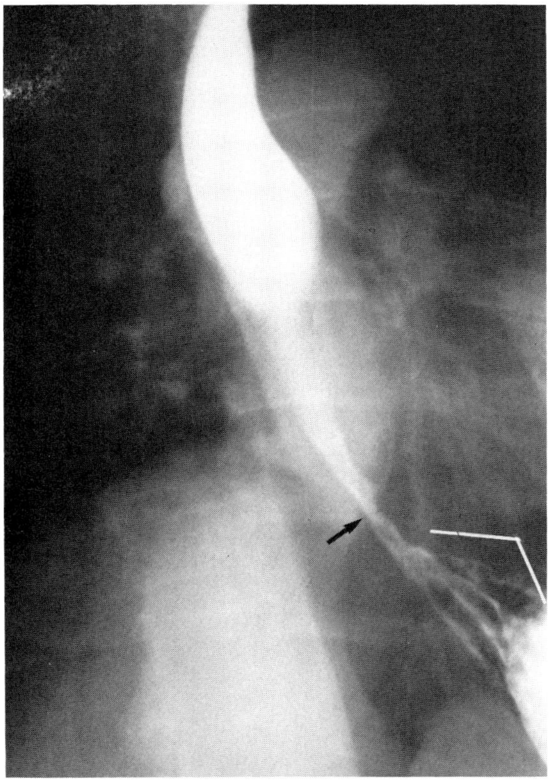

FIG. 1–1. A. Dilated upper esophagus, tapering slowly into a fixed circumferential stenosis above the diaphragm. Note gastric folds of hiatal hernia, prolapsing into thorax.

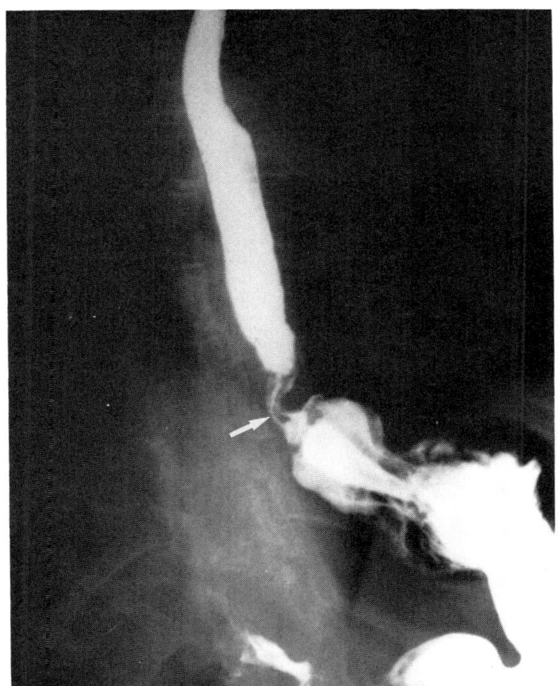

B. An early stricture of smaller length at the proximal end of a bulbous hiatal hernia.

PARAESOPHAGEAL HIATAL HERNIA

Occasionally, the portion of the stomach prolapsing upward into the chest is the fundus, specifically, the portion to the left of but not adjacent to the gastroesophageal junction. In the more common sliding (or axial) type, it is the cardia that herniates first, almost as though the esophagus pulled the uppermost stomach cephalad through the diaphragmatic hiatus. But, in the pure form of paraesophageal (or rolling) hiatal hernia, the fundus leads the way, shoehorning itself (Fig. 1–2A) through an enlarged diaphragmatic hiatus next to the body of the esophagus, while the gastroesophageal junction and the cardia stay where they belong (Fig. 1–2B). As the distal sphincter still straddles the diaphragm and its function typically remains intact, heartburn (esophagitis) or dysphagia (esophageal stricture) are uncommon. Symptoms, when present, are vague or nonspecific, such as retrosternal fullness after meals. Paraesophageal hernias are often found incidentally on a lateral chest x ray (Fig. 1–2C), where a large air shadow or horizontal fluid level suggests an enormous abscess or cavitary tumor. The amount of stomach capable of entry into the thorax can be astonishing, but the quiet presence of these hernias may be the prelude to a serious future.

Like its ligamentous attachment, the vascular supply to a large paraesophageal hiatal hernia is stretched excessively; painless GI bleeding from ischemic ulcers in the herniated fundus is the most common cause of anemia, rising from or in association with paraesophageal hernias. The hernias can also twist on their moorings, leading to volvulus. The only treatment of gastric bleeding or prophylaxis for volvulus, therefore, is surgical reduction of the hernia, which generally can be done successfully through the abdomen, with a low complication and recurrence rate. It should be remembered that this is not an antireflux procedure, but merely the pulling back of the stomach into the abdomen and the tightening of the diaphragmatic defect through which it passed, similar to the technique of inguinal hernia repair.

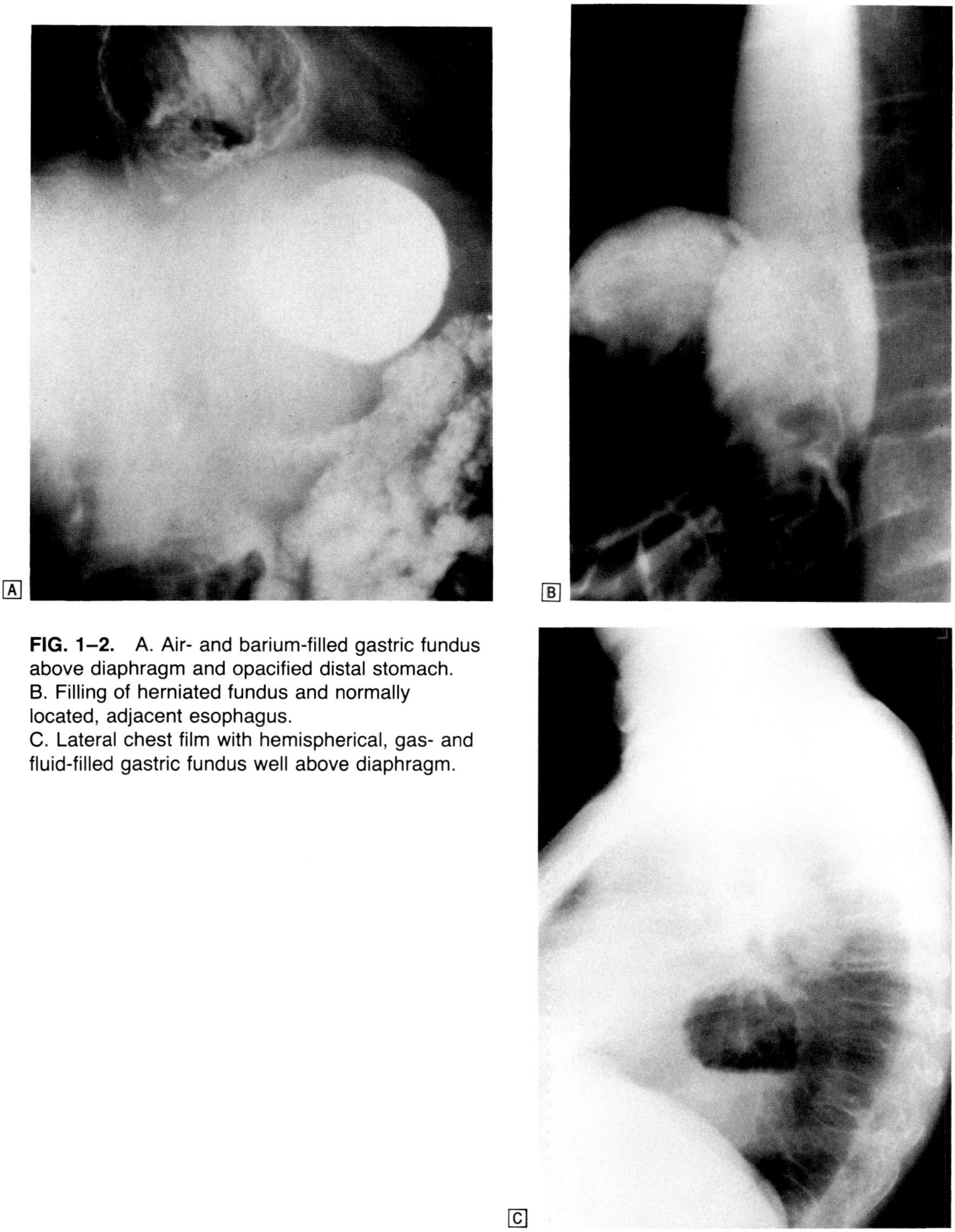

FIG. 1–2. A. Air- and barium-filled gastric fundus above diaphragm and opacified distal stomach.
B. Filling of herniated fundus and normally located, adjacent esophagus.
C. Lateral chest film with hemispherical, gas- and fluid-filled gastric fundus well above diaphragm.

BARRETT'S ESOPHAGUS

Often ulcerated, this mid or lower esophageal stricture is distinguished by a lining of columnar epithelium, resembling the glandular cells of gastric mucosa and, occasionally, that of the proximal small bowel. Typically seen in association with a sliding hiatal hernia, its mucin (not acid or pepsin) secretion may represent a mucosal adaptive response to chronic irritation of the lower esophagus. Dysphagia or odynophagia supervening on chronic heartburn therefore suggests the possibility of this fascinating stricture variant.

Radiologically, the lesions may look like carcinoma, and as any smooth or irregular esophageal stricture must be considered malignant until "proven" otherwise, esophagoscopy with brushings and multiple biopsies are mandatory. The rare adenocarcinomas of the esophagus probably originate from similar heterotopic glandular tissue. Because a small percentage of previously benign Barrett's lesions become malignant, the demonstration of benign columnar epithelium in a stricture, while temporarily reassuring, mandates continued careful observation. Even cellular atypia in Barrett's columnar epithelium is felt to be ominous.

Management includes accurate establishment of the diagnosis, full polytherapy of the esophagitis, and repetitive dilations of the stricture, all of which may be followed by regression of both symptoms and disappearance of stricture, columnar cells and all. Since comparison of stricture morphology using serial esophagograms is so important, one is well advised to have the patient retain his own films for review over the years. The propensity of radiology departments and physicians to mislay or "borrow" only the most critical films is a recurrent sad fact of the clinician's life.

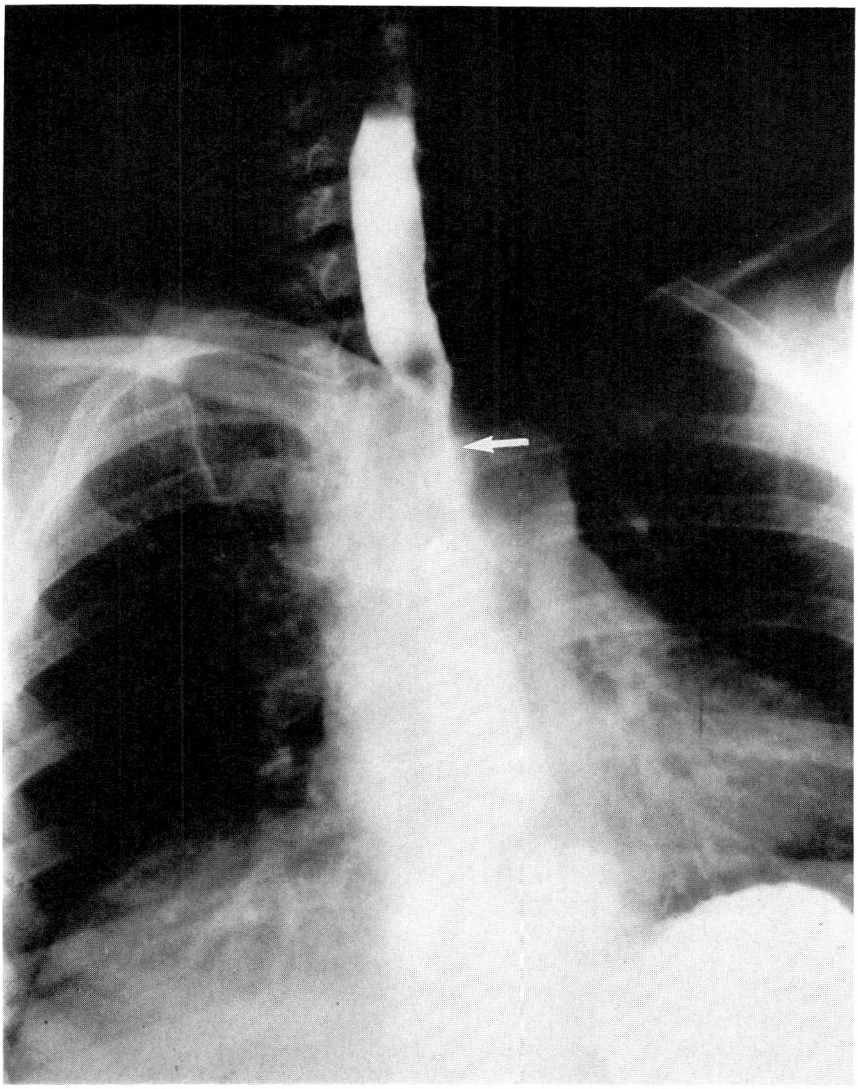

FIG. 1–3. Thickened, often ulcerated midesophageal stricture composed of benign columnar "gastric" epithelium. A sliding hiatal hernia is typically associated.

ESOPHAGEAL ULCER

Often located in the midst of or adjacent to regurgitant strictures, esophageal peptic ulcers are likewise a manifestation of severe or protracted esophagitis. They usually appear in the lower esophagus, typically with severe epigastric or retrosternal pain and odynophagia. The pain is more severe than in noncomplicated esophagitis and is relieved only fleetingly by antacids. Healing is commonly followed by stricture formation. These ulcers ordinarily follow a long history of regurgitation associated with a sliding hiatal hernia. The wise clinician also considers other underlying disease (gastric outlet obstruction, continuous vomiting, scleroderma), an antecedent event (protracted nasogastric intubation), or a gastric hypersecretory state (retained gastric antrum, Zollinger-Ellison syndrome).

Solitary ulcers of the esophagus may be infectious (herpetic) and occasionally appear in acquired immune deficiency syndrome (AIDS) patients, but not necessarily in association with candidiasis. Swallowed medication tablets adhering to the esophageal wall are increasingly recognized as caustic, producing an extraordinary focal mucosal disruption, and after healing, leaving a stricture. Patients with esophageal ulcers appearing de novo may relate a recent use of antibiotics in tablet form.

The distortion and edema of surrounding mucosa may resemble that of a typical stomach or duodenal ulcer, but this is a more serious disorder. The esophagus is thin, and transmural penetration (Fig. 1–4) can more easily occur in critical adjacent intrathoracic structures.

Since endoscopic biopsies of esophageal ulcers require a steady hand and a stout heart, cytologic brushings may seem preferable, particularly since they resolve the question of malignancy or virus almost as accurately as do biopsies, and are much safer. A link between chronic peptic esophagitis with ulcer formation and esophageal cancer is not established, except where adjacent biopsy shows columnar mucosa (Barrett's esophagus).

Antireflux surgery is more than justified in patients whose regurgitation is severe enough to produce ulceration, hemorrhage, or obstructive complications. However, this should be preceded by an attempt at maximum dietary medical management, to include promotility agents, antacids, H_2-receptor blockers, and mucosal protective agents in a demonstrably compliant patient. Despite the initial enthusiasm for infradiaphragmatic prostheses, the best antireflux operations still seem to mandate fundal plication and reduction of the hiatal hernia. Because of their inherent difficulty and formidable complication and recurrence rate, cases should be referred only to the most accomplished esophageal surgeons.

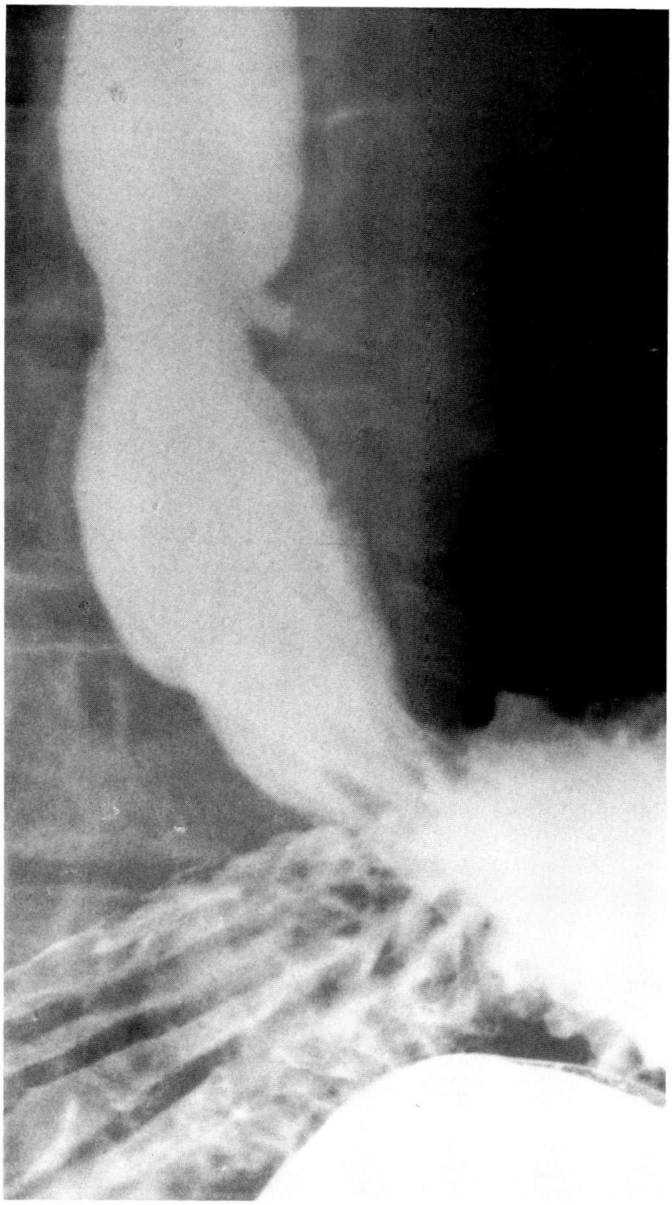

FIG. 1–4. Tiny, cylindrical collection of barium projecting out from the body of the esophagus, proximal to a hiatal hernia.

SCHATZKI'S RING

As originally described in the early 1950s, Schatzki's ring is a slender, circumferential narrowing of the most distal esophageal muscosa; the ring is probably the relatively less pliable squamocolumnar ridge at the junction of the stomach and esophagus. Its presence probably documents the intrathoracic displacement of a hiatal hernia (Fig. 1–5A). A more proximal, separate, and less clearly fixed "muscular" ring, which is clearly intraesophageal, does not necessarily connote a hiatal hernia, and may be seen with (Fig. 1–5B) or without its mucosal confrere. This ring may reflect only a localized, sustained hypertensive contraction.

Though not believed to be inflammatory, mucosal rings are often seen esophagoscopically beneath an inflamed or ulcerated esophageal mucosa, usually in an obese patient with a history of heartburn. They are demonstrated best on x ray, when the esophagus is filled with thick barium and the Valsalva maneuver is employed to force the upward prolapse of stomach. The typical symptom is intermittent, abbreviated dysphagia, particularly after hasty swallowing of poorly chewed, tenacious food. The sense of blockage usually passes after drinking liquids; occasionally, the bolus is regurgitated. The development of dysphagia in patients with either or both forms of this ring parallels the degree of luminal encroachment. If the distance between edges measures less than 12 mm, dysphagia is attributable to the ring.

In addition to the medical measures employed to manage esophagitis, the simplest therapy is bougienage, employing tapered, flexible dilators of gradually increasing diameter that, depending on the size of the patient, should widen to between 50 and 60 French (c. 17 to 20 mm). Restricturing occurs often; redilation can be done without significant risk, using gravity as a guide, with the patient lightly sedated and secured upright in an armchair. Laceration of the ring with biopsy forceps is rarely necessary. Pneumatic dilation conveys an unsupportable perforation risk.

Far more distressing is a food impaction, the culprit usually a wad of fibrous meat. Ineffective retching, salivation, and hiccuping are continuous. The agitated patient will often arrive at hospital emergency rooms at night, aware that something eaten has become "stuck" and able to point directly at its location. Episodes of food impaction often occur at banquets, perhaps relating to the quality of beef or the number of antecedent cocktails. Thanksgiving evenings are notorious.

Attempting to disimpact a food bolus by using endoscopic forceps to remove the meat or vegetable is laborious, time consuming, and rarely necessary. Swallowing a solution of meat tenderizer seems like a sensible approach; it almost never works. Gentle downward forcing of the impaction into the stomach by bougie is dramatically effective.

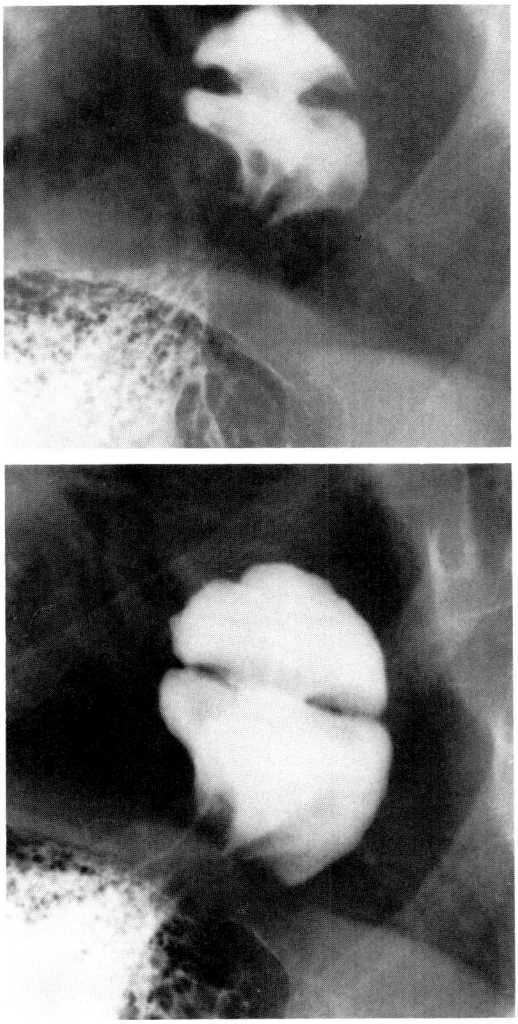

FIG. 1–5. A. Sequential spot films of circumferential, high grade, thin, mucosal stricture of the distal descending esophagus, demarcating its junction with a pouch of upwardly prolapsing stomach.

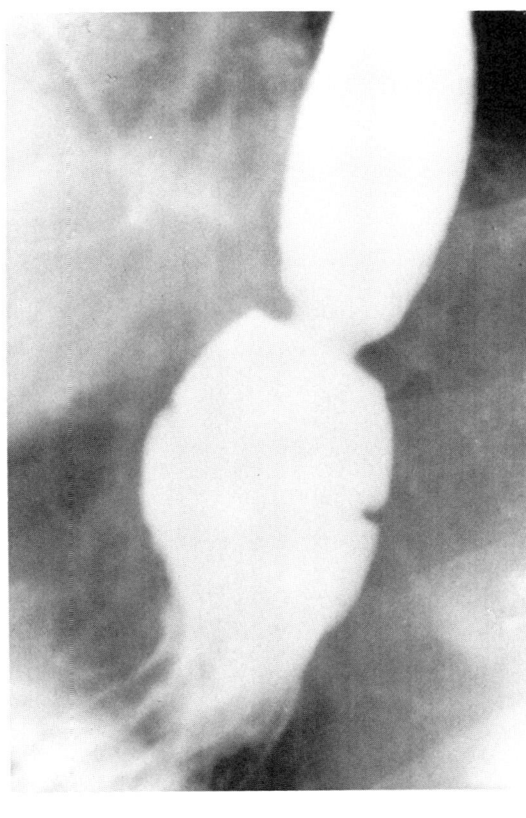

B. A slender, low-grade mucosal ring beneath superiorly located, thickened muscular ring. Slight irregularity of esophageal mucosa connotes esophagitis.

DIFFUSE ESOPHAGEAL SPASM

If compressive nonpropulsive GI motility is a cause of painful constipation, then diffuse esophageal spasm can be thought of as the irritable colon syndrome of the thorax. An almost exclusively physiologic (as opposed to anatomic) disorder, esophageal spasm as seen here (Fig. 1–6) may vary radiologically from a modest simultaneous rippling of the lower esophageal barium column to a highly convoluted, almost cork-screw deformity, almost as though a 20- or 30-fingered hand were rhythmically squeezing the gullet from without.

The clinical picture likewise varies widely. Often asymptomatic in longstanding diabetics and the elderly, hypertensive spasm from hypertrophied esophageal smooth muscle may produce intermittent disabling dysphagia and even esophageal obstruction. Most significant is its mimicking of acute coronary insufficiency, with central, squeezing chest pain, occasionally radiating laterally; partial or complete relief with nitrates; and prevention by calcium channel blockers. Its occurrence in the middle-aged or elderly and its potential induction by meals or emotional strain make this condition's symptom complex sufficiently worrisome to qualify it for a "Rule Out MI" ticket into a coronary unit. Even when the diagnosis of esophageal spasm seems established, coronary disease and cholelithiasis require consideration. The three conditions may also coexist; the prudent clinician must recall that only esophageal disease is guaranteed to be nonlethal.

Occasionally seen with hiatal hernia and regurgitation, spasm often follows gastric acid irritation of the esophagus. The actual motility abnormality is demonstrable by careful fluoroscopy using thick barium, while manometry shows sustained, high pressure, nonpropulsive contractions, and an occasional hypertensive gastroesophageal sphincter. Hyperresponsiveness to cholinergic stimuli (e.g., betanechol, methacholine) suggests an incomplete form of vagal denervation. Furthermore, in a significant portion of symptomatic patients, spasm progresses to achalasia, typically of the tonic or vigorous type, in which nonrelaxation of the lower esophageal sphincter and food retention are apparent. As achalasia responds to forceful pneumatic dilatation of the esophagus or surgical myotomy, the lesser muscular disruption accomplished by large bougie dilation is usually temporarily effective in esophageal spasm.

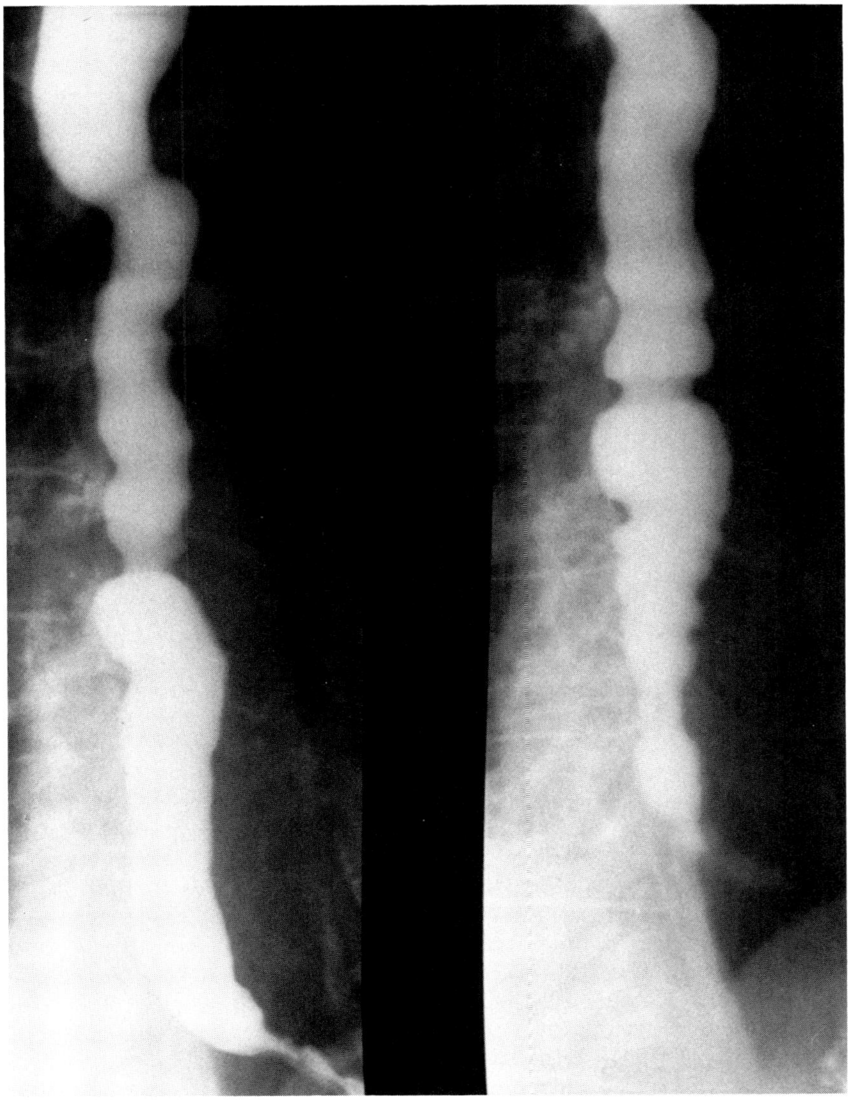

FIG. 1–6. Multiple broad ring-like constrictions of hypertensive, non-peristaltic waves.

ACHALASIA

Though its physiology is complex, the esophagus's missions are simple: orderly transport, impedance of gastroesophageal regurgitation, and accommodation to vomiting. It fails absolutely in achalasia, wherein peristalsis is lost in both smooth and striated muscle, and the gastroesophageal sphincter fails to relax with deglutition or emesis. Resulting from idiopathic degeneration or loss of the submucosal neural plexi, and resembling only the generalized smooth muscle motor disorder of Chagas' disease, the radiologic appearance of achalasia is never normal, with a full spectrum of disordered, always nonpropulsive motility, ranging from spasm to atony.

As this demented esophagus falls from an organ of transport to something akin to a vertical cistern, pneumonitis from aspiration may be revealed on the PA chest x ray; since air will perpetually float in the chest, untransmitted into the stomach in the upright patient, the same film may not show the typical gastric air bubble in the left upper quadrant, but rather a *cervical* air-fluid level and widening of the mediastinum. In advanced achalasia, the dilated esophagus kinks from side to side in the chest, assuming a "sigmoid" shape. Barium seen entering the esophagus here is dispersed amidst retained ancient food and saliva, trickling slowly in a thin stream down onto the gastric fundus. Yet, the tapering of the gastroesophageal junction in achalasia represents a *physiologic* stricture, and while potent enough to support a column of barium, it is gracefully smooth, unlike that of most fibrotic or tumorous stenoses. Gravity may protrude diverticula from the most dependent portions of the esophagus.

Though peristalsis is rarely restored, fluoroscopically observed dilation of the gastroesophageal junction by an inflatable balloon of fixed circumference is usually safe and provides sufficient sphincter muscle disruption to reduce or eliminate dysphagia in 70% of patients. Surgical vertical esophagomyotomy across the distal sphincter (Heller procedure) is more predictably successful, but the chest must be opened, and regurgitation may occur from too much incompetence. Also, once its serosa and muscle have been split by a scalpel, the esophagus can't be safely broached again by a balloon, should dysphagia recur. Either procedure should be preceded by thorough esophageal lavage. The use of calcium-channel blockers in esophageal hypermotility disorders has been advocated, as have been nitrates.

A few other points: the diagnosis of achalasia can be made with such certainty by x ray that esophageal motility testing is rarely required. Cancer of the esophagus developing in achalasia has been postulated, but its incidence is so low that multiple esophagoscopies or barium studies probably cannot be justified for reasons of early cancer detection. Conversely, an achalasia-like disorder can be seen when cancer of the gastric fundus involves and replaces adjacent esophageal neural plexi. Finally, I have never seen untreated achalasia and a sliding hiatal hernia coexist, and I'd love to know why.

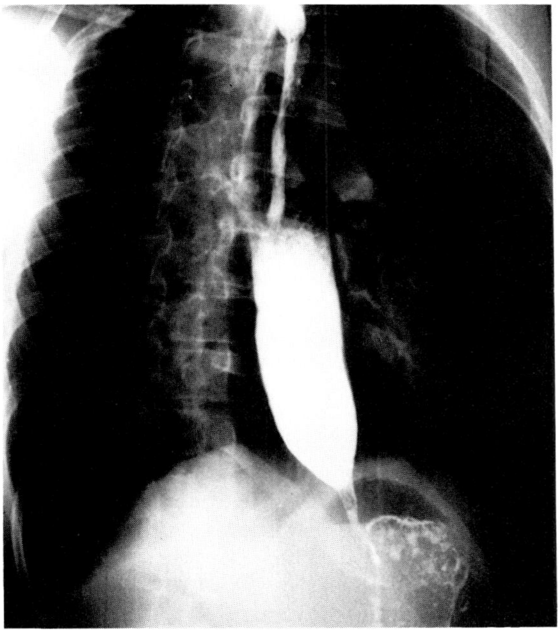

FIG. 1–7. A. Smoothly tapering, banana-shaped esophagus, with steady trickle of barium down posterior wall of the stomach.

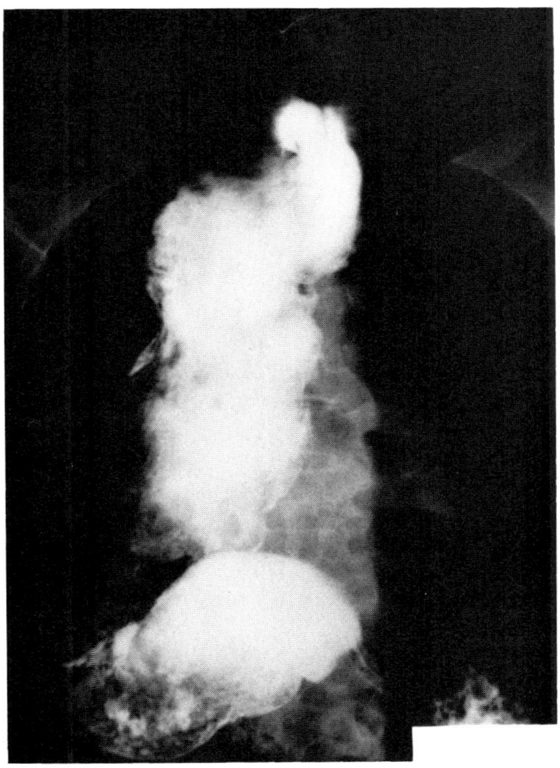

B. Sigmoid achalasia—markedly dilated esophagus, distended and kinked with the weight of chronically retained food.

SCLERODERMA

Dysphagia and pyrosis from esophageal hypoperistalsis is the commonest symptomatic digestive tract abnormality associated with progressive systemic sclerosis, and with the related CRST and Raynaud's syndromes. The atrophy of esophageal smooth muscle, characteristic of these diseases, diminishes propulsive motility, leaving the gullet's transport of food to unassisted gravity; the organ behaves much like the liquid cylinder of a carpenter's level. Atony of the gastroesophageal sphincter leads to regurgitation and intractable esophagitis, frequently resulting in organic-stricture formation, further worsening the dysphagia. While the barium esophagogram may show fine distal mucosal inflammatory serrations of peptic esophagitis with stricture or ulcer formation, usually only a smooth, modestly dilated, slow-to-empty esophagus is seen (Fig. 1–8) without the stasis of food, fluid, and saliva characteristic of achalasia.

Because progressive systemic sclerosis affects only smooth muscle, barium is cleared normally from the upper third and cervical esophagus. Retained contrast, when present, is seen in late chest films only in the distal two thirds, sometimes hours after swallowed. To make matters worse, hiatal hernias are commonly and inexplicably associated with scleroderma. To the careful clinician-radiographer, the ante barium chest x ray may show the scarred lungs of prior episodes of aspiration, intraesophageal air in the upright patient, or the associated pulmonary fibrosis, tissue wasting, and cardiomegaly of this multisystem disease.

While rarely necessary, esophageal manometric studies confirm the muscular hypotension by demonstrating feeble contractions, though invariably peristaltic, and little or no augmentation of resting pressure at the GI junction.

Because their smooth-muscle target organ has largely disappeared, promotility agents are of little value; on the other hand (and bright side), antacids are retained longer in the stomach and esophagus and probably afford better overall mucosal protection than if they were transported rapidly. H_2-receptor blockers in liquid or crushed-tablet form are a godsend.

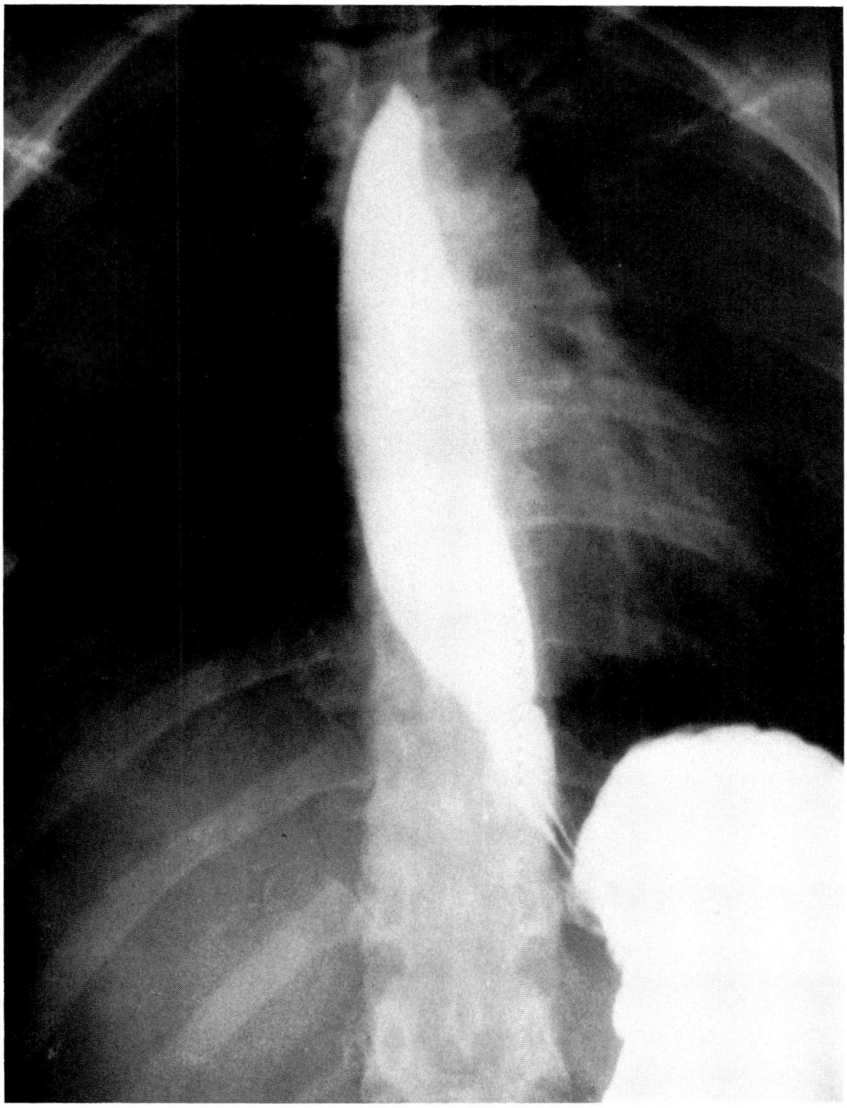

FIG. 1–8. Dilated featureless esophagus, slow to empty. Smooth contour denotes absent propulsion. Note small sliding hiatal hernia.

NEUROMUSCULAR DISORDERS OF THE ESOPHAGUS

These illnesses are typically manifested by cervical dysphagia, which results either in malnutrition or repetitive episodes of pulmonary aspiration. Etiologies, understandably, are multiple, relating either to the initiation, transmission, or completion of voluntary or involuntary swallowing. Accordingly, they may arise from dementia with brain infarction, bulbar polio, amyotrophic lateral sclerosis, any spinal muscular atrophic disease, myasthenia gravis, myotonic dystrophy, or inflammatory disorders of skeletal muscle. Apart from the history, the physical examination of the patient may provide valuable clues, which often include the following: muscle weakness or atrophy; fasciculations; an adenoid facies; a tentative, nasal voice; eyelid ptosis; foul breath; the pooling of oropharyngeal secretions; and retained food in the mouth.

On x ray, these disorders are frequently manifested by aspiration of barium into the trachea because of the inability of the epiglottis to occlude the respiratory tree. Because of defective muscular clearing, residual barium will appear in the pyriform sinuses, valleculae, and upper esophagus from minutes to hours after the x ray is done (Fig. 1–9). Diagnosis of these disorders is to be considered whenever dysphagia is present without an obvious organic stenosis.

Watching the swallowing efforts may be helpful. Most patients with skeletal muscle weakness will learn to avoid aspiration by throwing their head back, hurtling food into the esophagus across a paralyzed epiglottis and exposed tracheal orifice. Inability to perform this maneuver successfully with liquids makes patients with skeletal muscle weakness describe greater difficulty (i.e., cough) with liquids than with solids, unlike the patient with an organic stricture of the esophagus or upper stomach.

Weakened, backward propulsion of food by the pharynx (transfer dysphagia) is seen most commonly in the elderly patient with ischemic central nervous system disease, usually with a history of multiple strokes, pseudobulbar palsy, or senile dementia. Recurrent episodes of aspiration are often present, and food is often found retained in the mouth for hours. It is extremely difficult to manage. Feeding gastrostomy is almost always necessary; even that will not prevent aspiration of saliva. In the myasthenic (Eaton-Lambert) syndrome, the abnormal barium esophagogram may also show simultaneous bronchogenic carcinoma or pulmonary metastases.

Patients with globus hystericus will complain of a lump in the throat, but rarely of an actual difficulty in swallowing. Experienced clinicians will usually suspect psychogenic factors, particularly when the x ray reveals nothing abnormal. Patients rarely refuse to swallow barium, and most patients have no associated nutritional consequences.

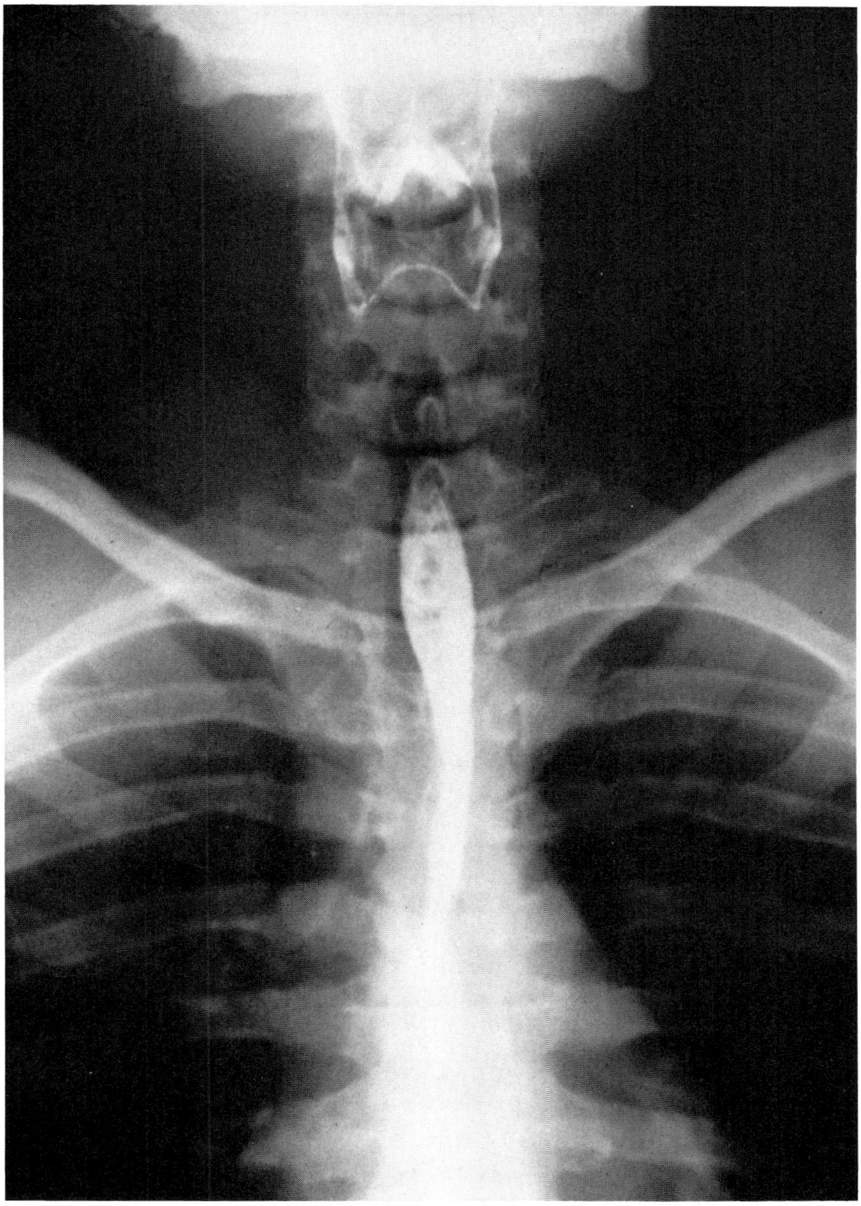

FIG. 1–9. Late film showing residual barium coating the skeletal muscle (upper third) portion of the esophagus, as well as the pharynx and valleculae.

CARCINOMA OF THE MID-ESOPHAGUS

This is an overwhelmingly fatal disease whose demographic and social implications seem as striking as the pathologic. Four to five times more common in blacks, particularly those in cities, and strongly associated with alcoholism and excessive, chronic tobacco use, epidermoid cancer of the esophagus, like pulmonary tuberculosis in earlier decades, can be thought of as a disease of poverty. The commonest symptom is dysphagia, which when brought to a physician's attention is almost always severe enough to effect significant change in alimentation, usually from foods of decreasing texture to liquids. Some patients present already unable to swallow their saliva. The frequently silent tolerance of worsening dysphagia remains one of clinical medicine's more conspicuous mysteries.

The disease is manifested radiologically first by decreased distensibility or peristalsis in the involved segment and then by the thinnest, usually irregular luminal ingrowth of tumor. Eventually they evolve into bulky, lobulated hemorrhagic and obstructive masses that can penetrate the mediastinum or tracheobronchial tree. Early diagnosis depends on vigorous pursuit of dysphagia of any kind, particularly when the patient admits to conscious alteration in the choice of food. Even if the initial endoscopy is visually negative, deep esophageal biopsies are reasonable on the chance that some retrievable portion of the tumor is submucosal.

The contemporary diagnostic approach is a "troika": barium swallow to identify dysphagia's cause as anatomic, endoscopy to obtain confirmatory tissue, later to aid in bougie dilatation, laser or heater probe ablation, and CT scanning for tumor staging, particularly to assess mediastinal invasion or periesophageal lymph node involvement. Tissue diagnosis remains relatively easy. Endoscopic esophageal biopsies and cytology are each positive in greater than 95% of patients.

In the first film (Fig. 1–10A), the tiniest tumor shoulder, measuring no more than 2 mm at the upper border of the lesion, is seen pushing inward. Though the lumen appears only a bit narrowed, esophageal stiffening has obliterated peristalsis, compounding the encroachment, permitting only a trickle of contrast past the tumor, and certainly preventing transport of a solid bolus. Relatively mobile, the esophagus is rarely penetrated by a bronchogenic lesion; the adjacent, fixed aorta and tracheobronchial tree (Fig. 1–10B) are likely targets of fistulous perforation by esophageal cancer.

Large, symptomatic tumors are nearly always incurable. Though palliation is the goal, resection is sometimes justified to restore the blessing of easy swallowing to a dying patient, even when local or distant metastases are found. Nonoperative palliation (drugs) is directed at a reduction of primary or metastatic tumor mass and the maintenance of luminal patency by x-irradiation, sequential bougie dilation, or tumor necrosis induced with bicap heater probe or laser therapy. As one cannot know exactly what is on the serosal side of the lesion, local tissue-destructive treatments may be followed by perforation.

Endoscopically placed, funnel-shaped luminal stents are best employed to straddle the tumor in patients with esophagotracheal fistulas; this is a difficult, painful, and frightening procedure. Moreover, once the stent is implanted (across the tumor, one would hope), it is almost impossible to adjust or retrieve, particularly if incorrectly located.

If the cancer is discovered while surveying the asymptomatic patient with "premalignant" Plummer-Vinson syndrome, Barrett's esophagus, or an old lye stricture, the chance for surgical cure is appreciably greater.

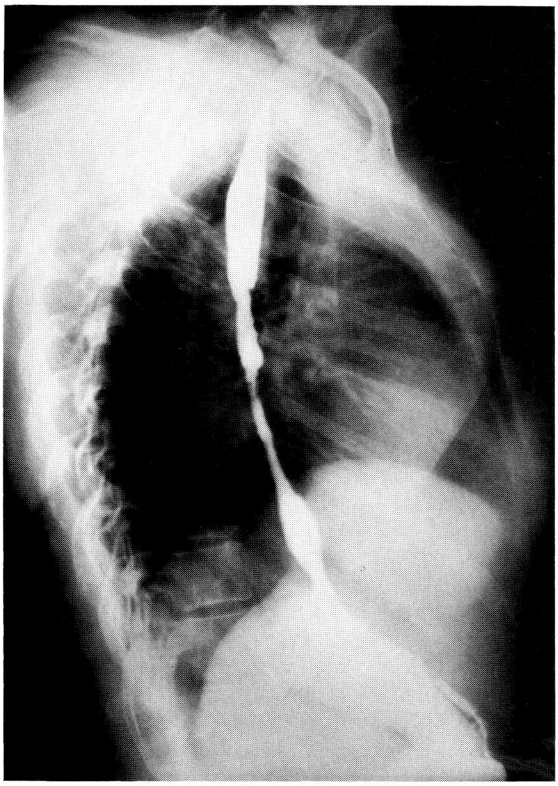

FIG. 1–10. A. Circumferential irregular stenosis allowing a mere trickle of barium below the lower edge of the tumor. Note the increased AP diameter of the thorax, consistent with a lengthy tobacco history, a risk factor in esophageal cancer.

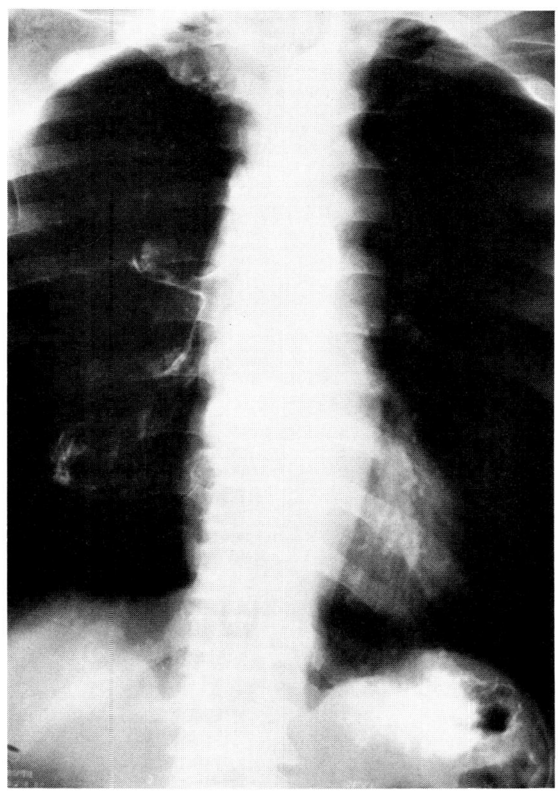

B. Barium swallow showing flow of barium into stomach with a substantial portion entering the right main stem bronchus and outlining the tracheobronchial tree on that side.

ADENOCARCINOMA OF THE GASTROESOPHAGEAL JUNCTION

Like other organic diseases that seem almost psychopathically murderous, this disorder's appalling qualities include surreptitious onset, deceptive progression, cruel symptomatology, therapeutic recalcitrance, and painful outcome. It often begins as a tiny primary tumor in the gastric cardia or fundus; while actively dissecting retrograde *under* the esophageal mucosa, this condition can be overlooked by a first upper GI series or endoscopy. Thus, persistent "distal" dysphagia, in the absence of an obvious esophageal obstruction, may argue for biopsies (with mucin stains) of an seemingly normal or minimally granular gastroesophageal junction or distal esophagus.

As seen here (Fig. 1–11), the first radiologic clues to diagnosis are fixation or rigidity of the distal esophagus or GE junction, followed by spiculation, centripetal luminal narrowing, and, eventually, gross mucosal irregularity. Because of its penchant to involve much distal esophagus before becoming symptomatic, the tumor typically is unresectable. If operative palliation is attempted, however, the surgeon must employ intraoperative frozen-section examinations to select a tumor-free proximal edge of esophagus for anastomosis. Because of the risk of postoperative aspiration from a gastric pouch lacking an upper sphincter, total gastrectomy seems advisable. Late dysphagia after operation is almost invariably a feature of local recurrent cancer.

Like carcinoma of the cervical esophagus, this is one of the most disappointing GI malignancies to manage. Surgical treatment is dreadful; radiotherapy adds vomiting and esophagitis to dysphagia, and chemotherapeutic regimens seem to shorten or worsen an already miserable, attenuated life. Maintaining a lumen by laser or heater-probe tumor necrosis, or with stent implacement, if possible, is valuable, as is feeding gastrostomy.

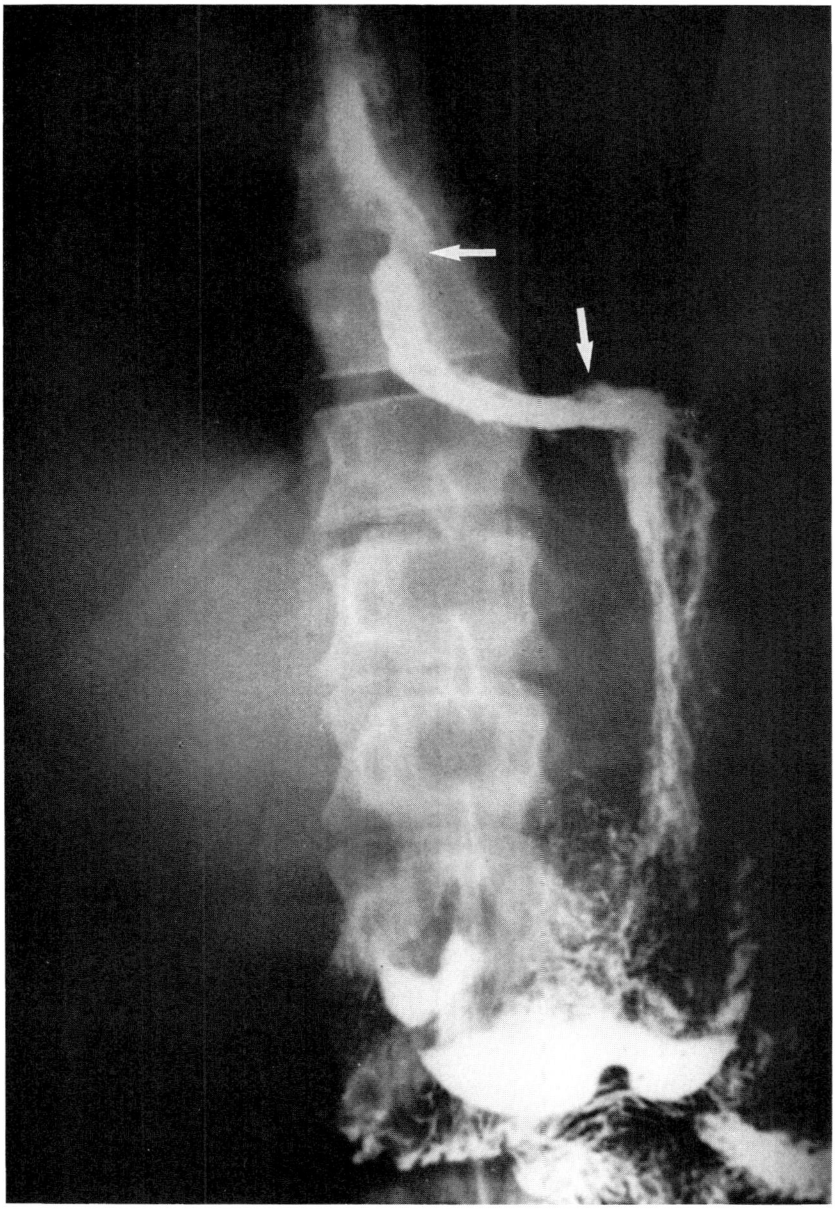

FIG. 1–11. Fixed, tubular transformation of gastroesophageal junction with irregular mucosal spiculation, extending above and below the diaphragm.

CARCINOMA OF THE CERVICAL ESOPHAGUS

Lacking the assistance of gravity, which would accrue to food passing through a filled, distended esophagus obstructed at its distal end, food can only be extruded past a proximal occlusion by the propulsive power of the patient's tongue. Another conspicuously cruel disease, one that is often accompanied by recurrent tracheal aspiration, epidermoid carcinomas of the cervical esophagus (Fig. 1–12) are almost all fatal; most clinicians will direct attention from the usual hopelessness of cure toward the several, sometimes significant, opportunities for palliation. Combined x-ray therapy and chemotherapy can be astonishingly effective, particularly when combined with regular tumor dilation by bougie. When the disease is recalcitrant, heater-probe or laser obliteration of tumor is used for luminal maintenance. The wide proximal edge of a luminal stent resting in the throat or cervical esophagus is generally too annoying to be tolerated.

Occasionally, the approach is so successful, the doctor directing traffic might find subsequent esophagectomy tempting, though the operative mortality may be 20 times the "cure" rate. The radical surgical removal of this lesion requires laryngectomy and near total esophagectomy, with the "swing-up" of an interposition of loop of colon, perhaps with a further prosthetic skin flap constructed from the patient's neck.

Successful conventional fiberoptic endoscopy of upper esophageal lesions is trying; obtaining the coughing patient's cooperation in swallowing is as difficult as it is necessary. Even if the patient can be intubated, the optical lens at the instrument's tip sometimes is conveyed flush against the obstruction, obliterating visualization.

Thus, after seeing an x ray like this many gastroenterologists will call on an otolaryngologist or thoracic surgeon, so that a proper examination can be done under direct inspection using general anesthesia. Bronchoscopy can be done at the same time, assessing for tracheal involvement by tumor, which, like CT scan or mediastinoscopy, will indicate inoperability.

Some upper esophageal cancers are extrinsic; these usually originate in the thyroid, circumferentially "strangling" the upper gullet. The barium column then tends to be smoothly, albeit dramatically, narrowed. These tend to be poorly differentiated, spindle-cell (not papillary) tumors, unresponsive to radioiodine and manageable only by feeding gastrostomy and salivary bypass via pharyngostomy. A benign substernal thyroid will deflect, but never invade, the esophagus.

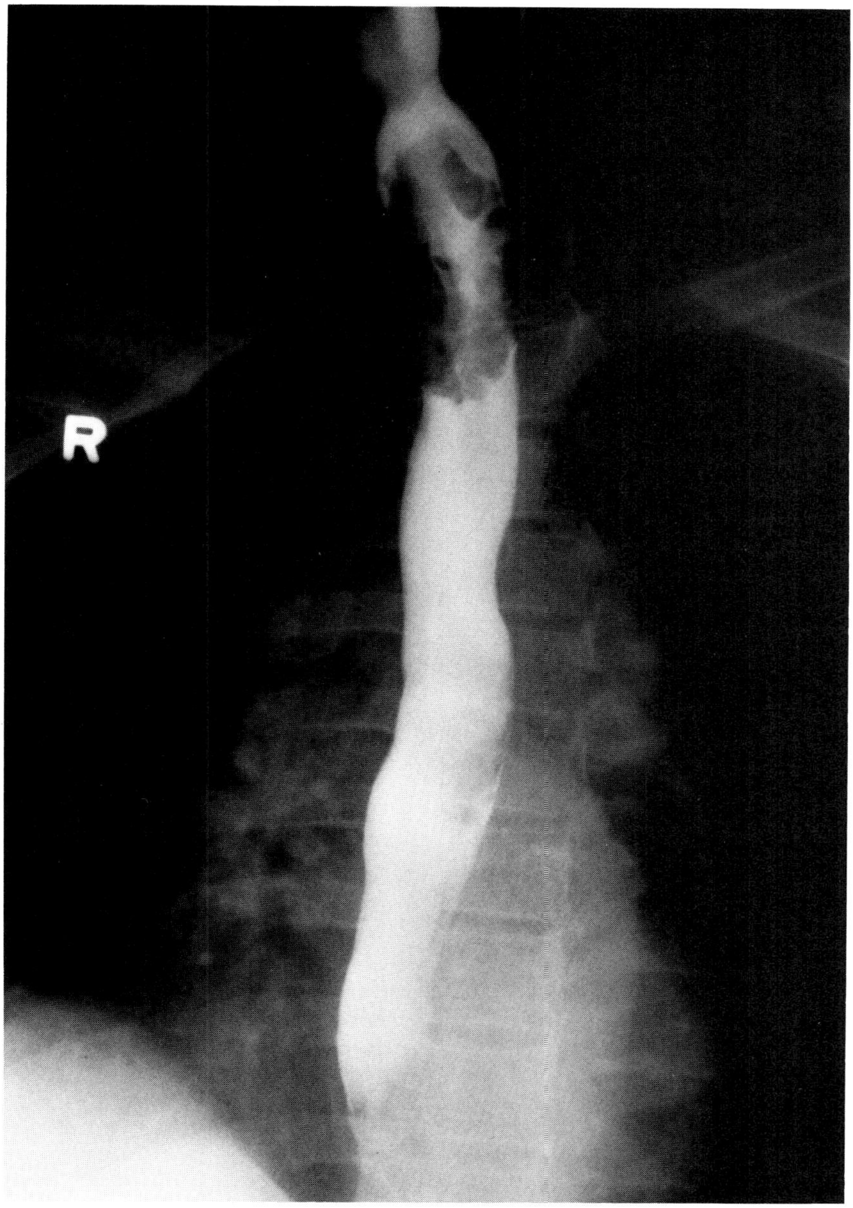

FIG. 1–12. Circumferential, well-demarcated, irregular mucosal destruction in the upper 25% of the esophagus. The extent of tumor above the clavicles indicates its proximity to the larynx and trachea.

PLUMMER-VINSON (PATERSON-KELLY) SYNDROME

Also called sideropenic dysphagia, PVS refers to the concurrence of iron-deficiency anemia and pharyngeal or upper-esophageal mucosal webs. These consist of fixed, slender, circular or semi-lunar folds of squamous epithelium extending perpendicular to the lumen. The anemia (or perhaps the iron deficiency) may also be associated with painful glossitis, hair loss, and angular stomatitis. Though the relationship of these webs to the anemia is uncertain, it is likely that the anemia and iron deficiency precede the mucosal hyperplasia. While it may be hypothesized that the dysphagia leads to a diminished intake of iron-containing foods, the anemia often precedes the appearance of dysphagia or the demonstration of webs. Moreover, the pharyngeal mucosa does not itself bleed; the lesions have been associated with multiple causes of hypoferremia, and both webs and dysphagia can recede after iron replenishment only. Since esophagitis is rarely, if ever, present at or around the webs, gastroesophageal reflux or induced vomiting probably play no role. Rare congenital mucosal webs have been described.

Probably due to dietary iron's increasing prevalence and availability as a nutritional supplement, tonic, or "vitamin," the frequency of this lesion is declining. The disorder was originally considered hysterical, suggesting a significant co-existence, and perhaps causative role, of neurotic disease in some patients. The syndrome seems to favor young females, developing in anorexia nervosa and other food or eating fetishes.

As in nearly all cases of cervical dysphagia, the best initial test is a barium esophagogram, with the radiologist instructed to spend considerable fluoroscopic time in the pharynx and upper esophagus. The webs are found as slender indentations of the barium column, best seen on lateral views, sometimes with an hourglass-shaped bulbous widening of uninvolved proximal or intervening esophagus (Fig. 1–13). Swallowing a large volume of thick barium or a contrast-impregnated marshmallow will disclose the subtler lesion.

In addition to oral or parenteral restoration of iron stores, the treatment is rupture or stretching of persistent webs by forceful bougienage. Sometimes passage of an endoscope alone will widen them adequately to eliminate dysphagia. Laceration of the webs by an endoscopic biopsy forceps may be required. It is important to note that if the patient's blood count does not return to normal after therapy, or if the lesions recur, the clinician should suspect continuing blood loss (menorrhagia, a silent tumor), a deceptive refusal to take iron, or, rarely, a defect in absorption of dietary iron (i.e., celiac sprue). Patients with Plummer-Vinson syndrome have a substantially increased incidence of proximal esophageal carcinoma and deserve continued endoscopic examination.

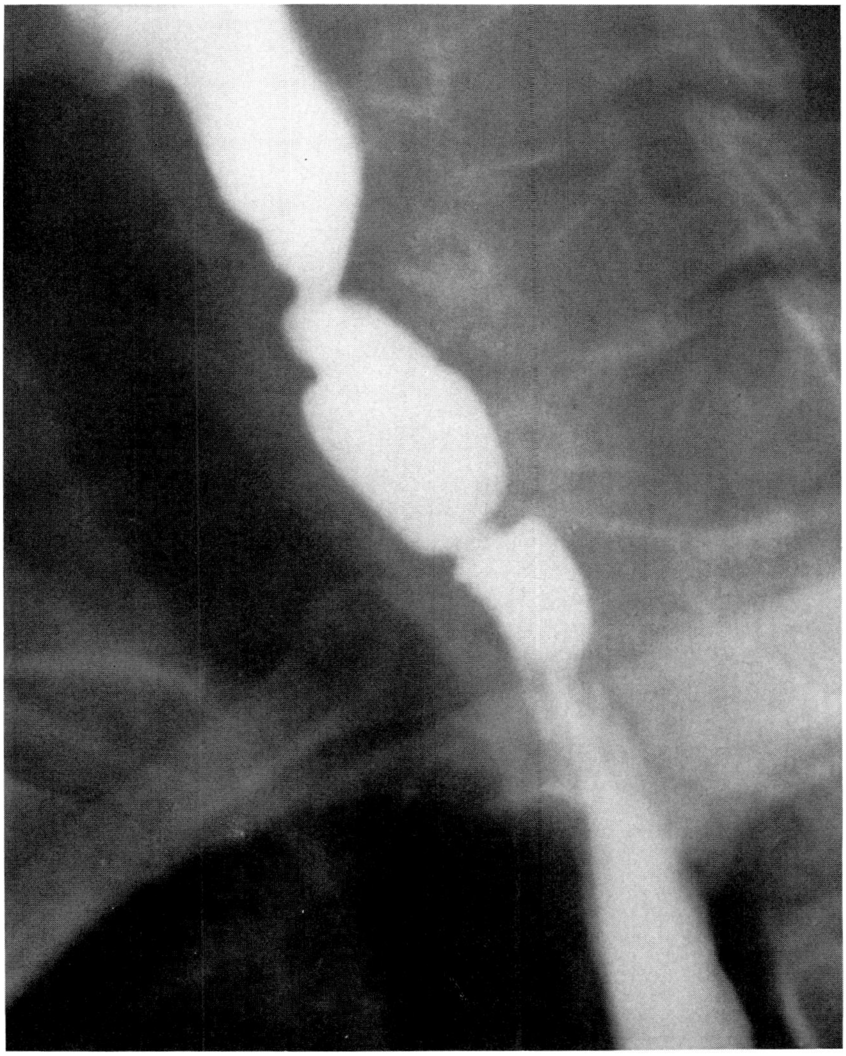

FIG. 1–13. Barium-filled view of the cervical esophagus revealing multiple, slender, horizontal constrictions of the lumen.

THE INTRATHORACIC STOMACH

Congenital short esophagus describes an abbreviated esophagus's distal termination in the midchest, joined "normally" to the gastric fundus, often with all of the stomach displaced upright above an unremarkable diaphragm. The gastroesophageal junction is fixed substantially above the diaphragmatic hiatus, and in Figure 1–14A this junction is easily visualized as a horizontal, radiolucent band, implying a normotensive, competent sphincter.

Despite its location in the "wrong" body cavity, the stomach is normal and generally not predisposed to gastroesophageal reflux or pyloric obstruction; the right diagnosis describes the anatomic abnormality present, i.e., a patient provided at birth with a too-short gullet. Though the dramatic x rays suggest a heroic thoracoabdominal operation to set matters right, the abnormality is typically benign. The filled stomach rarely compresses the left lung sufficiently to cause dyspnea or pain.

The intrathoracic stomach of the short esophagus is distinguishable from a paraesophageal hiatal hernia, in which usually only the gastric fundus is displaced upward through the wide esophageal hiatus of an otherwise normal diaphragm. Intrathoracic stomach contrasts further with eventration of the left hemidiaphragm, in which the stomach flips into an upside-down position with the greater curvature (Fig. 1–14B) topmost, pushing the left lung up toward its apex. The gastroesophageal junction remains fixed in cases of eventration often adjacent to the similarly immobile duodenal bulb. Though squarely in the chest, the stomach resides below the remnant of the left hemidiaphragm, and reflux is rarely an issue. When there is a major diaphragmatic defect in newborns, respiratory embarrassment may occur, while slow upward migration of the stomach is reasonably well tolerated in later life. Such patients breathe mostly with their right lung.

Other differential diagnoses of the visualized intrathoracic stomach include large sliding hiatal hernias and the upward retraction of the stomach into the thorax from a surgically resected lower esophagus (Fig. 1–14C), the latter almost invariably because of cancer of the distal esophagus. Absent the gastroesophageal sphincter, free reflux is typical. To prevent chronic acid or bile injury to the surgically shortened esophagus, a drainage gastroenterostomy, total gastrectomy, or enteroenterostomy may be necessary. Peptic esophagitis with eventual stricture development is common and, in this setting, often difficult to distinguish from recurrent gastroesophageal carcinoma.

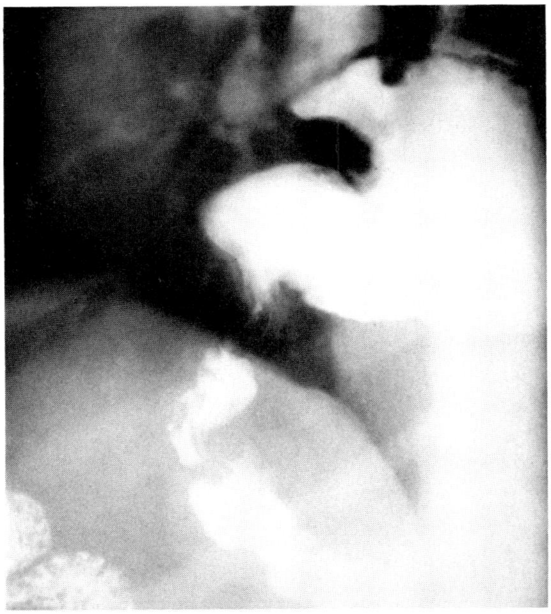

A

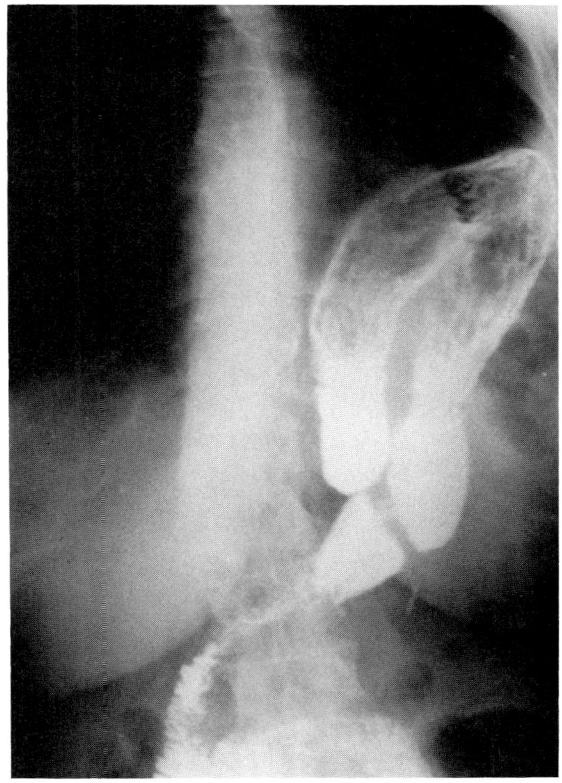

B

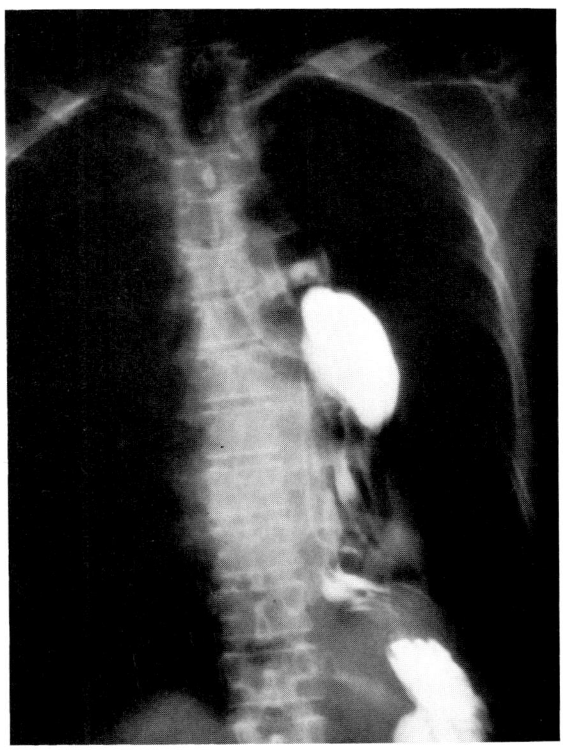

C

FIG. 1–14. A. Congenital short esophagus—entire stomach displaced upright into chest. There is no diaphragmatic eventration; radiolucent "ring" at gastroesophageal junction implies sphincter adequacy.
B. Eventration of the left hemidiaphragm. Led by the greater curvature, the stomach is herniated upward, compressing the lung.
C. Surgically resected distal esophagus, with upward retraction of the stomach.

CAUSTIC ESOPHAGEAL STRICTURE

The location of an esophageal stricture often suggests its cause. These unforgettable lesions are typically more dramatic in the upper or middle third, the areas first contacted where the swallowed poison is most corrosive. Large areas of mucosa are denuded and may appear shaggy and irregular on barium examination. The speed of stricture formation following ingestion is equally breathtaking; sequential contrast films show progressive, sometimes total obliteration of the esophageal lumen in hours to days. Absent a history, the severity and length of mucosal involvement and degree of stenosis suggests extensive tumor, fungal infection, or a disorder of squamous epithelium (e.g., pemphigus or epidermolysis bullosum). The luminal air-fluid level seen in the upper esophagus in this barium study implies the severity of obstruction.

Fortunately, long strictures of the esophagus are uncommon and, as suicidal lye-swallowing has fallen from fashion, this disease is encountered less frequently in adults, though accidental ingestion in children is still an important issue. Curiously, even with a history of other suicide attempts, confrontation with an opened or emptied container of drain cleaner, or simultaneous burns of their lips, tongue, and pharynx, these patients typically deny having ingested lye, and other causes of esophageal stenosis can be mistakenly considered. A high propensity for late malignant degeneration exists, suggested by worsening dysphagia in a stable lye stricture.

Once the diagnosis is established, immediate esophageal dilatations are called for to prevent total obstruction. Often these are unsuccessful. Intraoral and systemic steroids have been advocated as a mode of diminishing the inflammatory component of stricture formation, but their use is probably neither harmful nor helpful. Perhaps seen as one other painful penance, esophagectomy with colon bypass is often required.

Shorter strictures, often midesophageal, may be caused by local irritation from retained swallowed tablets, usually antibiotics. These may be acutely caustic, induce painful ulceration with odynophagia, and heal with smooth stenosis (Fig. 1–15B). The clinical approach is to rule out other potential etiologies, including some pre-existing anatomic or motor defect that delays peristalsis, and to employ antiulcer and bougienage therapy as necessary.

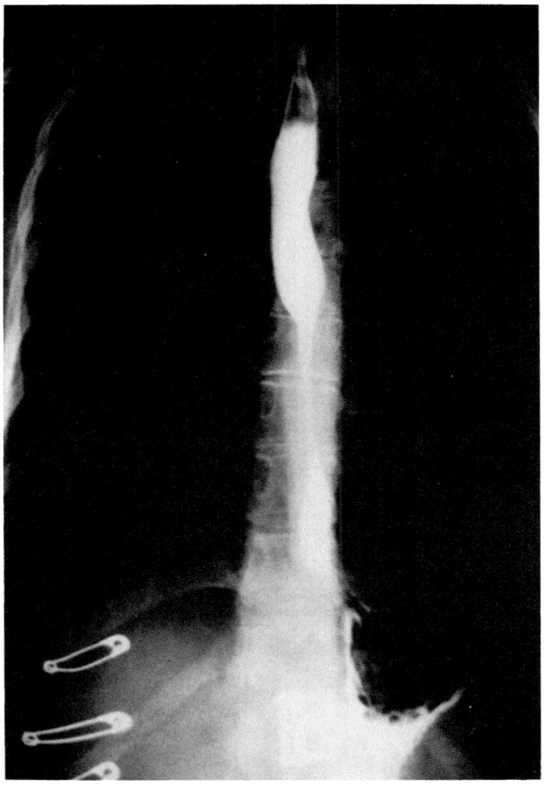

FIG. 1–15. A. Lengthy, fixed stricture with diffuse mucosal irregularity and rigid narrowing, secondary to lye ingestion.

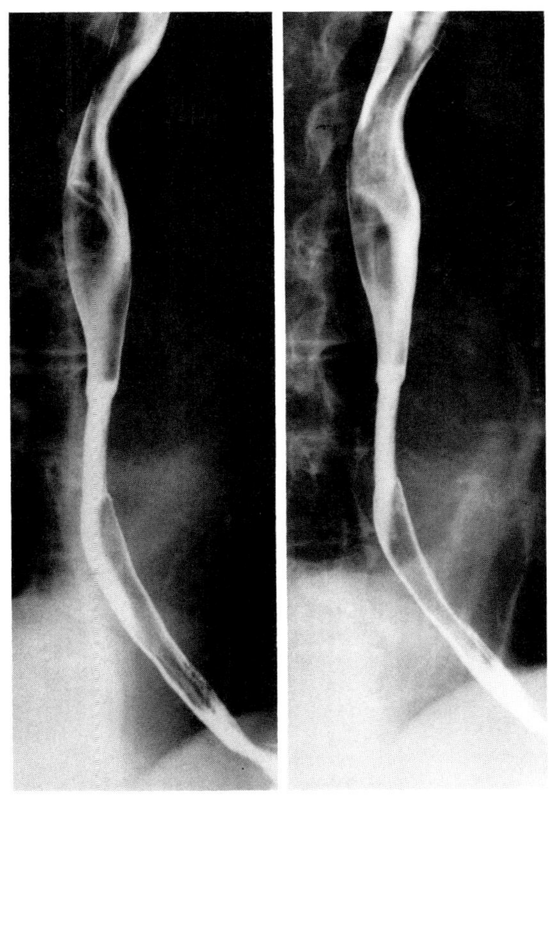

B. Well-demarcated, smooth, finite midesophageal stricture, probably resulting from adherent corrosive medication (a tetracycline tablet).

ESOPHAGEAL VARICES

Varices are simply collateral veins that protrude into the esophageal lumen while conveying blood cephalad, circumventing the hypertensive portal vein of hepatic cirrhosis. They appear here as multiple, smooth, submucosal, serpiginous lucencies, maximal in the lower esophagus. Filled only with flowing blood, they are rarely rigid enough to deform a barium-distended gullet or to affect transport, and are best seen in the barium-coated, air-filled esophagus after the first swallow of contrast has been partially cleared. Other features of portal hypertension visible on plain films may include hepatosplenomegaly, elevated diaphragms, ascites, or pleural effusion. Often widest in the gastric fundus, varices bleed there at least as frequently as from the esophagus; when burst, their potential for sudden, life-threatening hemorrhage is what they are all about.

But, and it is a big but, in the barium x-ray evaluation of upper gastrointestinal bleeding, the discovered varix *may not* be the bleeding source. Other hemorrhagic burdens of the alcoholic, such as duodenal or gastric ulcer, Mallory-Weiss tears, or gastritis, should be considered. Endoscopy and arteriography justify their conspicuous cost best in the bleeding cirrhotic.

The foolers, those x-ray "abnormalities" resembling varices, include normal, large esophageal mucosal folds, leiomyomas, and thick gastric rugae in an unappreciated sliding hiatal hernia. By pushing esophageal mucosa into the lumen, upwardly growing gastric carcinomas may mimic varices, but they usually create sufficient havoc with the overlying mucosa that fixation, stenosis, or spiculation of barium is evident. Noncirrhotic causes of portal hypertension do occur (portal-, hepatic-, or splenic-vein thrombosis), but rarely cause bleeding.

Because of the magnitude of variceal hemorrhage, treatment is urgent and must be instituted when the diagnosis is made and sometimes even when only strongly suspected. Therapeutic methods are directed at occlusion of the bleeding vein; these methods include (1) physical pressure on the vein by gastric or esophageal tamponade (Blakemore tube), (2) surgical variceal ligation, (3) diminishing the arterial component of the portal blood flow (parenteral pitressin), (4) direct-endoscopic-injection sclerosis of the varices, (5) lowering portal circulation by surgically shunting the portal vein or one of its tributaries into the systemic venous circulation (inferior vena cava or renal vein), and (6) repair, rarely possible, of coexisting bleeding abnormalities.

I am convinced that emergency shunt surgery's forbidding mortality is worsened by the clinician's understandable procrastination; indecision eventuating in a 20- or 30-unit blood exchange makes for poorer surgical candidates and a self-fulfilling prophecy.

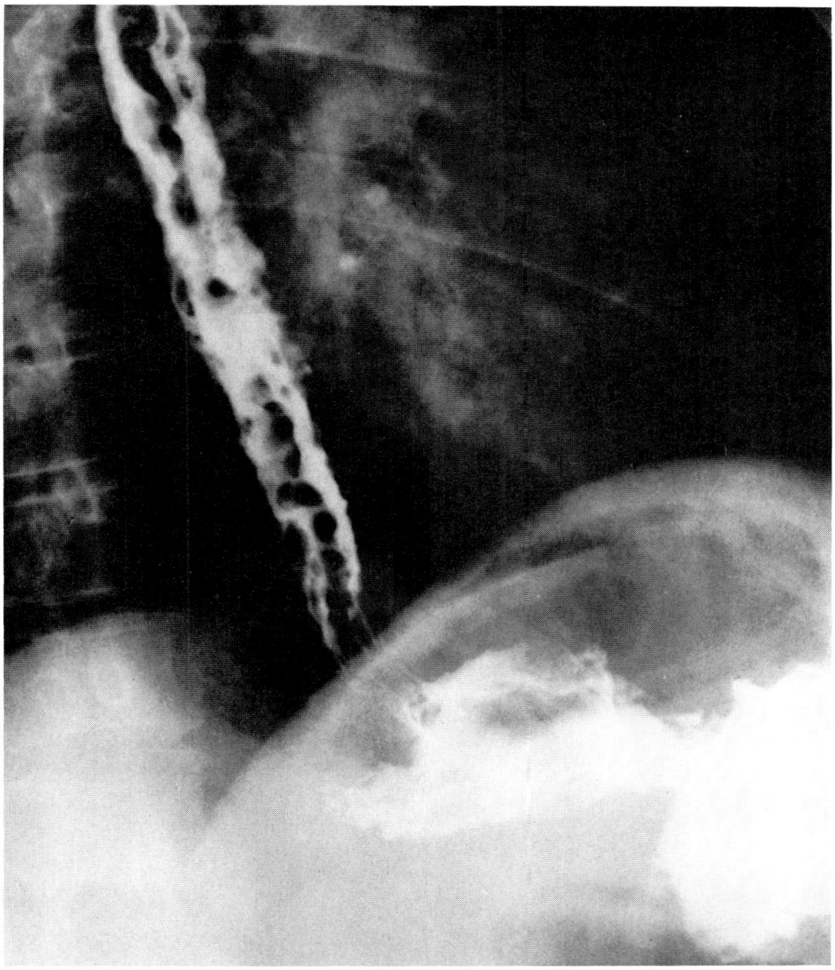

FIG. 1–16. Smooth, irregular submucosal lucencies, extending up the lower half of the esophagus in a patient with severe portal hypertension.

ESOPHAGEAL LEIOMYOMA

Esophageal leiomyomas are smoothly rounded, submucosal, and usually single tumors, typically in the mid to lower third of the esophagus. Though fixed in location and rubbery in texture, they are rarely circumferential, and the overlying, adjacent esophagus is mobile and pliable. Thus they infrequently produce more than mild dysphagia, unlikely to be modified by use of a dilator, and seemingly at variance with the often large size of the lesion seen indenting a barium column (Fig. 1–17). As esophageal mucosa is stretched over them, the lesions assume the ovoid or egg-shaped appearance seen on this film. Unlike their cousins in the stomach, these leiomyomas rarely ulcerate or bleed.

Distinguishing a leiomyoma from other "smooth" esophageal lesions (an upwarding prolapsing gastric fold or esophageal varix) is rarely difficult. The defects produced by an extramural, pulsatile, aberrant left subclavian artery ("dysphagia lusoria") or a thoracic aortic aneurysm are unlikely to suggest a fixed, submucosal tumor. Leiomyosarcomas are another matter. Though rare, they must be considered in the differential diagnosis, and the small amount of submucosal muscle tissue obtainable by endoscopic biopsy, even if seemingly benign, rarely calms the wise doctor. Accurate distinction between sarcoma and myoma usually requires more histologic material than a transendoscopic forceps can deliver.

The surgical extirpation of a leiomyoma is not difficult; it rarely requires segmental resection, necessitating only the shelling of the tumor out from between its muscular and submucosal layers. Thus most patients with an enlarging, symptomatic, or irregular lesion should undergo thoracotomy.

Alternative considerations in diagnosis of submucosal or extramural esophageal lesions include metastatic tumors to the esophagus (usual primary site: lung or breast) or pressure on the esophagus by a neoplastic mediastinal lymph node.

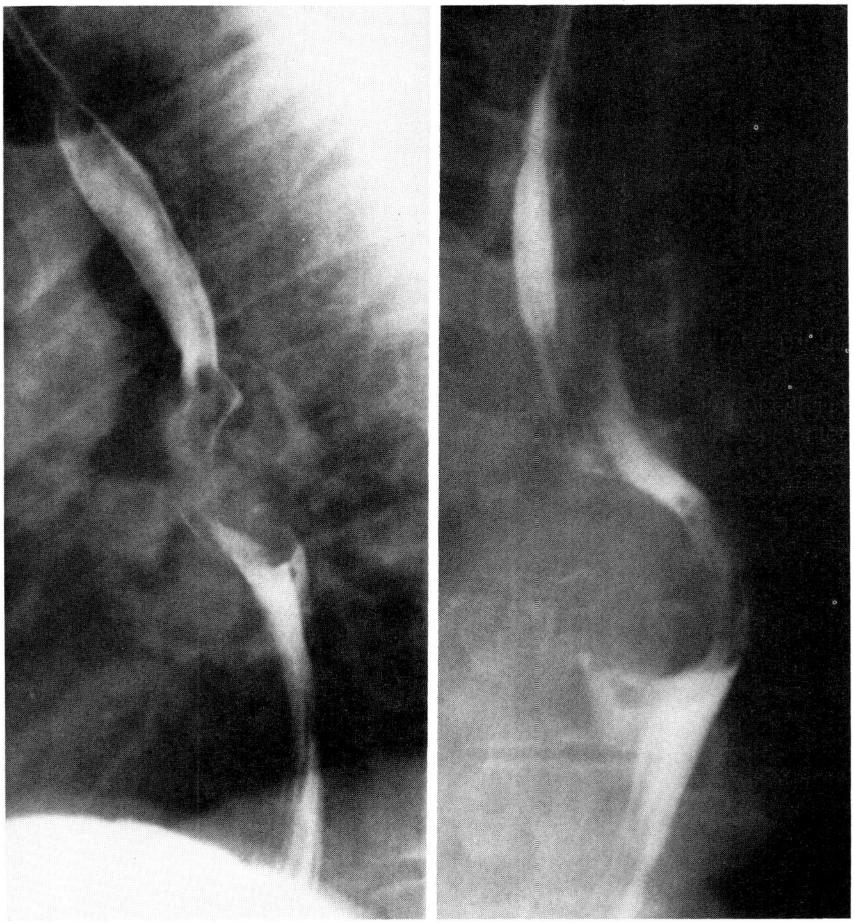

FIG. 1–17. Egg-shaped, rounded, smooth, fixed submucosal tumor, compressing the esophageal lumen, but not impeding barium.

MIDESOPHAGEAL AND EPIPHRENIC DIVERTICULA

Probably resulting from congenital muscle-wall defects, esophageal diverticula begin as hemispherical protrusions, but they empty poorly, if at all, and increasingly act as a saccular reservoir for swallowed food and saliva. They enlarge slowly and, through gravity, swing medially into the downward line of deglutition, allowing food to re-enter the esophagus only by overflow. They occur singly or in groups; when smaller they are insignificant and asymptomatic, but when large, their major implication is pulmonary. With recumbency, particularly with sleep, the cervical esophageal sphincter relaxes; the unobstructed upward drift of diverticular contents into the oropharynx permits predictable and potentially significant aspiration. With the patient on his back, gravity favors aspiration into the right middle and right lower lobe orifices. While an acute chemical pneumonia is likeliest, chronic adult onset asthma is occasionally traced to these esophageal cisterns.

As in Zenker's diverticulum, traditional fiberoptic esophagoscopy bears the risk of tearing a thin-walled outpouching with the instrument tip. However, this procedure is less hazardous with midesophageal lesions, because the optical head of the endoscope has passed the cervical esophagus and the true lumen or a diverticular orifice can be seen "on end" and distinguished. Since they rarely interfere with swallowing and never produce cervical dysphagia, the mid and lower esophageal diverticula only warrant surgery when accompanied by intractable or serious aspiration.

Because epiphrenic diverticula often actually rest atop the diaphragm (Fig. 1–18), they are less inclined to swing medially (which would produce dysphagia) and are often resectable from an abdominal approach, lessening their operative morbidity. Yet, they do tend to be more capacious than those in the midesophagus. The likelihood of aspiration is increased by diverticular size and diminished by the distance food has to migrate in recumbency. Traction diverticula, typically located opposite the tracheal bifurcation, are usually small and tent-shaped, little more than a radiologic curiosity apart from their known association with healed mediastinal granulomatous disease.

Occasionally described as a complication of achalasia, epiphrenic diverticula, if present, argue against conventional pneumatic dilation because of the risk of rupture of this nonmuscular sac.

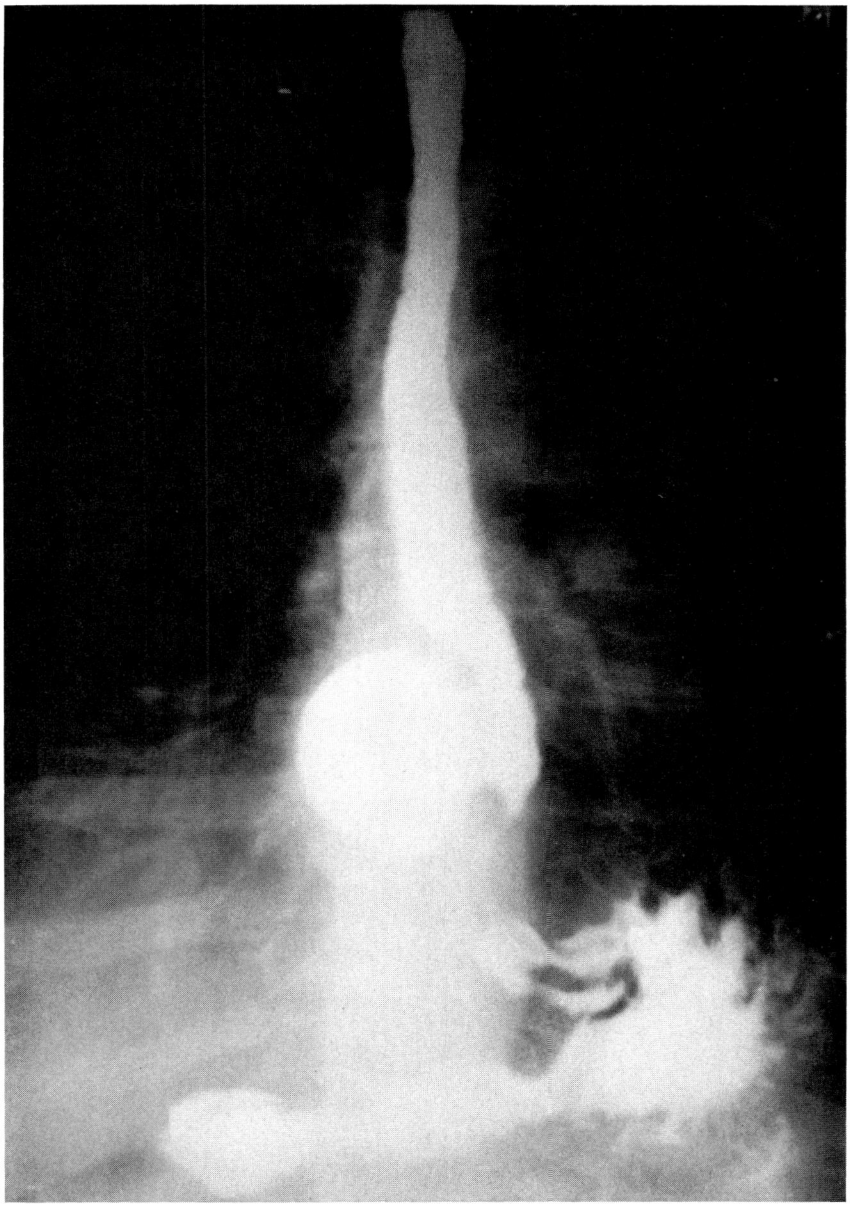

FIG. 1–18. Spherical supradiaphragmatic extrusion of esophagus creating a nonmuscular, intrathoracic reservoir.

ZENKER'S DIVERTICULUM

An important, treatable cause of cervical dysphagia in the elderly, Zenker's diverticulum is a saccular posterior protrusion of the nonmuscular pharynx, medial to the cricopharyngeus muscles. It is also a cause of late-onset asthma or acute pneumonia. Symptoms result from tracheal aspiration of swallowed but retained food and saliva, producing bronchospasm or pneumonitis. The disorder probably begins as a weakness or thinning of nonmuscular tissue surrounded by a cricopharyngeus whose resting tone is high. Protrusion commences, much like putty extruded from between fingers of a clenched fist.

Dysphagia produced by any esophageal diverticulum is a feature of their progressive expansion, for as the diverticulum enlarges, its dependent, saccular portion becomes the preferred route for food (i.e., pharynx to diverticulum to distal esophagus). The widened diverticulum then becomes a reservoir, whose unemptied contents make for further expansion. The diverticulum expands inferiorly, and gravity swings it into the line of deglutition, displacing the body and distal lumen of the esophagus laterally (Fig. 1–19A). A cervical air-fluid level sometimes is seen in the upright plain x ray, replaced by a rounded radiopacity remaining in the neck after barium is ingested. The ringed outline of the trachea is visualized (Fig. 1–19B) when the patient aspirates.

As the patients usually are aged, surgical treatment is risky and must be measured against the nutritional and respiratory implications of the lesion. Occasionally, reducing the pressure of its muscular periphery by simple myotomy decreases both the tendency for further protrusion and the volume of the diverticulum. Resection of the sac itself is surgically delicate, and ought to be left to a talented head-and-neck surgeon or otolaryngologist with a history of similar successful interventions. As some fluoroscopists think an upper GI series begins at the fundus of the stomach, the clinician must request attention to the cervical esophagus, with lateral views. Endoscopy is contraindicated, since "blind" introduction of a flexible endoscope is guided only by the patient's swallowing, and extra pressure on the instrument by the examiner can perforate the base of the diverticulum.

In patients who sense the neck as the site where food "sticks," barium or gastrografin x rays are the safest initial approach, even for patients with a history of aspiration or coughing after swallowing. If the diagnosis cannot be made with certainty, "straight" endoscopy is best, using general anesthesia where the neck can be adequately retroflexed, the patient is not swallowing, and the cervical esophagus is patent.

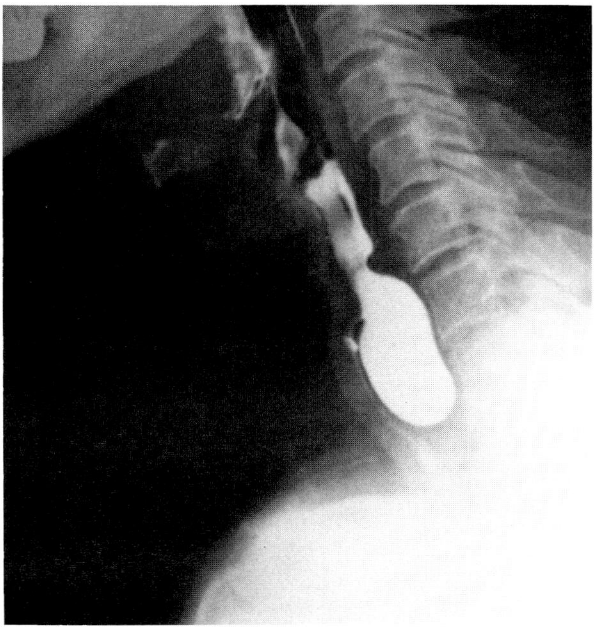

FIG. 1–19. A. Lateral view of cervical esophagus with dependent barium-filled sac anterior to vertebrae.

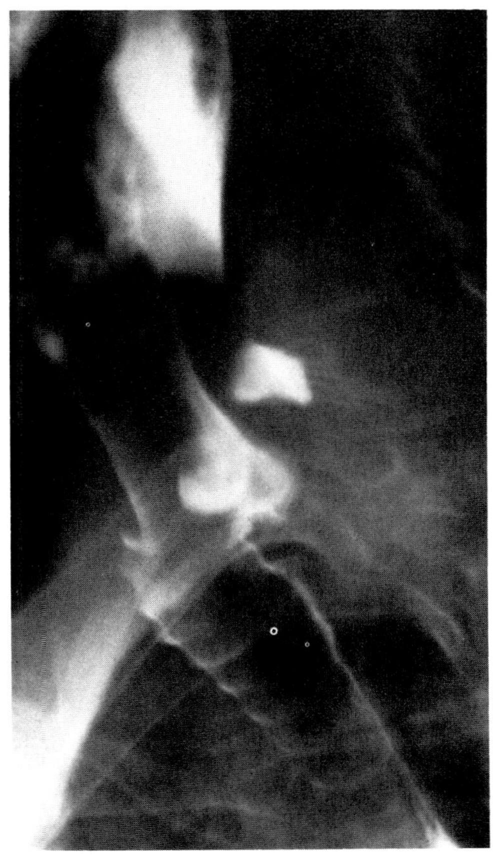

B. Aspiration from diverticulum. Contrast fills superior and posterior portions of diverticulum and ringed outline of trachea.

MONILIASIS

Once rare, and now an unhappy fact of contemporary medical life, moniliasis is a diffuse fungal infection of esophageal lining in the immunosuppressed, manifested on this typical barium swallow (Fig. 1–20) by innumerable fine mucosal spiculations covering a rigid, fixed esophagus. At esophagoscopy, these appear as multiple focal, occasionally coalescent exudative patches, which contain both budding and mycelial forms of Candida. Silver stains of directly applied brushings are preferable to biopsies, particularly if the patient is thrombocytopenic.

These fungal deposits may progress to a shaggy irregularity with diffuse, deep ulcerations, usually without a focal narrowing but still rendering the patient virtually unable to swallow. Deep, undercutting intramural ulcerations or "pseudodiverticula" represent serious infestation, often followed by stricture formation. Years ago, the common victim was either a debilitated diabetic on broad-spectrum antibiotics or a patient complaining of chest pain, vomiting, or odynophagia with a disease or medication (steroid or antimetabolite) affecting immunity.

Currently, this esophagogram is more characteristic of two "new" diseases, particularly that of the AIDS patient, whose peculiar susceptibility to myocotic infection hounds his or her shortened life, not only in the esophagus, but in the mid and distal bowel, as evidenced by heavy fecal infestation in diarrheal stools and occasionally in the blood stream, renal parenchyma, and CNS. The second group includes those receiving immunosuppressive therapy for cancer, but more typically the organ transplant recipient, as treatment with cyclosporin or azathioprine seems to partially mimic the T-lymphocyte abnormality in AIDS. Both predisposing conditions are often first manifested by mucocutaneous or oral moniliasis or "thrush," and the frequency of the illness is such that, in many centers, prophylaxis with oral mycostatin or ketoconazole is prudent and routine.

Though the diagnosis seems easily confirmed, *Candida albicans* appears in the esophagus of a modest number of normal persons; moreover, vesicular and ulcerative herpetic infections, as well as cytomegalovirus, are radiologically and clinically similar, and need consideration.

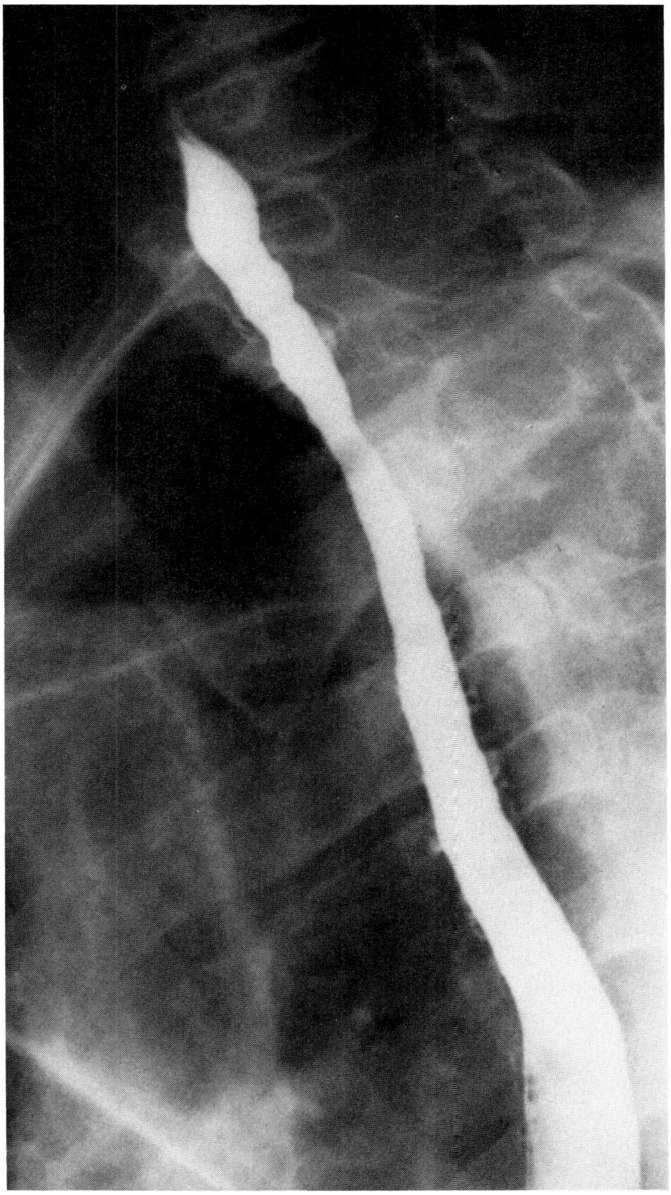

FIG. 1–20. The ordinarily smooth outline of the barium-filled esophagus is penetrated by multiple, perpendicular needle-like, and occasional intramurally dissecting ulcers.

MALLORY-WEISS—BOORHAAVE SYNDROME

Mallory (pathologist) and Weiss (clinician) first described these focal, linear tears of the distal esophageal or adjacent gastric mucosa in vomiting alcoholics with serious upper GI hemorrhage. Penetrating the submucosa, these rents develop when vigorous hyperemesis forces the gastroesophageal junction upward and inflates it centrifugally into the thorax. Because of its limited capacity for stretch, the cardia's lining splits, much like the center of a retracted lower lip. The diagnosis is suggested when continued, forceful vomiting or "dry heaves" suddenly produces blood. However, the syndrome can occur anytime after Valsalva maneuver, such as during defecation, labor and delivery, or grand mal seizure; these tears rarely occur spontaneously.

While usually negative, the barium x-ray examination may astonishingly demonstrate the tear itself, seen here (Fig. 1–21) as a long mural furrow, no more than 1 or 2 mm wide or deep, containing a thread of retained contrast on the esophageal side of the gastroesophageal junction. Increasing early endoscopy in acute upper GI bleeding shows these subtle lesions to be more common than previously appreciated.

Though the hemorrhage may be initially brisk, it usually subsides quickly, and the typical patient requires little beyond careful observation, fluid or blood replacement, gastric alkalinization, and sedation adequate to suppress additional vomiting. Continued bleeding means the tear has included a recalcitrant arteriole, and stitching the inside of an opened GE junction becomes the doctor's only choice. As most patients are alcoholic, a bleeding ulcer, hemorrhagic gastritis, or esophageal varices may coexist. But unless the blood is coming from a varix, treatment still is limited largely to monitoring, with acid neutralization or mucosal protection providing likely, but statistically unprovable, benefit.

The Boorhaave variant is a far more serious, occasionally spontaneous free perforation of the mid or lower esophagus, producing an immediate infective and chemical mediastinitis, which is usually associated with a large hemopneumothorax. Oral contrast provides a bone-chilling vision of dye extravasation into the chest or mediastinum, while on plain films, subcutaneous emphysema, pleural effusion (Fig. 1–22), or an air-fluid level in either thorax is evident. The lesion is often fatal, and can occur inexplicably in the absence of hyperemesis or the swallowing of a foreign body. Treatment, of course, is immediate open mediastinal and pleural cleansing and drainage, with hopeful repair of the esophageal rent. If the latter is considered impossible, esophagectomy with pharyngostomy, ligation of the gastroesophageal junction, and feeding gastrostomy are needed.

Still, most esophageal perforations are born of the marriage of a narrowed, inflamed, or ulcerated esophagus and an unlucky, insufficiently trained, or overzealous endoscopist. In instrumenting the high-risk patient, thought remains the superior prophylaxis.

FIG. 1–21. Persistent 2-cm filamentous streak of barium across gastroesophageal junction.

FIG. 1–22. Obvious collection of pleural fluid in a patient with acute hematemesis and mediastinitis.

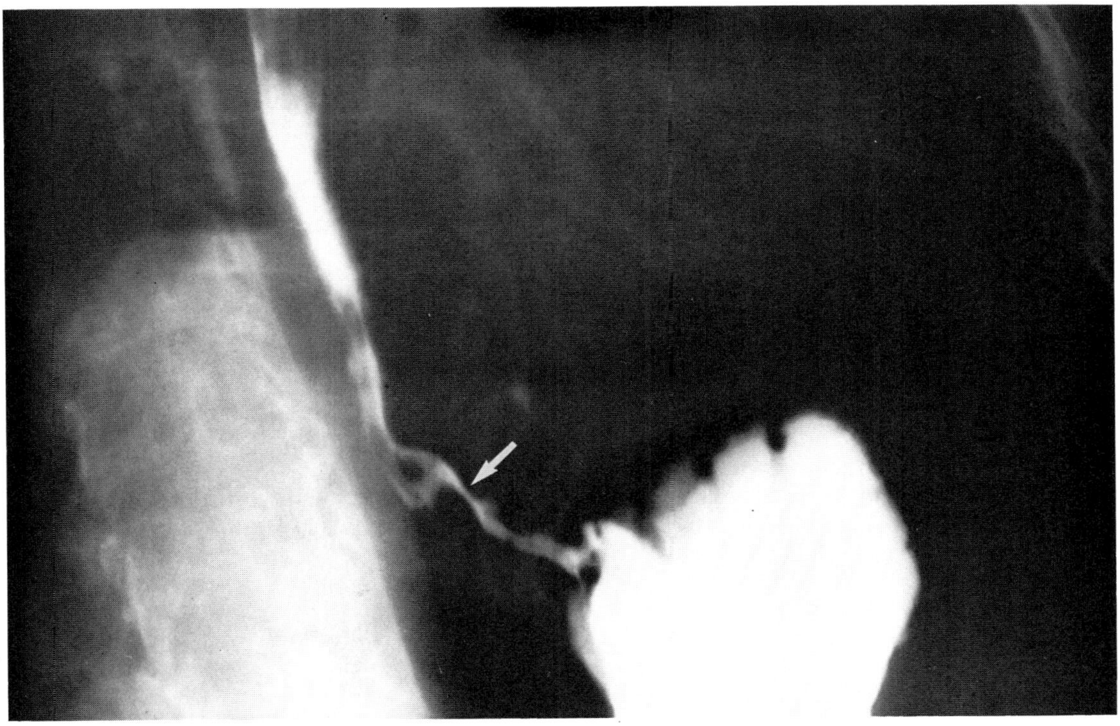

FIG. 1–21.

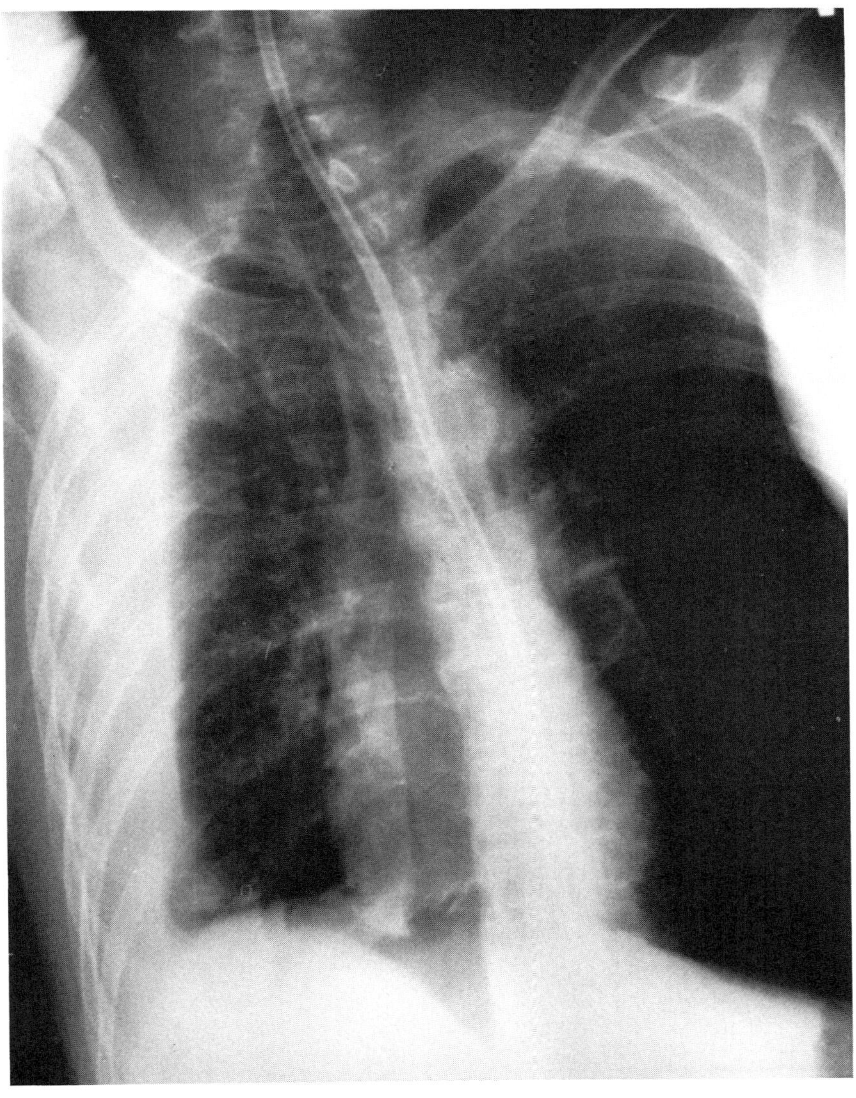

FIG. 1–22.

EXTRINSIC COMPRESSION ON THE MIDESOPHAGUS

Intrusions on the esophageal lumen from without are typically vascular or tumorous, and rarely inflammatory. The vascular lesions almost never cause serious dysphagia and are now uncommon, mostly originating in the late phases of diseases now cured or prevented by penicillin, including aneurysms of the ascending aorta (syphilis) or left atrial hypertrophy (rheumatic mitral stenosis). Far less commonly, a congenital, aberrant subclavian artery, crossing left to right, traps the esophagus between itself and the aorta (dysphagia lusoria). Simple chest x rays will disclose an aortic aneurysm, compressive tumorous defects (Figs. 1–23A and B), and left atrial enlargement. Malignancies are usually in the lower or middle third of the esophagus; they are most commonly bronchogenic, less often lymphoproliferative, and rarely of distant metastatic origin.

Esophagoscopy reveals a static or pulsatile compression defect, which is covered by elevated mucosa and is stretched and sliding over and around the intruder. Unless there is circumferential entrapment, dysphagia is uncommon. The gradual tenting displacement of esophageal mucosa around the defect usually distinguishes an extraluminal from a more finite, sharply circumscribed, fixed submucosal defect, such as leiomyoma. In the cervical esophagus, circumferential compression usually reflects advanced thyroid cancer, which has an appearance similar to prostate cancer when wrapped around the rectum.

A history of bronchogenic or neck cancer, lymphoma, or lymphocytic leukemia often solves what is rarely a dilemma. In contrast to epidermoid esophageal cancer, which commonly perforates into the mediastinum, tracheobronchial tree, or thoracic aorta, extraesophageal tumors rarely burrow fistulous openings into the gullet. Treatment of the problem, if any, is naturally treatment of the underlying disease.

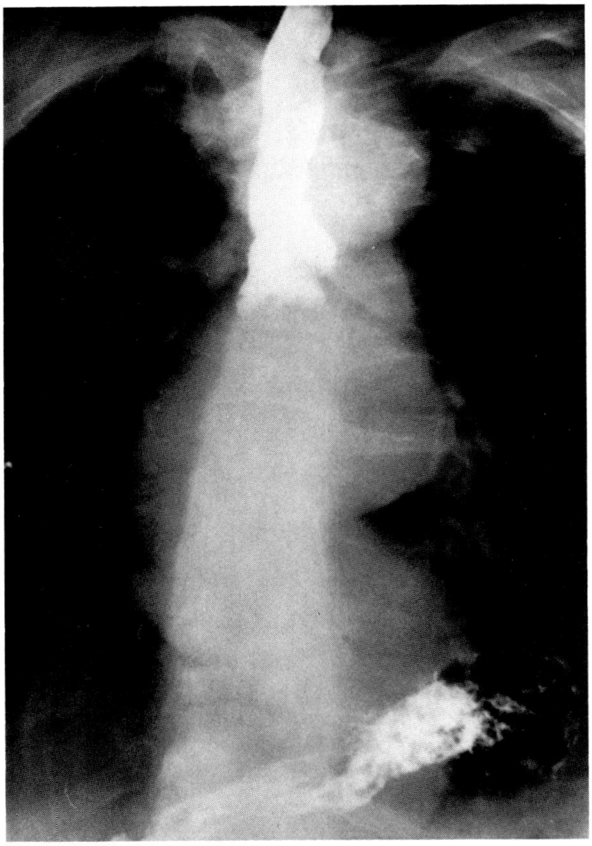

FIG. 1–23. A. Near complete "holdup" of a barium-filled esophagus, compressed by an aortic arch aneurysm.

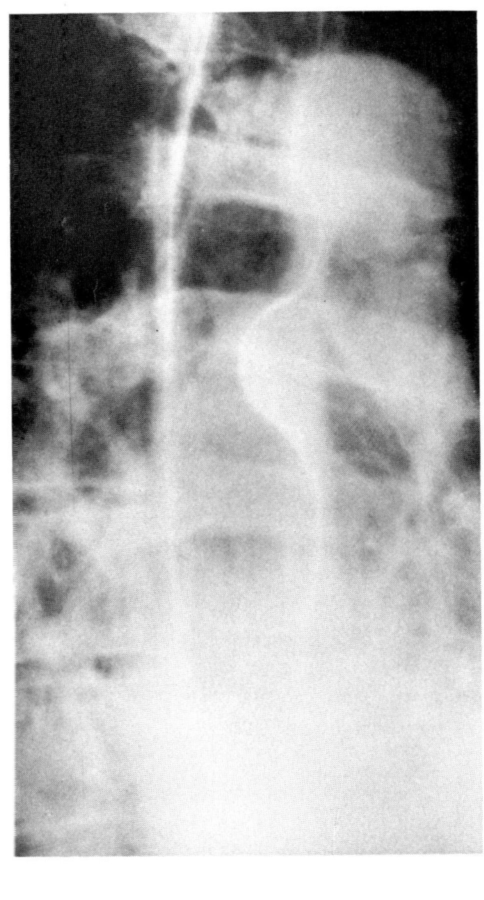

B. Enlarged mediastinal lymph node deflecting esophagus in patient with lymphocytic leukemia.

EXTRINSIC COMPRESSION OF THE CERVICAL ESOPHAGUS

Apart from weakness of the muscles of deglutition or intrinsic lesions (tumors or webs), cervical dysphagia can arise from direct anatomic compression by lesions adjacent and extrinsic to the esophagus. One classic example includes compression on the posterior wall of the upper esophagus by intervertebral discs or osteophytes. This generally produces a mild cervical dysphagia, which can be identified best on lateral views (Fig. 1–24A) of the barium-filled esophagus. These sequential indentations extending anteriorly define the multiple compressive defects. Barium esophagogram is usually the preferred and safest diagnostic test. Straight or flexible fiberoptic endoscopes are dangerous; pressing a thin esophageal wall between bony vertebral prominences and a man-made instrument risks laceration. Despite the obvious temptation to chisel away the external obstructions revealed by this esophagogram, treatment is best left to the choices of a softer diet and admonitions to chew one's food well. Inadequate dentition or poorly fitting dentures may compound the dysphagia associated with this generally benign abnormality.

A more pernicious extrinsic compression of the cervical esophagus results from progressive growth of thyroid cancer, which in more malignant, nonpapillary, spindle-cell forms often encircles the upper esophagus, occasionally progressing to total obstruction (Fig. 1–24B). The esophagogram often reveals a high-grade stricture without mucosal irregularity, typical of extraluminal GI compressive disease anywhere in the tract. These strictures are extremely rigid and, like most intrinsic or extrinsic obstructions of the upper esophagus, are difficult to visualize while employing conventional esophagoscopy. Moreover, attempts at bougie dilatation also risk a through-and-through tear of the esophagus. Responsiveness to treatment is measured by improvement in swallowing, generally limited to the effects of radiation, local surgery, or chemotherapy. If dysphagia outpaces the other features of the tumor, a bypassing cervical esophagostomy may be required, particularly when patients are unable to swallow their saliva.

Along with the dysphagia accompanying neuromuscular disease or scleroderma, that accompanying thyroid carcinoma is one of the rare instances in which the bedside examination aids in the diagnosis of dysphagia. The usual nontoxic goiter or thyroiditis may be associated with modest difficulty in swallowing, while the intrathoracic, substernal goiter will rarely involve, but rather only deflect, the upper thoracic esophagus, producing mild dysphagia, if any.

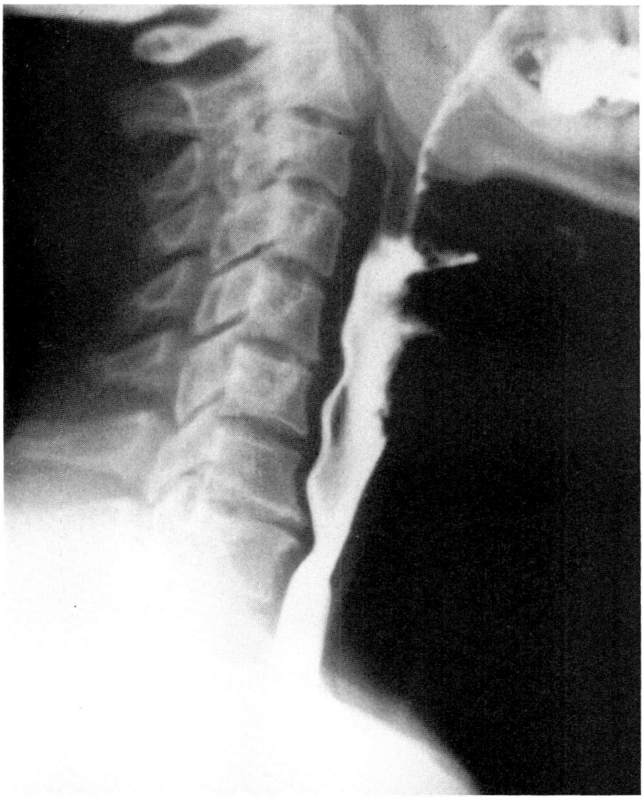

FIG. 1–24. A. Cervical osteoarthritis—indentations on posterior wall of cervical esophagus, corresponding to hypertrophic cervical spine interspaces and osteoarthritic spurs.

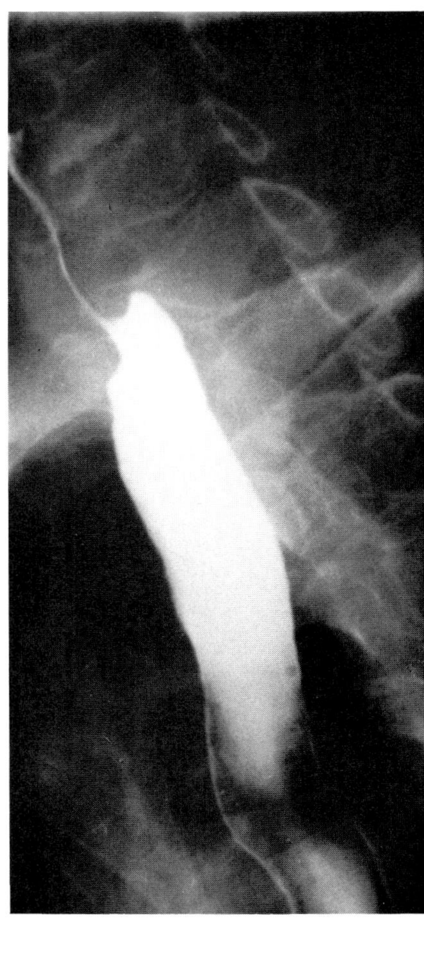

B. Carcinoma of the thyroid involving the esophagus—extremely high-grade, filiform, but smooth, near-total occlusion of cervical esophagus, reflecting circumferential entrapment by a slow-growing thyroid cancer.

CHAPTER 2

THE STOMACH

BENIGN GASTRIC ULCER

What must strike one first on examining this x ray is that the ulceration is both dramatic, enormous, and obviously deeper than the normal gastric wall is thick. Hence, its base, while consisting of exudate and digested blood, must rest somewhere against the liver, pancreas, or mesentery. Indeed, deep gastric ulcers can be thought of as confined penetrations, rarely stopping at, but often extending through, the serosa. Their strong clinical association with the use of nonsteroidal anti-inflammatory agents reinforces the clinical conviction that they arise more as a function of diminished resistance to gastric acid and enzymes than as the hypersecretion of either. Thus, in contact with their duodenal relations, ulcers of the stomach resist healing through acid inhibition or neutralization, particularly when they occur in the elderly. Small gastric ulcers must be more common than ordinarily appreciated, as gastroscopic examinations reveal transitory hemorrhagic or inflammatory changes in a substantial number of otherwise healthy people.

When pain or bleeding is investigated radiologically and an ulcer of this type is found, the issue of its histology dominates. This lesion exhibits a classic benign appearance: residing on the lesser curvature, with a regular, ovoid contour, smooth edges, and hyperplastic folds, radiating to or from it like spider legs. In profile, a radiolucent rim (Hampton's line) is seen.

Yet, despite all x-ray arguments, any gastric ulcer can be cancerous. Generalist or specialist, physicians must remember that no patient's disease is obliged to follow the anatomic rules in textbooks. The location, shape, and size of cancerous ulcers can be misleading. Admittedly, ulcers in the fundus or cardia are more likely to be tumerous than those in the body or antrum. While a malignant ulcer is the necrotic center of a mural tumor, many cancers have a smooth, "hyperplastic" edge. Yet, on direct or endoscopic examination, most malignancies still resemble an inverted clam shell, often surrounded by atrophic or polypoid gastric mucosa.

In all cases, good judgment and conservatism overlap. An ulcer that does not heal quickly with treatment, one that looks radiologically or endoscopically "suspicious," or an ulceration developing in the absence of demonstrable gastric acid (should one still be doing acid secretory testing) needs removal. Finally, the more endoscopic ulcer biopsies provided a pathologist, the more accurate the diagnosis is likely to be. A slightly bad egg is a bad egg, and carcinoma cells may be present only over 5 to 10% of a lesion's circumference.

Finally, a word about bleeding: Because gastric ulcer bleeding tends to accrue in the elderly, whose sclerotic vessels include those in the ulcer, bleeding tends to continue unless surgery is performed. Endoscopic heat or laser therapy is usually only a temporizing measure; if an operation is likely to be inevitable, early decision for surgery is always superior.

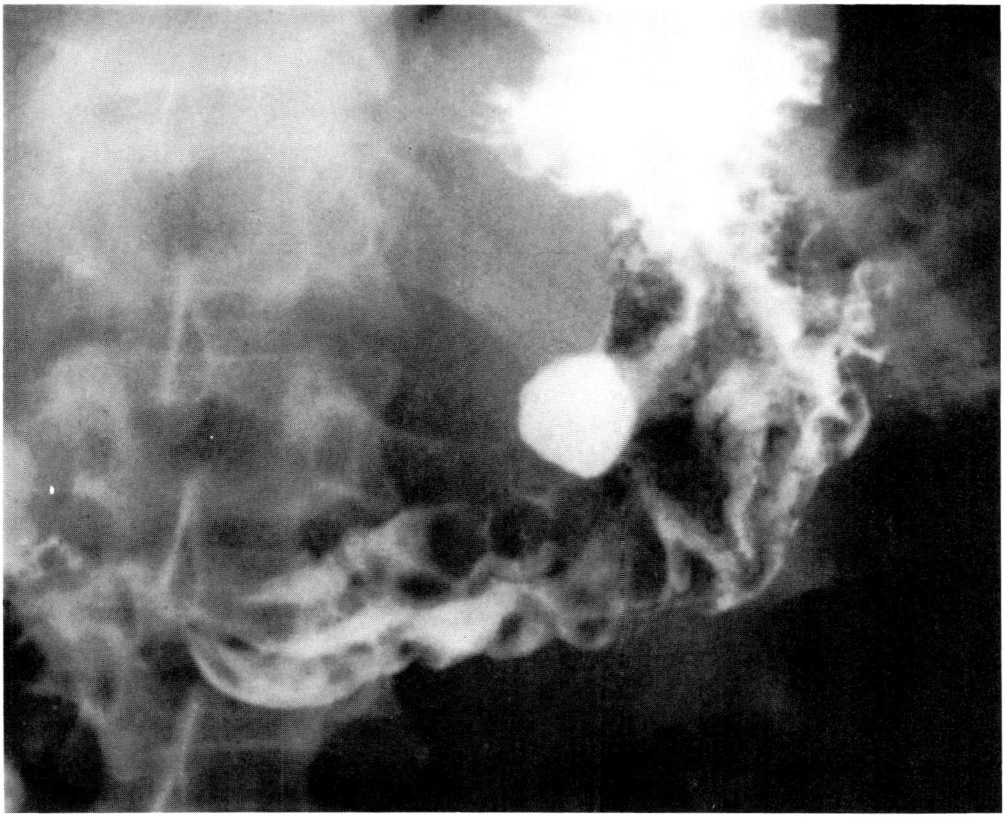

FIG. 2–1. A 3-cm lesser curvature, circular barium collection, opposite thickened, "hyperplastic" gastric folds that appear to radiate to or from the ulceration. There is no evidence of obstruction.

MULTIPLE GASTRIC ULCERATIONS

Upper digestive tract ulcerogenesis can be thought of as a staged battle. Attackers are acid and pepsin; defenders include gastric mucus along with duodenal and pancreatic bicarbonate. In patients with multiple gastric ulcers, gastric hypersecretion probably plays a small role; defective resistance is the probable etiology. Other significant factors affect mucosal resistance, including the use of steroids and nonsteroidal anti-inflammatory agents, concurrent stress, and a setting of overwhelming illness (crush injury, burns, head trauma). Typically, they are shallow and hemorrhagic, and occur on both greater and lesser curvature, generally accruing in the distal stomach.

Multiple large ulcerations are easily seen in the upper GI series of Fig. 2–2A. The patient, a rheumatoid arthritic, presented with several days of melena that followed administration of high-dose oral salicylates. Marked osteopenia on x ray correlated a history of earlier, lengthy steroid use.

The treatment of drug-induced ulcers is usually successful following withdrawal of the offending agent and the ancillary liberal use of traditional antiulcer agents. The role of prostaglandins for gastric mucosal protection deserves and will receive further attention and debate.

Figure 2–2B illustrates an interesting subdivision of this problem. Probably of a different etiology, these multiple, tiny ulcers resemble the aphthous lesions of oral mucus membranes; while possibly peptic in origin, these ulcers also suggest early Crohn's disease. Similar tiny ulcers are frequently found in the rectal mucosa on careful proctoscopy. Their appearance in the mouth, tongue, or gingiva often parallels development of lower bowel symptoms.

Visualizing shallow ulcers radiologically requires an intrepid radiologist, parsimonious with barium and liberal with air. The lesions generally show up as tiny (1- to 2-mm), opaque, superficial circles surrounded by radiolucent halos. When they appear as a satellite manifestation of a systemic disease, their treatment with antacids and acid-inhibiting agents are less clearly effective. There may also be a more specific role for oral mucosal protective agents (sucralfate or synthetic prostaglandins) and topical corticosteroids in managing aphthoid ulcers.

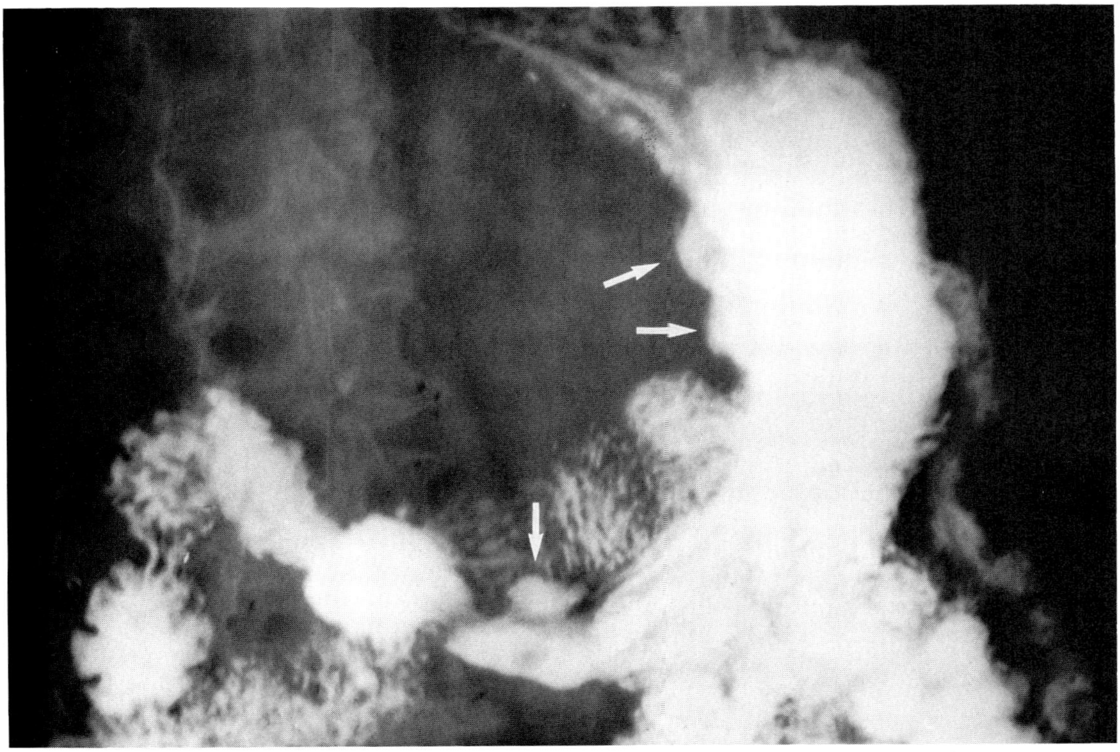

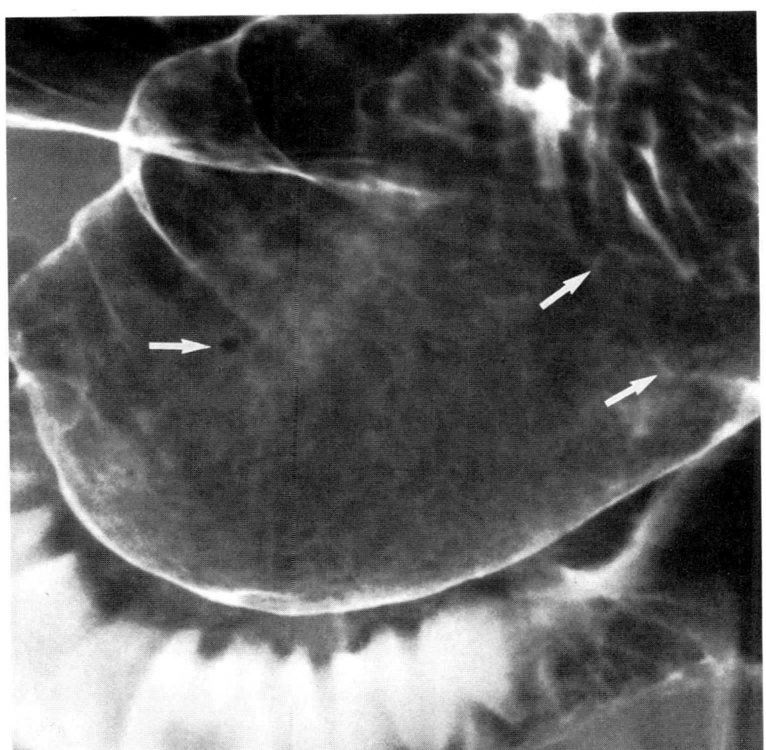

FIG. 2–2. A. Multiple, large, benign-appearing ulcers seen best along both curvatures. B. Note tiny, 1- to 2-mm barium-filled erosions with edematous halos, resembling aphthous lesions of oral mucous membrane.

GASTRIC FUNDAL ULCER

This is a typical disease in an atypical location, one that does not differ in any anatomic or biologic form from conventional ulcers in the body or antrum of the stomach. Yet, their medical features and surgical implications are sufficiently noteworthy to deserve special mention. Like leiomyomas or the occasional proximal gastric cancers, fundal ulcers are often difficult to diagnose by both x ray and endoscopy, unless particular attention is paid to the possible presence of these lesions. Barium x-ray visualization requires that the fundus be mostly emptied of dye and re-expanded in the typical air-contrast technique. Also, because they are frequently located lateral to or behind the tip of a front-viewing endoscope, the instrument has to be maneuvered into a J-shaped position, looking back on itself, to identify these lesions.

Probably because the fundus is the site of acid production, it is amply supplied with blood vessels, and these ulcers may appear with severe bleeding. As antacids and mucosal protective agents exert their topical effects in the stomach's most dependent areas, proximal ulcers are more medically refractory; this is particularly important because, when deep, they may penetrate into the adjacent spleen or pancreas. Like proximal gastric cancers, these ulcers require sacrifice of a substantial amount of stomach to be adequately excised. This carries the important consequences of a diminished gastric reservoir and the potential for mechanical damage to the gastroesophageal sphincter, increasing the postoperative risk of regurgitation and aspiration. Figure 2–3A illustrates a typical, benign-appearing gastric fundal ulceration. The usual radiologic signs of a benign lesion, such as radiating hyperplastic folds or a hyperplastic radiolucent mucosal ridge at its edge (Hampton's line), are not regularly seen in this area. Like other gastric ulcers, they need not be associated with acid hypersecretion, and their presence probably reflects an equivalent defect in mucosal resistance. Apart from contrasting them with an ulcerated malignancy, their primary distinction is from gastric diverticula (Fig. 2–3B), which are typically located in the fundus. However, in the case of diverticula, a funnel-shaped neck is usually evident.

The point at which the esophagus enters the gastric fundus can be seen subdiaphragmatically as a stellate collection of barium whose margins conform only to rugae. Gastric fundal cancers may, however, confuse the inexperienced viewer, as they often resemble the edematous folds of some benign ulcerations.

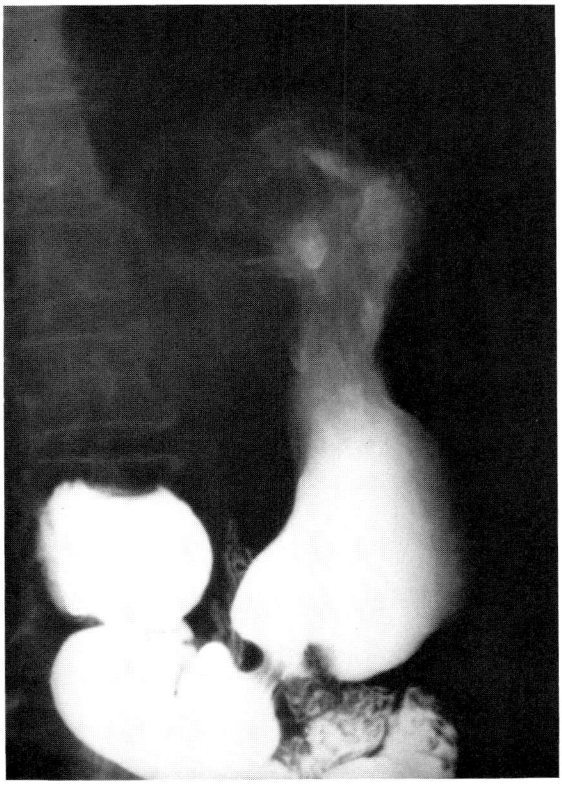

FIG. 2–3. A. Ovoid superficial collection of barium in the gastric fundus in a patient with intractable pain who was previously considered hysterical. Note conspicuous absence of rugal folds.

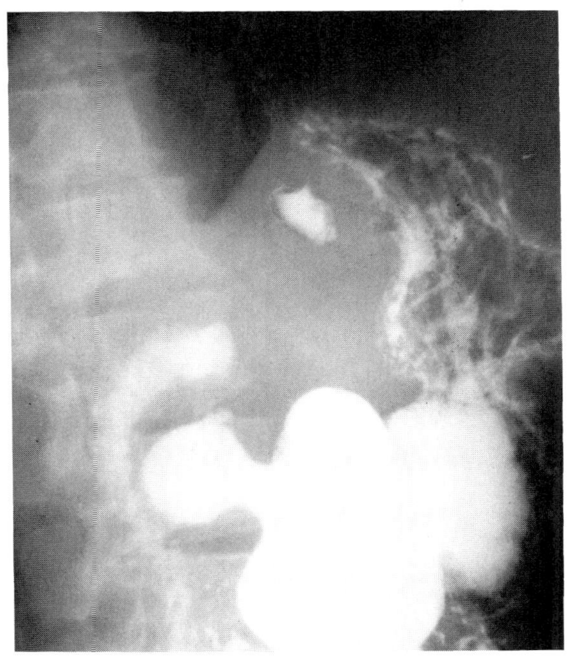

B. A fundal diverticulum, which can be mistaken for a deep ulcer. Note the slender neck connecting it with the stomach.

POSTGASTRECTOMY (ANASTOMOTIC OR MARGINAL) ULCER

A conspicuous surgical treatment failure, the posthemigastrectomy ulceration's hallmark is bleeding, often as massive as it is painless. The lesion results both from acid secretion continuing after antrectomy and its direct exposure onto jejunal mucosa, without prior neutralization by duodenal or pancreatic bicarbonate. This lesion was obviously more common in the period prior to H_2 receptor blocker therapy (i.e., there were more operations then for ulcer disease), particularly when either distal gastrectomy or simple gastrojejunostomy was not combined with truncal or selective vagotomy. The lesions are almost always on the jejunal side of an end-to-side Billroth-II-type gastrojejunostomy. Intestinal bile's regurgitation further diminishes the gastric mucosa's usual resistance to acid injury, promoting additional peristomal tissue damage, while the unavoidable surgical separation of bicarbonate from acid at the jejunal portion of the anastomosis additionally increases the caustic insult.

Conventional acute medical therapy is generally unsatisfactory, and while tempting in the vagally intact patient, "chemical" (anticholinergic) vagotomy inhibits acid less than surgical division. Moreover, treating a bleeding patient with agents that can induce tachycardia sacrifices one clinical parameter (pulse rate) of circulating blood volume. If done alone, even emergency surgical vagotomy, whether abdominal or thoracic, still leaves behind a bleeding point and the risk of reoperation. Accordingly, ulcer excision and modifying or moving the gastroenterostomy seems to be the most conservative management overall.

If searched for properly, the ulcers are relatively easy to see, often as elliptical or triangular barium collections (Fig. 2–4) adjacent to or just separate from the gastric pouch. The patient is best examined using a small amount of barium, which is necessary only to coat the gastric remnant and adjacent midgut. An ulcer should be searched for early after barium ingestion, as loops of contrast-filled proximal jejunum may obscure the anastomosis, while dye filling the abbreviated stomach may approximate the collection in the ulcer crater. If rugal folds are thickened or proximal jejunum edematous, an unrecognized acid hypersecretory state (Zollinger-Ellison syndrome?) needs consideration. Plain abdominal x rays should be searched for metallic clips at the gastroesophageal junction, indicating the surgeon has done, or at least attempted, truncal vagotomy.

The culprit crater may be visible endoscopically only when the tip of the endoscope is maneuvered into either afferent or efferent loop, beyond a usually erythematous, circumostomy gastric mucosa. A pool of blood obscuring a suspicious area may be mobilized by placing the sedated patient gently into a semiseated position. Physically manipulating a clot, like performing a biopsy on a recently bleeding ulcer, risks rehemorrhage.

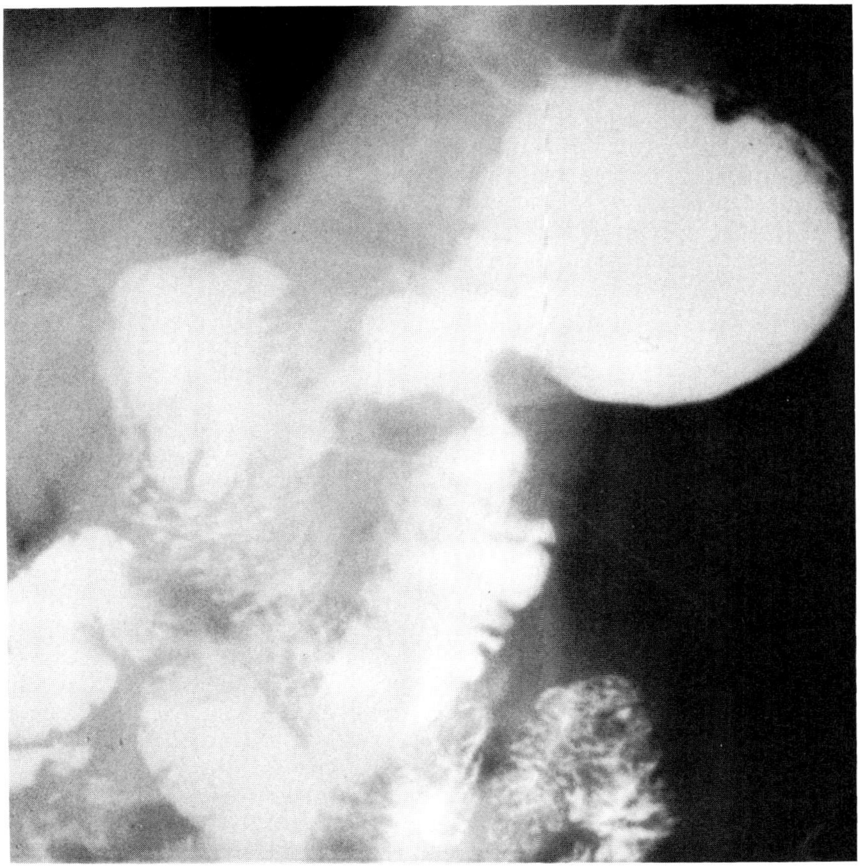

FIG. 2–4. Rounded collection of barium at the junction of gastric pouch with afferent and efferent jejunal loops, an ulceration on the intestinal side of a gastroentrostomy. No vagotomy clips are seen.

GASTRIC POLYPOSIS

Gastric polyps are focal or diffuse, single or multiple; as in pernicious anemia and most gastric cancers, the development of polyposis reflects a diffusely abnormal gastric mucosa, often associated with achlorhydria and intrinsic-factor deficiency. The presence of polyps may indicate concurrent or future gastric carcinomas and thus are considered premalignant. Scattered or in clusters, they are almost always true adenomas when large enough to be seen radiologically. Since they are often achlorhydric, patients with bleeding adenomatous polyps cannot be expected to respond to attempts to decrease gastric acid.

Patients with familial colonic polyposis have a higher frequency of adenomatous polyps of the stomach. Unlike the lesions of familial colonic polyposis, the gastric varieties are not hereditary. However, their discovery mandates continued gastroscopic or radiologic surveillance, or both, unless one opts for a hazardous and often debilitating prophylactic total gastrectomy. Performing gastric cytology is cumbersome, time-consuming, inaccurate, and probably useful only in a center where it is employed as a particular researcher's hobby.

Some gastric polyps are pedunculated, and their transection is thus made easier. However, in contrast to the case of colon polyp retrieval, the speed of antral peristalsis risks the gastric lesions being swept into the small intestine immediately after separation from the gastric wall. Hence, if they are to be retrieved for histologic analysis, the lesions usually have to be grasped by a separate endoscopic snare prior to their being transected by cautery.

Because most gastric polyps are sessile, endoscopic snare polypectomy remains difficult. Reliance on Japanese inventiveness has usually been rewarded, suggesting that gastric polypectomy may eventually become popular, particularly in the poor-risk patient.

Hyperplastic "polyps" are small, have little association with gastric carcinoma, rarely bleed, and are usually seen only at endoscopy. Clearly, they are the most common gastric "neoplasm," probably accounting for as much as 90% of all isolated, benign, polypoid lesions of the stomach. They are usually under 5 mm in diameter, are typically sessile, and probably represent an innocent transformation of otherwise normal gastric mucosa. They tend to persist, occasionally increasing and decreasing in number, often remaining in the same location when re-examined endoscopically.

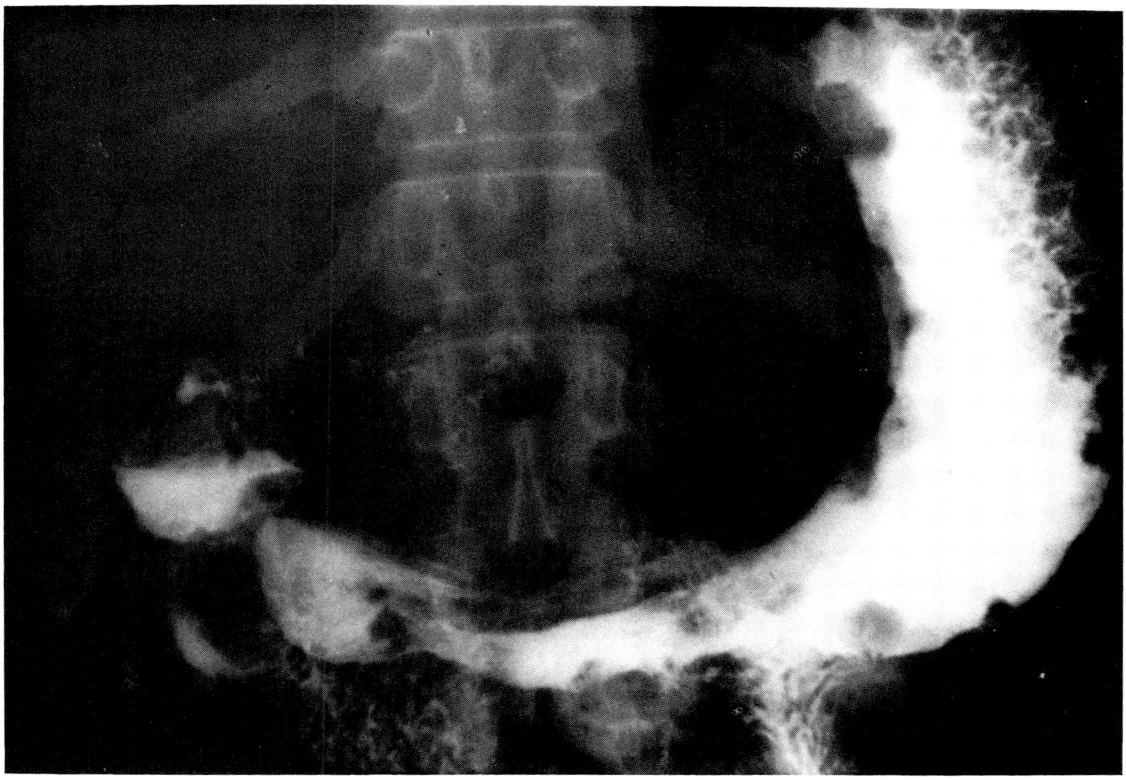

FIG. 2–5. Multiple 5- to 15-mm lucent nodules along greater and lesser curvature of fundus, body, and antrum. Lesions appear sessile, with short, thick attachments.

CARCINOMA OF THE GASTRIC FUNDUS

Like similar malignancies in the cecum, an adenocarcinoma beginning in the concave, upper reaches of the proximal stomach can grow to considerable size before becoming symptomatic, particularly if it does not involve the gastroesophageal junction. Because of their high, left upper quadrant location, they are rarely palpable. And since they rarely hinder gastric emptying or block the downward passage of food, their first appearance is almost invariably a function of metastasis or bleeding from a substantial mass. As centrifugal growth parallels that into the lumen, extension through to adjacent organs (e.g., diaphragm, pancreas, or spleen) may be found at CT scan or surgery.

For the same reasons that proximal gastric ulcers or leiomyomas are often overlooked, fundal malignancies can be obscured. The fundic reservoir pools contrast, and barium studies that do not employ air-contrast technique will bypass serious lesions. A similar danger accrues to gastroscopy. Most endoscopes are straight viewing, and though their tips contain wide-angle lenses, they pass forward from the esophagus into the body of the stomach and may overlook a lesion that is literally 150 to 170° posterior, behind, or above the cardia. Employing the so-called J-turn instrument maneuver, the careful endoscopist will fully retroflex the tip of the instrument back upon itself to better inspect this underside. But this takes time, as does the proper coating and air-filling of the upper stomach. The issue of obscure GI bleeding is often resolved in the gastric fundus.

On x ray, the tumors are usually visualized as irregular nodular excrescences of the upper stomach (Fig. 2–6A). Occasionally, they may be seen on a plain film of the chest, indenting the gastric air bubble (Fig. 2–6B). Similarly, a widening space between the stomach and the diaphragm can imply a thickened mucosa.

Management almost always necessitates total gastrectomy, with intraoperative examination and resection of as much distal esophagus as is required to extend above the tumor's upper edge. The cancers are often found when advanced; therefore, local palliative resection is sometimes indicated, particularly for chronic bleeding. The same is true for laser or BICAP fulguration. Yet, removal of even a portion of fundus often sacrifices a segment of gastroesophageal sphincter or impairs its function, leaving the patient at risk for recurrent aspiration. Then, the most conservative procedure is, paradoxically, total gastrectomy and esophagojejunostomy.

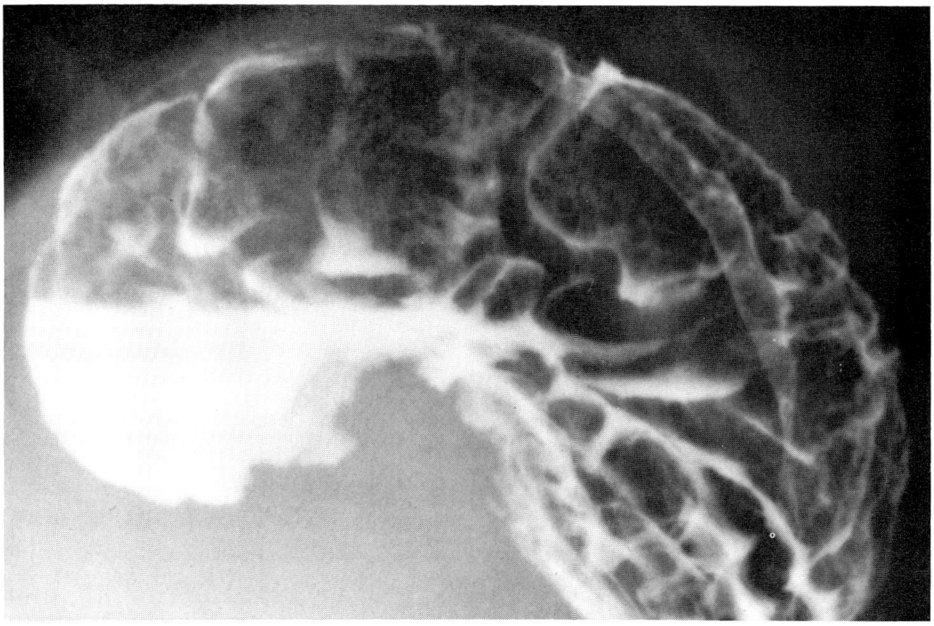

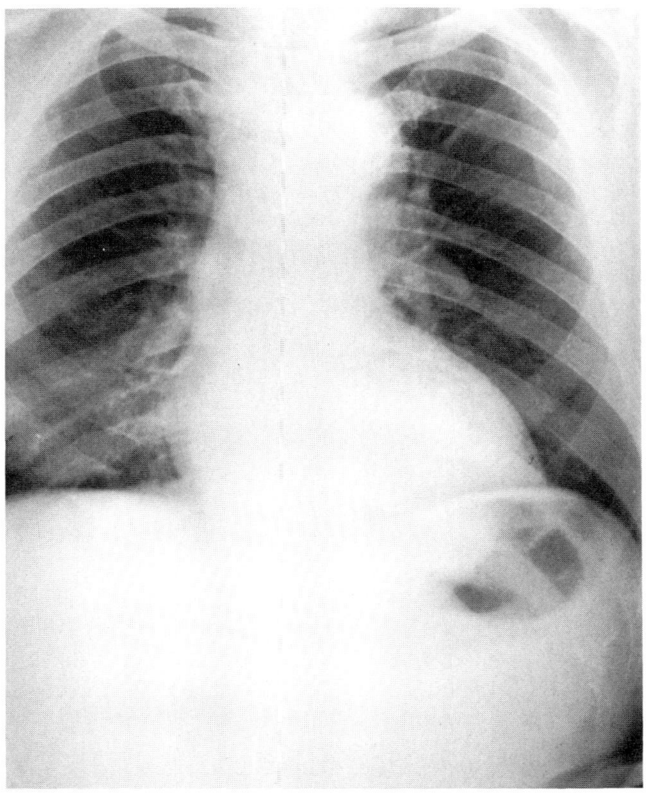

FIG. 2–6. A. View of distended, contrast-coated fundus. Tumorous involvement suggested by enormous, irregular mucosal thickening.
B. Chest x ray revealing gastric air bubble indented medially by a large spherical mass in the left upper abdominal quadrant.

MALIGNANT GASTRIC ULCER

The tumor is seen here as a primarily negative shadow in the form of an archer's bow, indenting the upper greater curvature of the stomach (Fig. 2–7). Its central depression reflects cavitation necrosis within the mass, whose expansion is outstripping its blood supply. In contrast to benign ulcers, which enter a gastric wall of relatively normal caliber, cancerous ulcers constitute penetration into a tumor mass. Its greater-curvature location and abrupt "shoulder" at upper and lower edges also argue for the lesion's tumorous nature. Located in the most capacious portion of the stomach, it is unlikely to cause obstruction, yet given the evident large ulceration, continuous, usually low-grade bleeding is a certainty. Perhaps atypically, this tumor appears to emerge from a radiologically healthy gastric mucosa. The rugal pattern appears normal; no associated gastric polyps appear, and barium flows unobstructed. The proximity of the upper fundus and the left hemidiaphragm suggests there is no significant transmural extension, making the tumor appear resectable, though perhaps not curable. Yet, its high gastric location argues that prudent surgical removal will mandate total gastrectomy, since attaching an acid-producing gastric remnant to an esophagus unprotected by a sacrificed gastroesophageal sphincter risks severe regurgitant acid injury, regurgitant bile injury, and pulmonary aspiration.

The mass-like configuration of this typically shaped gastric cancer contrasts with those of the Orient, particularly Japan, where they tend to be smooth and superficial, extending across the mucosa like an oil slick. The late development of deeper penetration and nodal involvement render these tumors more surgically curable, though their rapid centrifugal extension necessitates wider excision.

Apart from Japanese ancestry, factors favoring gastric cancer development seem to include antecedent adult celiac disease, living in Northern climates, possessing blood type A, concurrent gastric mucosal atrophy or polyposis, and a prior gastric ulcer or distant subtotal gastrectomy performed for acid-peptic disease.

Even though metastases may be demonstrable at the bedside, on CT scan, or on routine plain films, hemigastrectomy usually proves the most effective palliation, eliminating a transfusion requirement or reducing dysphagia while retaining some gastric reservoir capacity. No convincing evidence of the value of chemotherapy or x-irradiation has yet emerged. Less dramatic endoscopic palliation by tumor-debulking through laser or heater probe may prove valuable in selected patients.

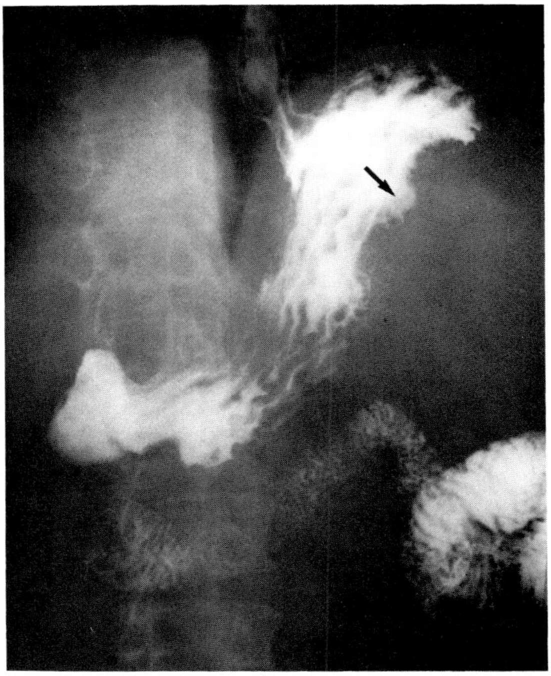

FIG. 2–7. Note doubly rounded negative shadow encroaching on the lumen from the greater curvature of the fundus. A central depression ↗ reflects ulceration within the tumor. The duodenum is obscured behind the pylorus, but gastric outflow appears unimpeded, and the rugal pattern is otherwise normal.

OBSTRUCTING ANTRAL CANCER

Without the reassurance provided by an antecedent history of peptic-ulcer disease, the insidious development of gastric outlet obstruction argues for tumorous encroachment. Regardless of its etiology, antral obstruction displays a fairly standard history: early satiety without dysphagia, followed by upper abdominal distention and copious, generally painless vomiting of food recognizable from the last meal or meals, with rapid return of appetite. Physical examination may disclose pallor, wasting, an epigastric mass, left upper quadrant distention, or evidence of metastatic disease, such as a large liver or ascites. Even hours after meals, a so-called "succussion splash" may be audible from the to-and-fro cascade of trapped gastric contents while rocking the recumbent patient laterally on the examining table or bed with the stethoscope on the upper abdomen.

If the first surgical option, which is radical hemigastrectomy with gastroenterostomy, is considered impossible, high, simple gastroenterostomy is next best, making the anastomosis wide enough to forstall occlusion by any future tumorous growth. Shrinking the distended stomach by several days of constant, adequate nasogastric suction will restore its tone and decrease the postoperative time required for a gastroenterostomy to begin functioning. Though there are some advocates of endoscopic balloon dilation, use of the heater probe, or laser tumor ablation, the best decompressive treatment is always surgical. The problem of obstructing gastric cancer seems to be an instance in which enthusiasm for therapeutic endoscopy still exceeds its technical capability.

Figure 2–8 discloses the anatomic correlates of the physiology suggested by the symptoms. There is circumferential narrowing of the distal 3½ in. of stomach, with a more or less "applecore" configuration, representing the narrowed lane for gastric contents into the duodenum. The proximal edge of the tumor appears as an irregular shoulder on the barium column, distinguishable from the smooth, usually focal narrowing of a typical postinflammatory scar. The body and fundus are enormously distended, the most inferior portion of the greater curvature falling well below the pelvic rim. The mottling of barium confirms its contamination with retained food, gastric mucus, and saliva.

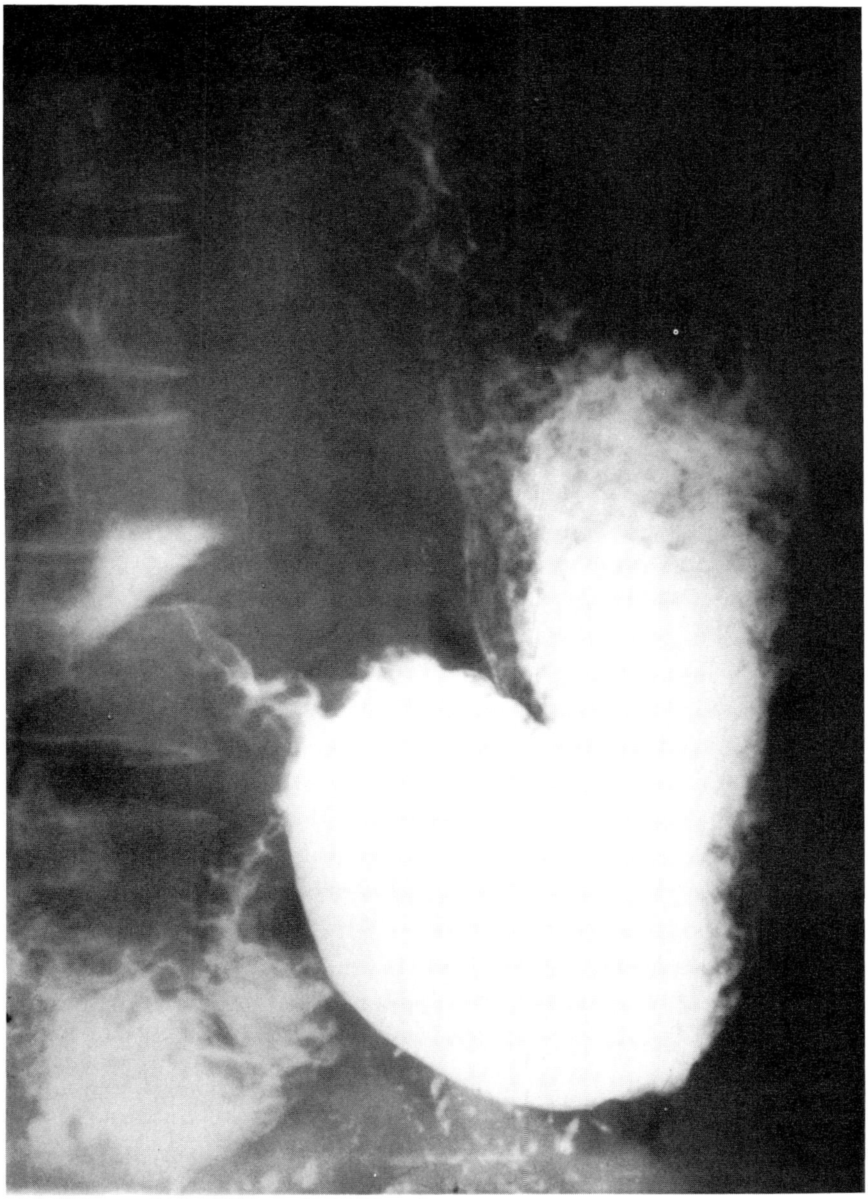

FIG. 2–8. Extraordinary proximal gastromegaly leads to a thin trickle of barium through an irregularly stenotic antrum. The gastric rugal pattern is effaced by gastric distension. Barium flocculates amid a dispersion of old retained food and secretions.

ZOLLINGER-ELLISON SYNDROME

The clinical hallmark of this classic tumor-humor (usually pancreatic, always gastrin-related) syndrome is intractable, recurrent, often bleeding peptic ulcers, sometimes in unforgettably atypical locations such as the esophagus, the distal duodenum, the midgut, and (rarely) the colon, but most often in the duodenal bulb or stomach, just like the ulcers of nonhypergastrinemic states. The first visual clues on the barium x ray include a fasting, unobstructed stomach filled with fluid and exhibiting generalized thickening of its mucosa, both of which are responses to a profound hormonal secretory drive. Coarsening of duodenal and jejunal folds reflect both their irritative inundation with high volumes of concentrated stomach acid and the edema resulting from secondary albumin loss. More than half of pancreatic gastrinomas are malignant; hence, widening of the duodenal C-loop or hepatomegaly may be evident. Esophageal strictures are common, and barium flocculating in the flooded small intestine often suggests sprue.

Typically, Zollinger-Ellison syndrome is belatedly identified in a patient who returns with peptic-type symptoms after undergoing ulcer surgery. This typical x ray (Fig. 2–9) shows an anastomotic ulcer on the small-bowel side of a Billroth-II-type gastrojejunostomy. The adjacent jejunal mucosa is typically spastic or irritable, and its sprue-like appearance correlates the patient's usual diarrhea and cachexia with blunting of villi seen on intestinal biopsy specimens. Indeed, the x ray and bedside combination of a "malabsorption pattern" and peptic-ulcer disease strongly suggests the hormonal cause.

The diagnosis is confirmed by the demonstration of an elevated fasting serum gastrin, and is further augmented by intravenous secretin infusion along with a markedly increased basal acid output, or the angiographic disclosure of a vascular tumor of the pancreas or gastric wall. Medical management often requires many times the dosage of H_2-receptor blockers employed for ordinary peptic ulcers. Prior to their availability, treatment was total gastrectomy, still needed when medication is incompletely effective or poorly tolerated. As the ulcers are aggressive and the tumors slow-growing, patients stay sick or die more frequently from their ulcer disease than from cancer. Hence, when required, gastrectomy surgery must remove every vestige of acid-secreting epithelium at the risk of anastomotic perforation by another peptic ulcer. Thus, the proximal and distal edges of the resected specimen should be proven by frozen section to be esophageal and duodenal mucosa respectively. A curious, unexplained regression or stabilization of metastatic gastrinoma has been reported in some patients following total gastrectomy.

Because gastrin elaboration is stimulated normally by alkalinization of specific antral cells, a similar ulcer syndrome can be produced when the surgeon, operating for ulcer, fails to properly identify the junction of stomach and duodenum and mistakenly creates an afferent loop whose proximal edge contains a nubbin of antral mucosa chronically bathed in duodenal bicarbonate.

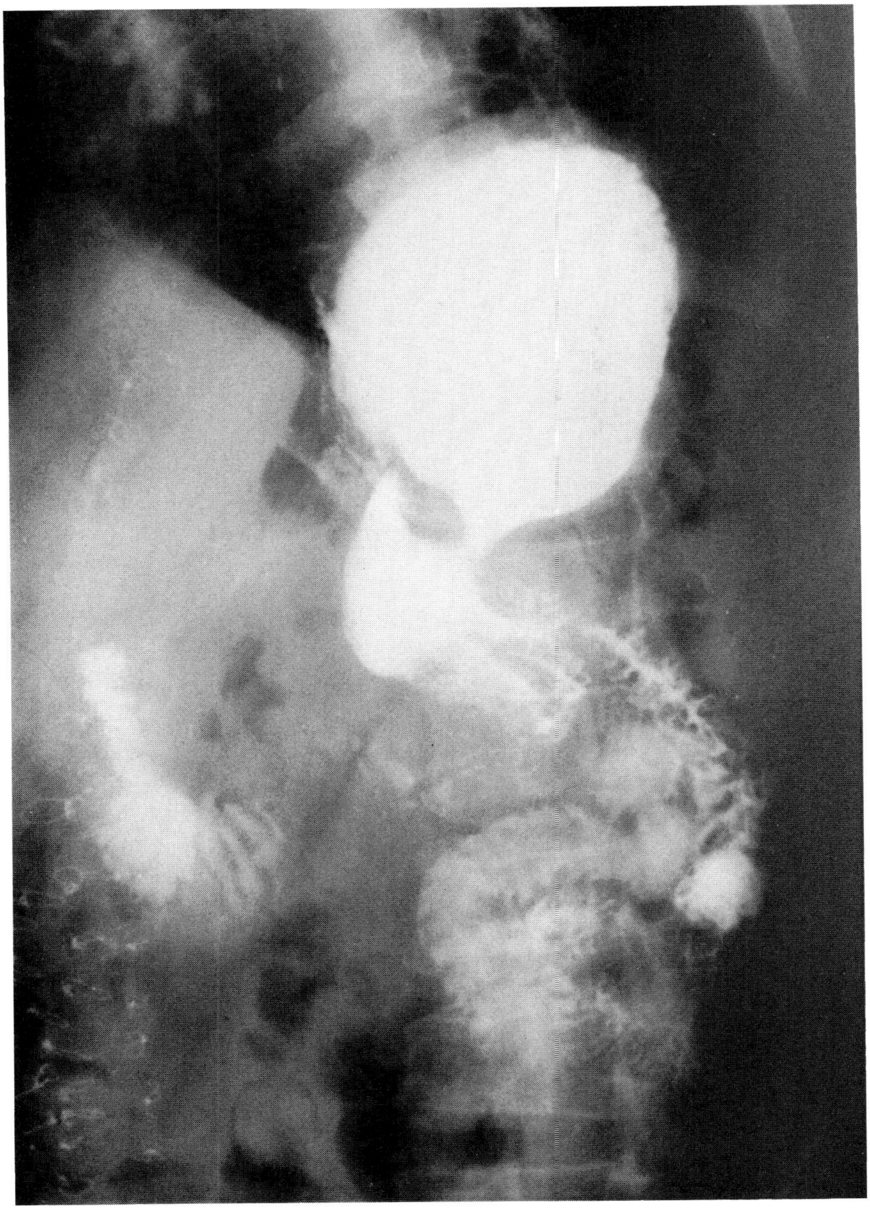

FIG. 2–9. Upper GI showing Billroth-II-type hemigastrectomy and a large jejunal ulceration with an "ace-of-spades" contour. Spiculated mucosa of the efferent loop argues for a jejunitis, typical of massive gastric hypersecretion.

BENIGN INFILTRATIVE DISEASES OF THE STOMACH

In the rarer benign (or perhaps better stated, noncancerous) gastric infiltrations (including a radiologically exuberant, but healthy gastric mucosa), either the clinical history or the multisystem nature of a disease provides the useful clues. While the upper GI series merely raises the curtain on a panoply of disorders, only a careful history or well-used clinical laboratory, endoscopy with biopsy, or even a full-thickness surgical specimen are definitive. Yet, while staring at the viewbox, there are still some useful facts to recall.

Eosinophilic gastroenteritis (Fig. 2–10A) typically involves and obstructs an edematous gastric antrum. This condition is seen rarely with ascites, and often includes a diarrheal enteropathy and an extraordinary circulating eosinophilia, sometimes with pruritis and bronchospasm. It remits dramatically with corticosteroids and recurs without obvious provocation, though food allergies are occasionally implicated.

Menetriere's disease, an idiopathic, rare, hyperplastic, noninflammatory disorder of gastric mucosa (Fig. 2–10B), is typically confined to the proximal two-thirds of the stomach, constituting a focal but not readily resectable cause of protein-losing enteropathy. Symptoms include painless anorexia and hypoalbuminemic edema. While the thickened proximal stomach suggests cancer, deep gastric biopsies just show an increase of large mucus cells, which occasionally coalesce into cysts or penetrate the muscularis mucosae. Some patients do eventually develop adenocarcinoma in the involved area; thus, while a correct diagnosis excludes cancer, the risk of eventual malignancy mandates continued endoscopic and radiologic surveillance.

Primary Crohn's disease or sarcoidosis of the stomach are rare, except as relatively trivial satellite features of a dominant intestinal or pulmonary disease. Gastric syphilis is one feature of Internal Medicine's ineradicable bad penny. Pseudolymphoma is probably a pseudodisease, only an extravagant but mature lymphocytic and other acute and chronic inflammatory cell reaction to an indolent gastric ulcer.

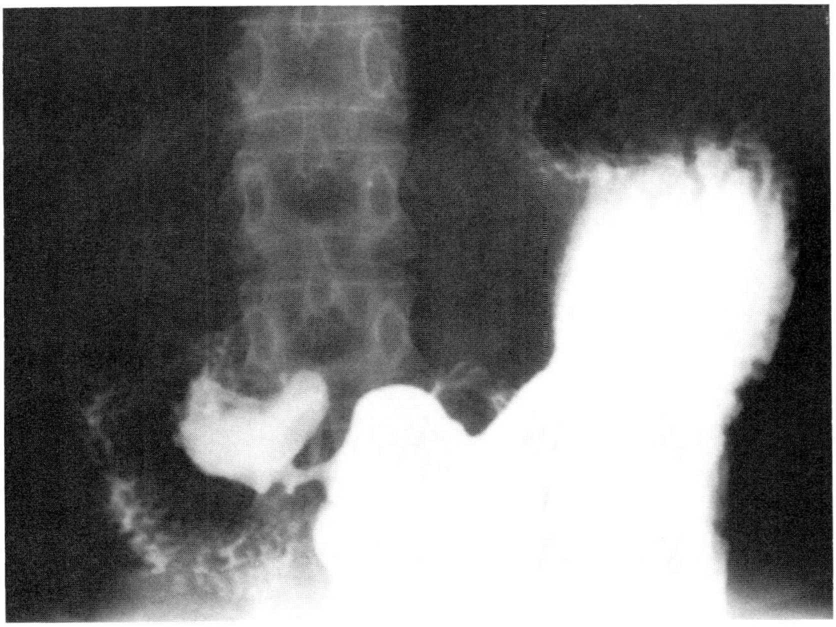

A

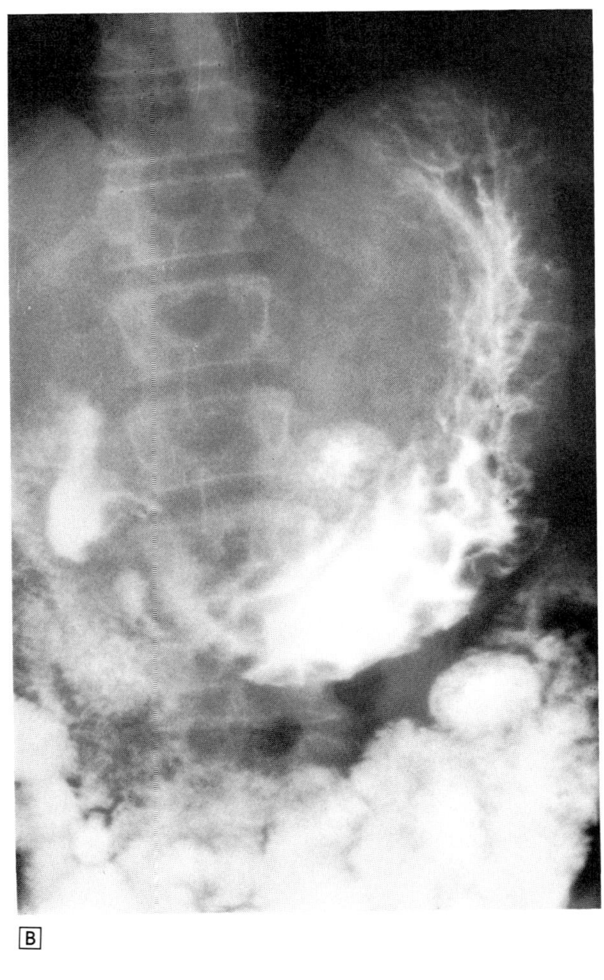

B

FIG. 2–10. A. Eosinophilic gastroenteritis—a smooth, discrete stenosis of the gastric antrum, proximal to the duodenal bulb and indistinguishable from an antral web, stricture, or even an atypical smooth adenocarcinoma. The stomach is distended.
B. Menetriere's disease—prominent, coarse, regular hypertrophy of gastric rugal folds in the proximal two thirds of the stomach with relative antral sparing.

MALIGNANT INFILTRATIVE DISEASES OF THE STOMACH

Collectively, these usually transmural gastric disorders display segmental or diffuse rugal hypertrophy, often with mucosal ulceration and delayed emptying. Responsible are both primary gastric lesions and generalized malignancies involving the stomach. Though diagnostic considerations vary widely between these and the noncancerous gastropathies, the x rays are often similar, one thickened stomach pretty much resembling another.

The more common malignant infiltrative diseases include gastric lymphoma, leiomyosarcoma, and the so-called "linitis plastica" (or leather-bottle) distribution of submucosal gastric adenocarcinoma. When symptomatic, the latter tumors (Fig. 2–11A) are often locally advanced, and cancer is already clinically suspected. Patients complain of early satiety, and even if the gastric reservoir seems undiminished at fluoroscopy, fixation is apparent, particularly when later films show near identical outlines, thus implying that the stomach neither expands, empties, or moves. The diminished gastric pliability, peristalsis, and reservoir capacity of advanced malignant diseases may occur without large intracavitary excrescences. Carcinoma's tendency to metastasize, and lymphoma's often multicentric nature, provide other radiologic clues (e.g., small-bowel obstruction, lytic bone lesions, pulmonary nodules).

Typically, the non-Hodgkins type, the usual gastric lymphoma displays exuberant, often distorted or irregular rugal folds (Fig. 2–11B). As the commonest "nonhematologic" organ involved, the stomach is sometimes the sole site of lymphoma, which may be cured by gastrectomy and is often sensitive to both x-ray therapy and chemotherapy. Gastric lymphoma's treatment, therefore, should be vigorous and approached with a view toward cure, even beyond surgery.

Gastric leiomyosarcomas usually appear with chronic pain followed by vigorous bleeding. They are typically radioresistant and rarely cured by surgery, responding only to wide, but usually only palliative, excision. They may resemble unusually large leiomyomas with the characteristic central ulceration, but centrifugal infiltration often distinguishes them from their benign relations.

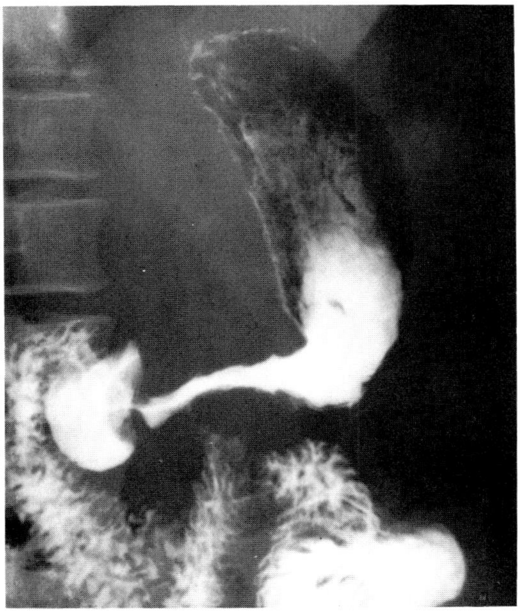

FIG. 2–11. A. Linitis plastica. Fixed semicircular deformity of the gastric antrum, with mucosal spiculation throughout and tissue protuberance leftward into the duodenal bulb; only partial obstruction is present. Congruence of the gastric outline on repeated films of the same area indicates nonpliability.

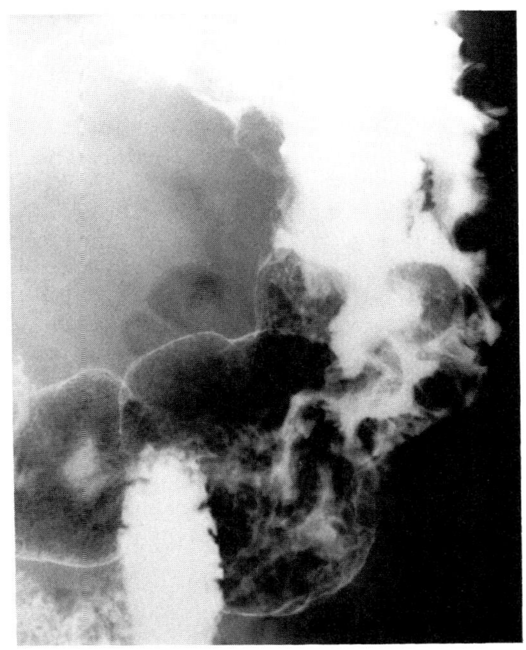

B. Massive, irregular rugal hypertrophy of advanced lymphoma. The gastric wall is replaced by a tumorous nodularity, comprised of clusters of mature and immature lymphocytes.

ATROPHIC GASTRITIS

Atrophic gastritis can be thought of as the radiologic opposite of both benign and malignant gastric infiltrative disorders. Generally speaking, it is a disease of the elderly, though a variety of antibodies, including those to intrinsic factor, parietal cells, and thyroglobulin, have been described in patients of any age with idiopathic gastritis. The low but unquestionable incidence of an immunoglobulin deficiency in certain patients with atrophic gastritis also suggests an immunologic role. Though etiology remains speculative, the physiologic and clinical implications are clear and important. While there is no motor abnormality associated with mucosal atrophy, and hydrochloric acid is not necessary for adequate digestion of foodstuffs, deficiency of intrinsic factor will lead to B-12 malabsorption and eventually to classic, pernicious anemia. The earlier the onset of gastric atrophy, the likelier is the effect on erythropoiesis.

The gastric mucosa on upper GI series is generally flat and featureless, losing the normal rippling rugal pattern of an exuberant, secretory mucosa to be replaced by a bland, featureless, seemingly effaced wall. This correlates gastroscopically with mucosal thinning and transparency, as well as the visual emergence of multiple, blue submucosal veins, ordinarily obscured by a healthy mucosa. On occasion, the gastroscopist or the radiologist may be the first to suspect early pernicious anemia.

Though the mucosa seems quiescent, it is microscopically active. Inflammatory infiltrates, fundic-gland disappearance, intestinal metaplasia, and cellular dysplasia may be seen. As a precursor of gastric carcinoma, the late mucosal atrophy of gastritis should be followed by regular endoscopies, which are superior to air-contrast x rays in detecting small lesions. Gastritis, eventual atrophy, and carcinoma are also described in the postgastrectomy stump of patients who have undergone an operation for peptic-ulcer disease.

Though the term "gastritis" is often used by patients to describe a sense of bloat, fullness, upper abdominal pain, nausea, or vomiting, the phrase is as meaningless and nonspecific as "gas." There is no identifiable symptom pattern that can be attributed to gastric mucosal inflammation, atrophy, or both. Some form of dyspepsia may prompt the upper GI or gastroscopic examination that reveals an anatomic diagnosis. Certainly, the doctor who ascribes abdominal pain to gastritis is well advised to keep looking.

Apart from their debatable academic interest, acid secretory tests in gastritis are rarely useful, except in documenting pentagastrin-fast achlorhydria. The widespread, usually inappropriate administration of vitamin B-12 for its presumed tonic-like effect has probably lessened the clinical appearance of pernicious anemia in gastritis patients in much the same way as oral antibiotics, given for all respiratory diseases, have fortuitously decreased the frequency of rheumatic heart disease.

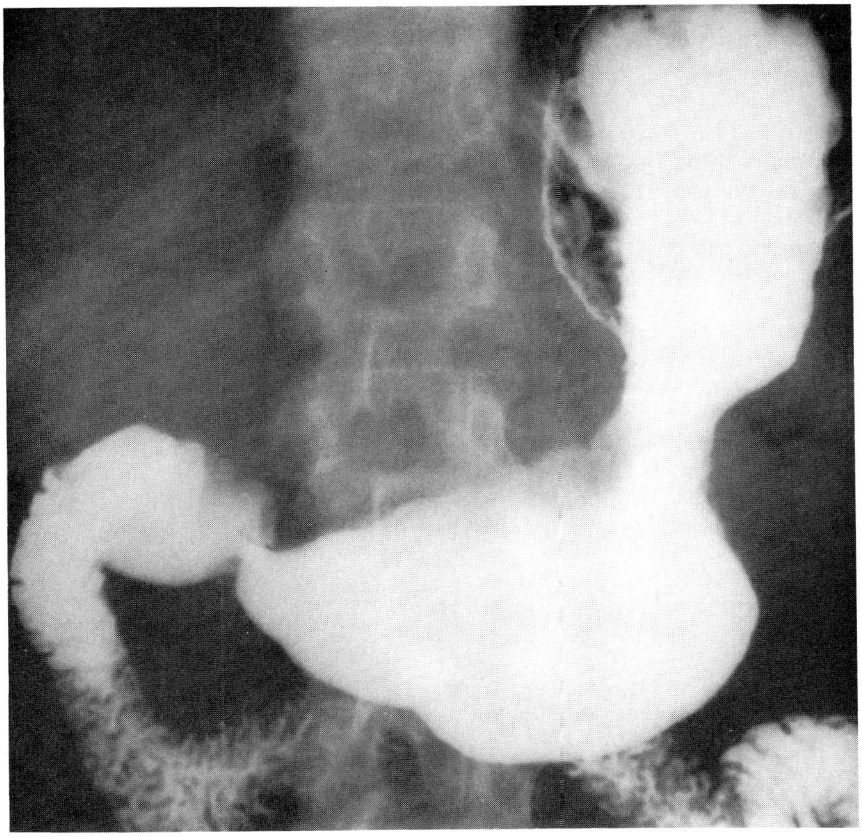

FIG. 2–12. Smooth, featureless stomach, showing virtually complete absence of rugal folds. Indentation on the greater curvature is the tip of the spleen.

SUPERFICIAL SPREADING GASTRIC CARCINOMA

Previously thought to be a Japanese medical monopoly, the superficially spreading form of gastric cancer is increasingly recognized in Western populations, probably as a function of gastroscopy's wider employment and despite a decrease in the overall occurrence of adenocarcinoma of the stomach. Since these carcinomas possess such small actual mass, most are discovered "incidentally," when the patient's x ray or endoscopy are performed for symptoms likely to arise from other causes. These malignancies tend to spread web-like along the mucosa of the stomach, rarely penetrating more than two or three cells deep until late in the course of the illness. The malignancy is well treated by wide excision with nodal dissection and, true for the Far East as well as the West, survival rates for this form of tumor are superior to those of the remainder of the gastric cancer population. Whether this malignancy is a special tumor with a history of slow local growth and late distant metastasis or merely an artificial subselection of less malignant gastric cancer is unknown. The gastric cancer problem in Japan is addressed by public education and the widespread availability and employment of high-quality radiology and endoscopy, doubtless further accounting for Japan's impressive surgical success.

X-ray examinations are likely to be profitable only when double-contrast technique is utilized and the patient is rotated, coating the air-filled stomach with a thin layer of barium. There are few instances in medical gastroenterology when cooperation of the referring physician and radiologist is as critical; if unprepared for these subtle changes, even the best radiologists are not likely to find them.

Representative films of two different patients are shown. Figure 2–13A reveals faint mucosal thickening, elevation, and nodularity, involving a 2- to 3-in. portion of the greater curvature of the stomach. In Figure 2–13B, superficial tumor at the junction of fundus and body is manifested again by only the most seemingly trivial irregularity. In this second patient, biopsies of an area of benign-appearing mucosal erythema discovered at endoscopy disclosed adenocarcinoma, and this upper GI series was performed, in part, to help the surgeon considering gastrectomy to locate a likely proximal resection line. Easily missed in a barium-filled stomach, the size of these tumors may also be underestimated by gross inspection at surgery. Intraoperative frozen-section microscopy is a valuable guide to avoiding an inadequate excision and reoperation.

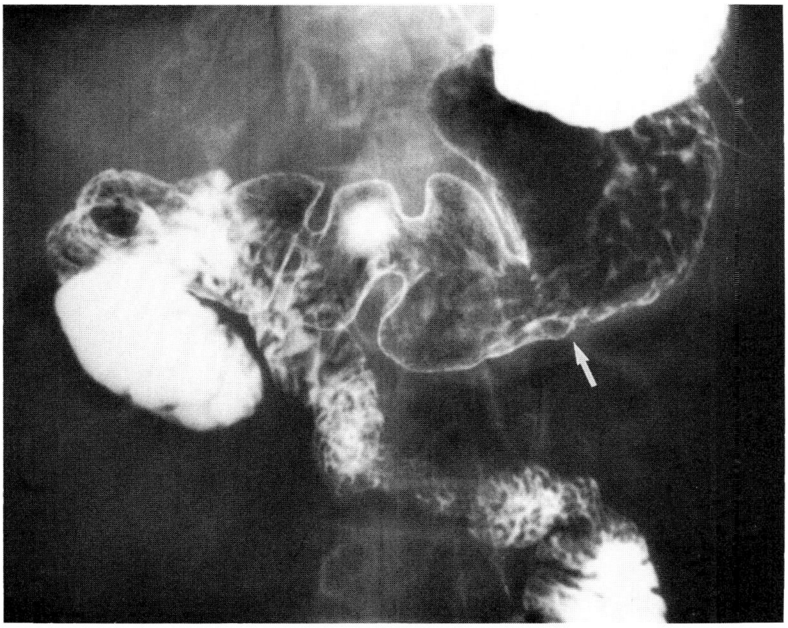

FIG. 2–13. A. Modest straightening and fine nodularity of the greater curvature of the body and antrum of the stomach, but no significant loss of reservoir capacity. This lesion can be easily missed if the stomach is filled with barium.

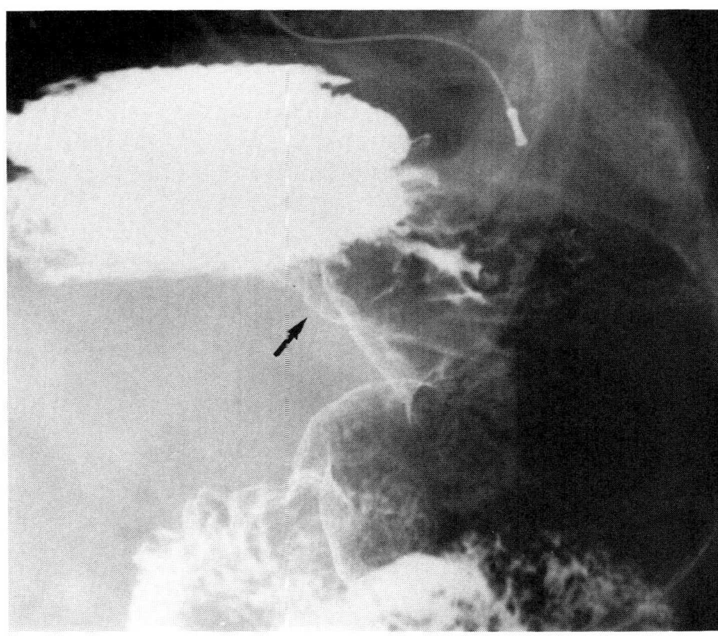

B. Minimal degree of mucosal elevation seen at the junction of fundus and body of the stomach on the lesser curvature. This extremely subtle finding is disclosable only when the radiologist is forewarned and air-contrast views are performed.

GASTRIC METASTASES

Uncommon when compared with primary gastric tumors, metastases to the stomach usually occur from certain highly malignant tumors, of which melanoma is the classic, demonic example. In addition to the usual sites of secondary deposit, such as liver, lung, bone, and brain, melanomas have an almost lunatic penchant for involving viscera; metastases occur in unpredictable and clinically significant ways to such unlikely areas as orbit, gallbladder mucosa, pancreatic bed, ureter, skin, and genitalia.

Involvement of the GI tract by melanoma is fairly common. The rate at which these tumors grow partly accounts for their exuberant size and cavitary necrosis, producing the typical so-called "bull's-eye" or "donut" metastasis, which is also radiologically characteristic with midgut metastases. This lesion (Fig. 2–14) was the solitary reappearance of a melanoma removed years earlier from the shoulder of a 34-year-old white male. The study was performed following his presentation with painless GI bleeding and early satiety. The patient with melanomatosis may likewise demonstrate evidence of hypermetabolism with continuous, non-infectious fever, tachycardia, and rapid weight loss, which derive more from the lesion's biologic overactivity than to the patient's anorexia or diarrhea.

The x ray itself (Fig. 2–14) reveals the greater curvature of the fundus of the stomach invaded by a large spherical mass, which elevates the gastric mucosa circumferentially and contains a deep central ulceration over the tumor's necrotic center. Several factors—an ongoing transfusion requirement from this solitary, demonstrable GI bleeding site; the youth of the patient; and the opportunity for palliation from tumor debulking—argue for gastrectomy, which may yield complete, albeit temporary, remission. As alternative considerations, tumor-necrosis therapy by laser or heater probe seems unlikely to effect hemostasis, and high-dose irradiation to the stomach is certain to induce debilitating nausea.

A lesion in this location and of this shape may represent other dismal, alternative considerations, such as a large, atypical primary gastric carcinoma, leiomyosarcoma, or local invasion by a pancreatic tumor.

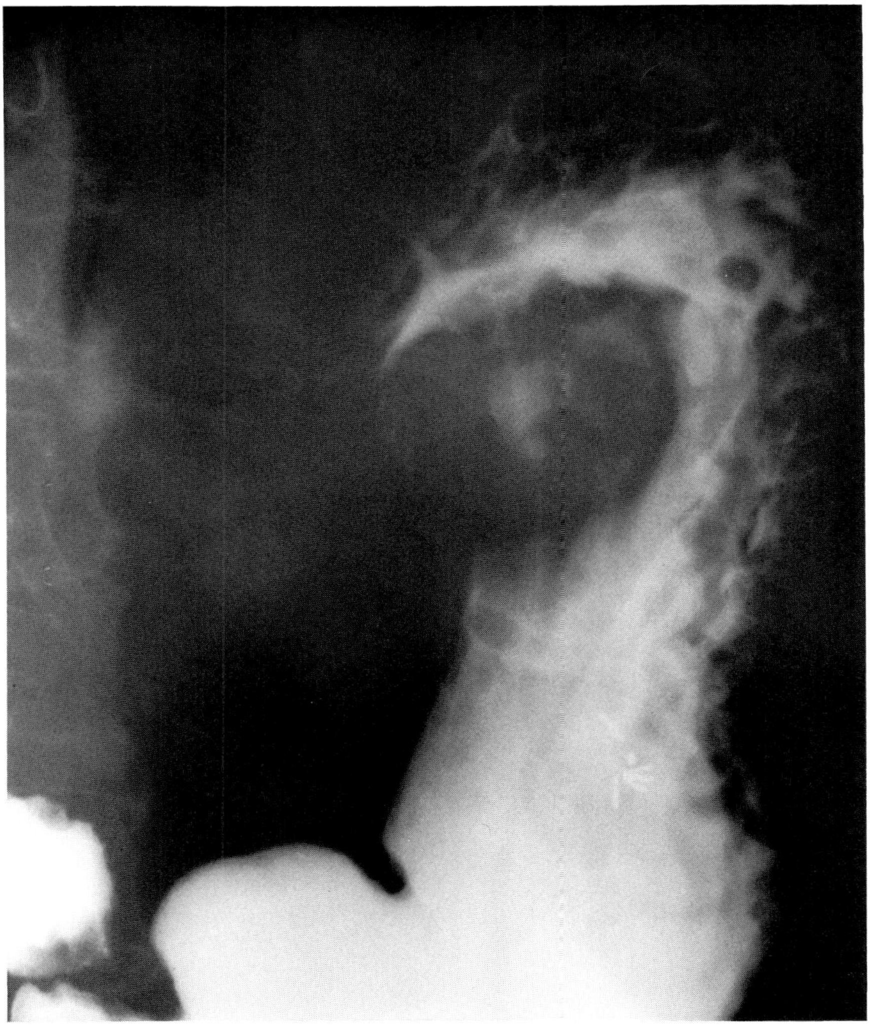

FIG. 2–14. A large radiolucent halo of tumor tissue in the upper 25% of the stomach surrounds a central, barium-filled ulceration. Exuberant elsewhere, the gastric rugae covering the tumor are effaced.

GASTRIC LEIOMYOMA

Not all gastric tumors are malignant, and apart from the usual adenomas or hyperplastic polyps, the commonest benign neoplasm is a leiomyoma. Invariably submucosal, most are rarely more than 1 to 2 cm in diameter and are clinically quiescent. Their slow growth correlates with the tedious microscopic similarity of the composition of the smooth-muscle cells. Mitoses are rare, and when present suggest the less common leiomyosarcoma. Assuming an egg-shaped or hemispheric contour, leiomyomas are pliable, with a rubbery-to-soft texture, and are rarely obstructive. But even benign tumors can continue growing, and while the gastric wall is mobile, its mucosa over the tumor becomes fixed as it is progressively stretched thin and smooth. Eventually, like the seam of a too-tight pair of trousers, it ruptures or ulcerates, either from pressure or ischemia; painless, often vigorous bleeding ensues.

And they can be missed. Most leiomyomas arise in the fundus, and because upper gastrointestinal bleeding usually originates from lesions of the distal stomach and duodenal bulb, casual radiologic investigations may overlook these tumors. Moreover, with the patient supine or recumbent, swallowed barium pools first in the fundic reservoir, often obscuring its mucosa. An example is noted in Figure 2–15A. The barium-filled stomach seems normal, but its uppermost portion is "amputated" by the top of the x-ray film plate. Understandably occupying the fluoroscopist's attention, the stomach's remainder does not appear abnormal, and the study was reported negative. With the patient's rebleeding, endoscopy confirmed that the hemorrhage was arising from just below the gastroesophageal sphincter. Performed with attention to the upper stomach, and with the thinly coated fundus largely emptied of barium, a repeat x ray (Fig. 2–15B) clearly outlines a well-demarcated, smooth, spherical tumor.

Excisional surgery in this area risks damage to the adjacent spleen and to the gastroesophageal sphincter; even limited resection may mandate a simultaneous antireflux procedure. If this involves folding the fundus about the distal esophagus, the resulting deformity makes it useful to obtain another contrast x ray several weeks later. It may be desirable to have the patient retain the films. Changes identified from the early postoperative gastric contour suggest development of new or recurrent tumor.

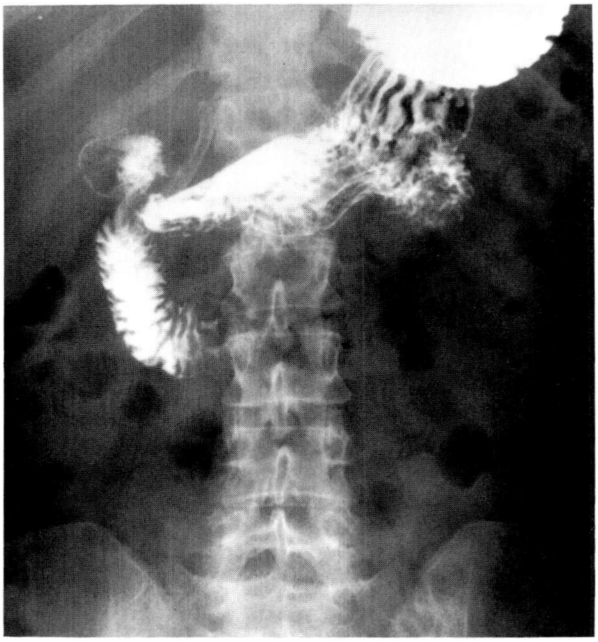

FIG. 2–15. A. Barium filled gastric fundus, whose upper third is cut off by the x-ray. The remainder of the stomach is normal.

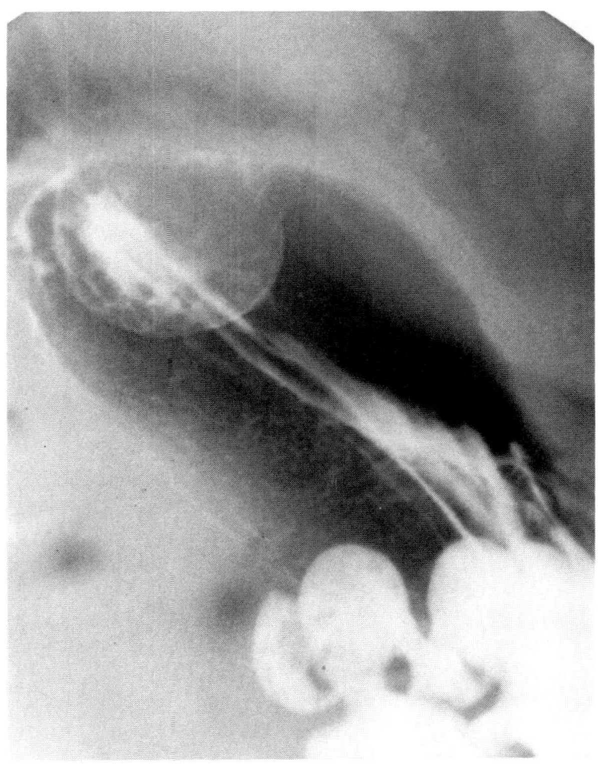

B. In the same patient, the upper film now includes the diaphragm, the left lower lung, and a barium-coated mucosa, containing a well-demarcated hemispherical tumor with a benign, but far from insignificant, appearance.

GASTROPARESIS DIABETICORUM

Gastric dilation with delayed emptying is a serious additional feature of diabetic autonomic neuropathy, attendant to long-standing insulin-dependent disease. Erratic insulin control of blood sugar can be a first sign, due, of course, to retarded calorie absorption. Here, as always, the radiologic clues of gastroparesis (Fig. 2–16) include a dilated, hypoperistaltic stomach that lacks anatomic evidence of gastric-outlet obstruction, suggesting to the fluoroscopist that the patient has eaten prior to examination or taken an anticholinergic. Gastric stasis is typically profound, and barium entering the stomach will be seen to flocculate with retained secretions, previously ingested food, or mucobezoars. The plain x ray may show an isolated fundic air-fluid level and mottled gastric contents in the left upper quadrant, without small-bowel distension, as well as other diabetic "fellow travellers" (e.g., calcified pancreas, aorta, seminal vesicles, and gallstones).

An ominous finding in those whose nutrition is already precarious, symptomatic gastroparesis is typically accompanied by other neuropathic abnormalities, including noctural fecal incontinence, mixed peripheral neuropathy, orthostatic hypotension, bladder and renal dysfunction, and diarrhea with steatorrhea. These should temper the impulse to perform gastrojejunostomy, but in this illness, two openings from the stomach may be better than one. Treatment with cholinergic agents or metoclopramide is often initially useful but eventually disappointing. The clinical examination therefore may show wasting, an abdominal succussion "splash," nausea unrelieved by vomiting, and feces-stained bedclothing.

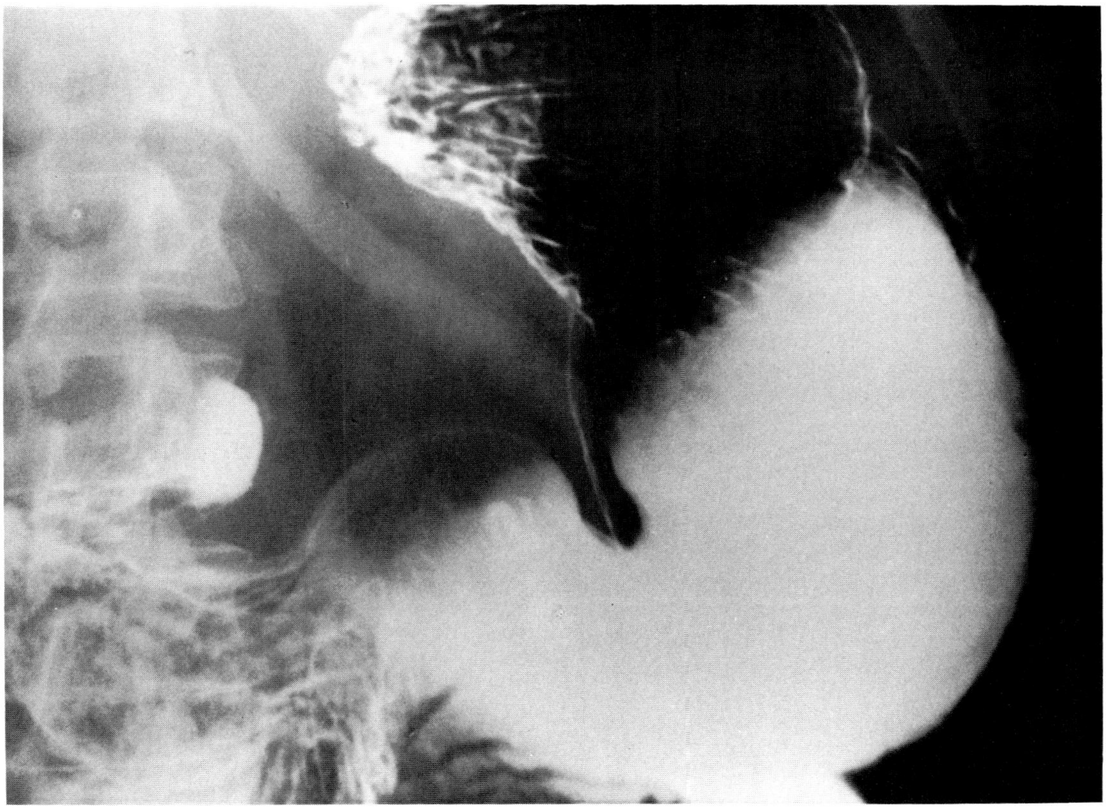

FIG. 2–16. Extraordinary gastromegaly, a filled stomach, and a patent antrum imply sluggish gastric emptying, without anatomic obstruction. Rugal folds are flattened because of gastric distention.

GASTRIC VOLVULUS

This surgical emergency is most commonly seen in elderly patients with a large, pre-existing paraesophageal hernia with ligaments stretched flaccid by years of a gastric fundus slipping freely upward through a widened diaphragmatic hiatus. A type of closed-loop obstruction with occlusive twists at the pyloric channel and cardia, gastric volvulus is caused by rotation of the stomach around its horizontal axis. Blocked proximally and distally, the body of the stomach becomes an expansile balloon. Swallowed air may continue to enter, while acid and mucus are retained in the volvulus itself, threatening imminent rupture.

Figure 2–17 discloses the characteristic "two-step" distended stomach, with air-fluid levels both in the left upper quadrant and further left and superiorly, in the intrathoracic paraesophageal hernia. The proximal gastric twist in the chest not only prevents decompression by vomiting but also blocks passage into the stomach of a nasogastric tube, here seen deflected laterally around the hernia.

Immediate surgical gastrotomy and gastric derotation are needed. To prevent recurrence, the stomach is stitched onto the inside of the abdominal wall or diaphragm, the transverse mesocolon is shortened, and the diaphragmatic hiatus is narrowed.

The larger the paraesophageal hernia, the greater the likelihood of volvulus; also increased is the frequency of ischemic ulcerations within the dislocated fundus. Thus, if bleeding from the herniated portion of the stomach can be demonstrated or volvulus is threatened, surgery is mandated.

Gastric volvulus is to be distinguished from the "upside-down stomach" of a congenital or traumatic diaphragmatic eventration, in which the most superior portion of the intrathoracic stomach is its greater curvature. Operation for eventration is employed mostly in newborns or infants, when respiratory embarrassment is caused by the stomach's upward compression onto the left lung.

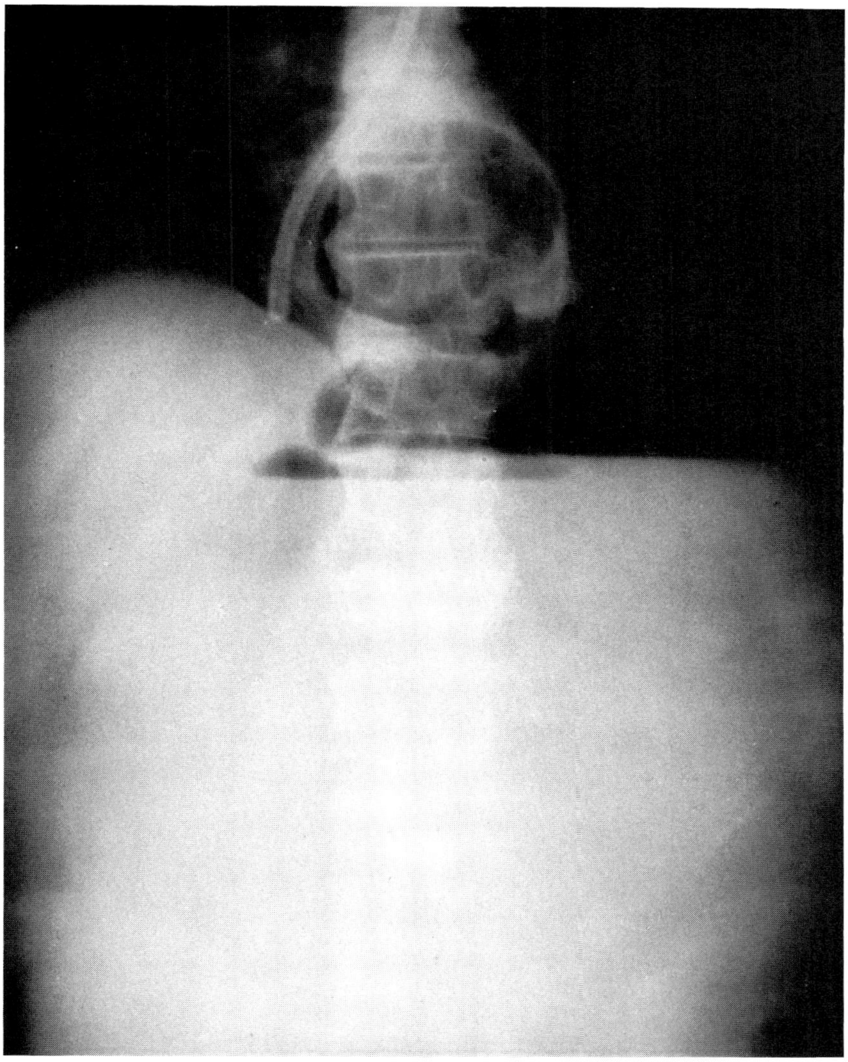

FIG. 2–17. Acute, closed loop, obstructive twist of a paraesophageal hiatal hernia. The large infradiaphragmatic portion of obstruction displays a broad air-fluid level. Note deflection of nasogastric tube to the right of the upper portion of the two-step blockage.

CHAPTER 3

THE SMALL INTESTINE

DUODENAL ULCER

While declining in frequency, certainly as a cause of hospitalization, the duodenum remains the commonest location for peptic ulcer. Perhaps as much a disorder of parietal-cell population as of small-bowel mucosa, the most reliable hypothesis on its cause continues to be an increased, acid-secreting cell mass. However, other etiologies may occupy additional, important roles, including the following: cigarette smoking; major organic and psychiatric stress; use of nonsteroidal anti-inflammatory agents; genetic predisposition; altered pepsinogen secretion; and associated endocrine, pulmonary, rheumatoid, or alcoholic disease.

Alongside the occasionally indeterminate radiologic and endoscopic observation rests the sentiment that duodenal ulcer is a clinical entity, whose typical hallmarks include burning, central, food-relieved and then-induced abdominal pain, often occurring at night, with consistent though temporary improvement after antacid use. To some, these hallmarks establish the diagnosis and justify treatment. Admittedly, though, peptic esophagitis, cholecystitis, or so-called non-ulcer dyspepsia may imitate and be imitated by ulcers. Moreover, as ulcers may provoke considerable mucosal deformity, they become obscured radiologically. Even under the best of circumstances, endoscopic visualization within the bulb itself is imperfect.

The upper GI series remains the diagnostic gold standard. In it, the bulb is first filled with and then emptied of barium by approximating its anterior and posterior walls through manual or paddle compression on the epigastrium. Contrast is thus retained within any crater, often accentuated by a perimeter of mucosal edema (Fig. 3–1A). As in benign gastric ulcers, folds radiating about the crater may be seen. The x ray may disclose more. Edematous distal duodenal, jejunal, or gastric folds suggest Zollinger-Ellison syndrome; nephrolithiasis can reflect hyperparathyroidism. Significant arthritic change implies antecedent therapy with nonsteroidal anti-inflammatory agents, just as a corticosteroid history is inferred upon finding osteoporosis. In chronic or recurrent ulcers, the scarred bulb may contract (Fig. 3–1B) or assume a cloverleaf configuration, making visual identification uncertain.

Though society seems to float equally on fossil fuel and antacids, the latter's ulcer-healing power remains debated, while the value of H_2-receptor blockers, sucralfate, prostaglandins, and the substituted benzimidazoles is unquestioned. Oral bismuth has exciting possibilities, particularly as it helps eradicate a possibly causative bacterium, Campylobacter pylori, now implicated in many cases of erosive gastritis and gastric ulcer.

In the uncommon patient with refractory pain, partial gastric-outlet obstruction, or continuous bleeding, surgery still has a role. Most patients who want to stop smoking can't, and too many of those under chronic stress are powerless to overcome it.

FIG. 3–1. A. Close-up view of pylorus and proximal duodenum showing collection of barium in the center of the bulb, with a "cloverleaf" halo of surrounding edematous mucosa. The bulb is normal in position and contour; radiating streaks of retained barium point to (or away from) the crater.
B. Close-up view of pyloric channel, with constricted and eccentrically curved duodenum, scarred from chronic ulcer disease. The normal "ace-of-spades" contour of the bulb is completely lost.

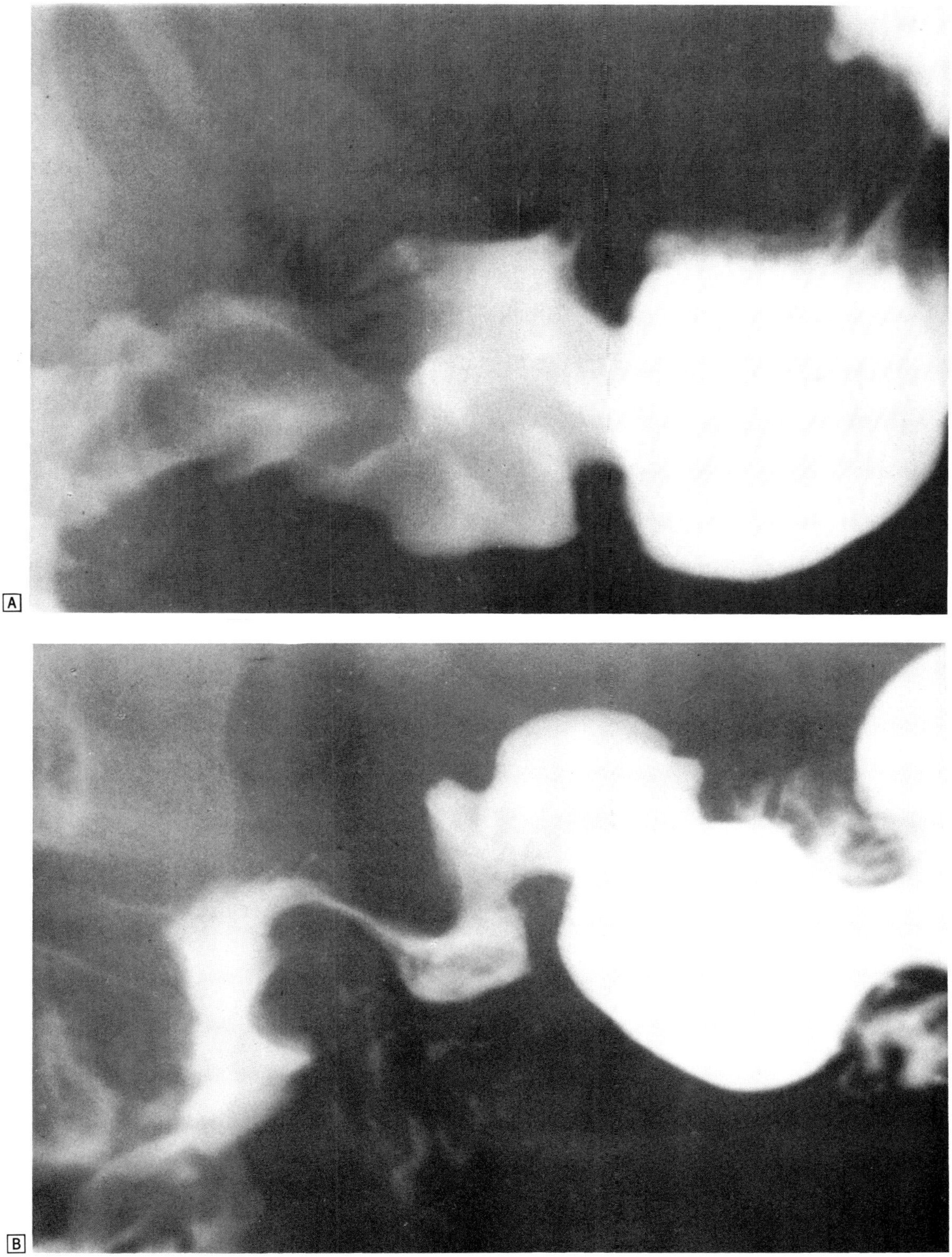

FIG. 3–1.

GIANT DUODENAL ULCER

Though the pain and disability accompanying peptic ulcers rarely correlate with their size, their ultimate clinical significance may. Larger ulcers seem to heal less rapidly, are more likely to bleed or recur, and often eventuate with scarring to the point of partial or complete gastric-outlet obstruction. Giant duodenal ulcers are those greater than 3 cm in transverse diameter. Their diagnosis is often missed simply because a large ulceration can be mistaken for a normal, perhaps eccentric duodenal bulb that may not seem deformed. Barium retained within the crater may conform to the normal bulb contour. Though its base is well through the mucosa, an ulcer of this size is often as deep as it is wide, and some penetration beyond serosa into the pancreatic bed, liver, or retroperitoneum can be inferred. Duodenoscopy and biopsy might seem valuable in distinguishing a giant ulcer from an atypical duodenal diverticulum or a large sacculation resulting from a previous, healed ulceration. Yet the virtual absence of primary malignant lesions of the duodenal bulb and the risk of inducing free perforation with the instrument are strong contrary arguments.

Often felt following the use (sometimes surreptitious) of non-steroidal anti-inflammatory agents, symptoms may not disappear following their withdrawal, since complete healing involves not just re-epithelialization but actual regrowth of the duodenal bulb wall. Considering the genesis of atypical (including giant) ulcers, a hormonally induced acid-hypersecretion (Zollinger-Ellison syndrome, multiple-endocrine neoplasia, parathyroid adenoma) requires consideration. Even in this age of varied H_2-receptor-blocker and mucosal-protective therapies, duodenal stricture may develop and pain may become chronic.

In the x-ray opposite (Fig. 3–2), the ulceration can, at first glance, be overlooked, as it is large enough to be mistaken for an atypically shaped bulb. The hammock-like inferior barium collection, in truth, is the bed of the enormous crater, extending from the pyloric channel to its apex. The descending limb of the duodenum seems to begin about 2 cm to the left of and proximal to the most distal portion of the crater.

Understandably, the surgical removal of a lesion of this size is difficult, risking defective duodenal-stump closure.

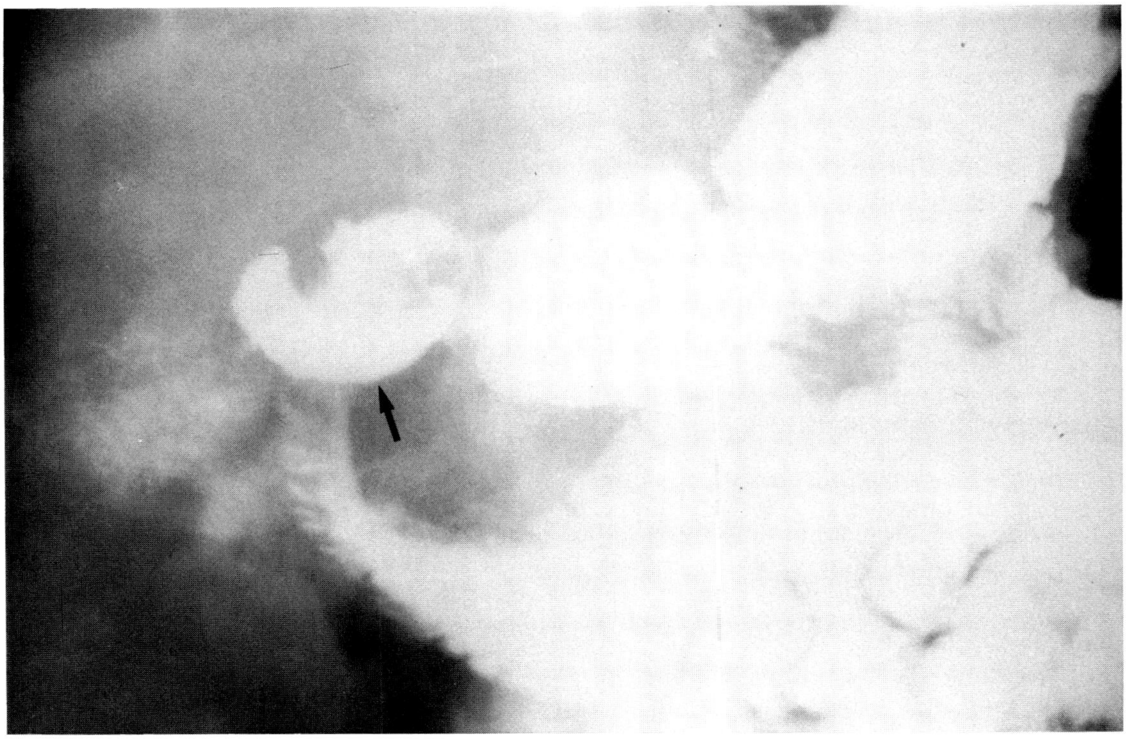

FIG. 3–2. Hammock-like, crescentic collection of an enormous duodenal bulb ulcer. The descending limb is clearly posterior to this perforative lesion.

PERFORATED DUODENAL ULCER

While giant ulcers of the duodenal bulb are described as local, confined perforations, the transmural penetration of a duodenal ulcer into the free peritoneal cavity is less an issue of speculation than a call to some immediate action. The majority of these ulcers occur following a prodrome of protracted, burning abdominal pain and progressively ineffective antacid use. The perforation is an extremely acute event, suspected by the patient's sudden perception that "something happened." Progressive, noncolicky abdominal pain and distention are followed by voluntary and involuntary abdominal-wall guarding, hypoperistalsis, and typically diffuse and often rebound tenderness. Pneumoperitoneum may be suggested by loss of dullness to percussion on the lower right lateral chest wall over the liver. In most cases, the upright chest x ray (Fig. 3–3A) will reveal intra-abdominal air that has risen to outline the undersides of both diaphragms. Thus identified, free perforations require nasogastric suction, IV fluids, and multiple antibiotics, along with an immediate call to more than one surgeon, retaining the first available responder.

Because barium is an intense, peritoneal irritant, upper GI series is contraindicated unless the evidence for perforation is incomplete. Absorbable iodinated contrast is a blander substitute and, like barium, may flow freely out of the pyloroduodenal area, layering over visceral serosa, about the liver, or into the pelvis. Sometimes, contrast will be found confined in a paraduodenal sac (Fig. 3–3B). Vigorous, repetitive peritoneal lavage, oversewing and patching the leak with omentum or serosa, and placing multiple drains are necessary. A second operation to prevent recurrence is almost always required. Despite fashions in pyloroplasties and vagotomies, the old mousetrap, antroduodenectomy and truncal vagotomy, still works best. Anything less than definitive surgical management of the ulcer disease, including reliance on medical management, risks recurrence.

Under exceptional circumstances, including perforation in the aged or catastrophically ill, a decision for operation may be tantamount to a death sentence, and medical "treatment" must suffice. Scrupulous chart documentation of the decision-making process (and the surgeon's concurrence) are employed, along with vigorous nasogastric drainage, maintenance of intravascular volume, nutritional support, observation for bleeding, and treatment for presumed polymicrobial infection. When fortune smiles, the perforation seals over, intraperitoneal gas resolves on sequential x rays, and sepsis is held back.

Ulcer perforations into the lesser peritoneal sac are more confined, and are suspected by identifying central, loculated extraintestinal air anterior to the area of the pancreas (Fig. 3–3C) without evident subdiaphragmatic gas. This less-commonly identified emergency is equally significant, as is the likelihood of sepsis originating from it.

If either form of intraperitoneal soilage undergoes unsuccessful operation or is inoperable, an abscess may eventuate. These abscesses are often subhepatic or subdiaphragmatic, and are suspected on an upright chest film by a half-moon shaped, right upper quadrant air-fluid collection. Ideal surgical drainage is extraperitoneal, sometimes managed by an interventional radiologist's catheter placement or sequential guided-needle aspirations. When ulcers perforate the gallbladder or common duct, biliary air will be seen on plain abdominal film, and the ducts outlined with contrast (Fig. 3–3D) will be seen during conventional upper GI series.

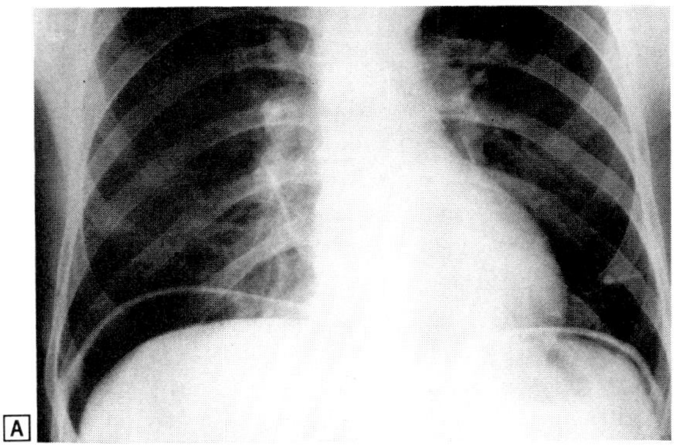

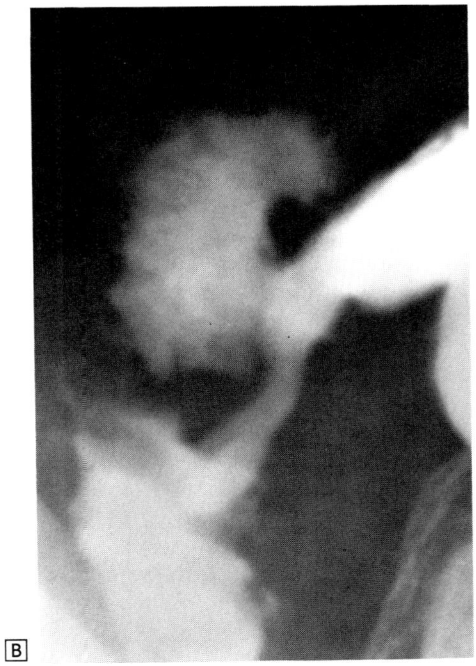

FIG. 3–3. A. Upright chest film revealing bilateral subdiaphragmatic crescentic airs shadows of free perforation. Gastric and small bowel air (and juices) have violated a once sterile peritoneum.
B. Mushroom-shaped extravasation of barium extending superiorly and leftward from area of deformed duodenal bulb.
C. Lesser sac perforation. Triangular collection of confined gas above and medial to stomach and transverse colon.
D. Barium is filling the right and left main hepatic ducts via ulcer perforation into choledochus.

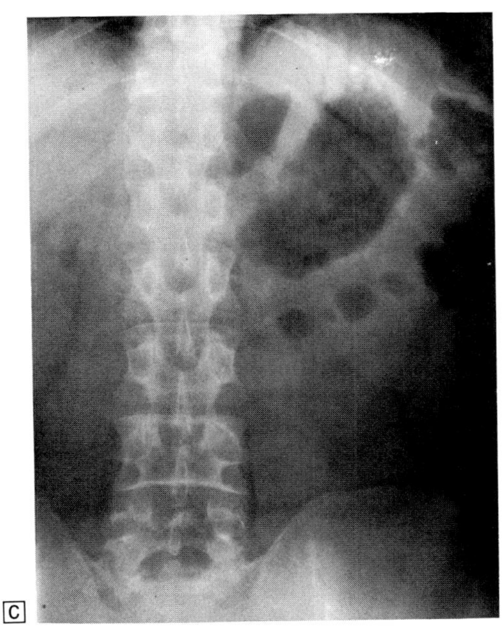

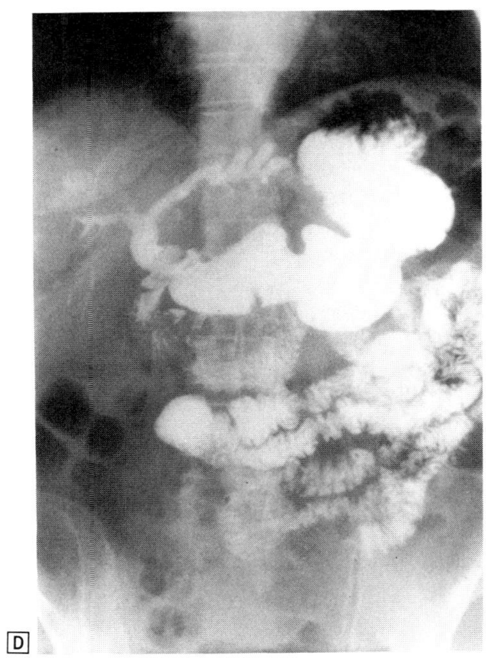

DUODENITIS

The proponents of duodenitis as a distinct disease have had their difficulties, among which is its recognition only as some variable intermediate between normal mucosa and full-fledged ulceration. In truth, its causes are multiple, including not only acid-peptic and Crohn's diseases but celiac sprue and infiltration by various parasites, among them Strongyloides, Ascaris, Necator, and Giardia lamblia.

When the duodenal mucosa is inflamed from either hyperacidity or defective defense against acid, it is typically edematous and friable; at endoscopy or on barium x-ray evaluation, its folds appear thickened to resemble gastric mucosa. A cobblestone mucosal nodularity on x ray (Fig. 3–4A) may reflect hyperplastic Brunner's glands. Their mucinous bicarbonate secretions, stimulated by secretin, are of indeterminate purpose. Present submucosally in the bulb and postbulbar duodenum, their enlargement may imply only gastric hypersecretion. A similar appearance of the opacified distal small bowel or colon suggests Crohn's disease.

Duodenitis symptoms are similar to those of actual ulcer, and as they often coexist, it is difficult to know when the patient has "crossed the line." However, major bleeding in isolated, nonulcerative duodenitis is unlikely. The duodenum does possess its share of arteriovenous malformations, although bleeding then represents more of a vasculopathy than a mucosal disease.

Duodenal infiltration by parasites is common. Giardia is an almost ubiquitous protozoan. While making a home in the gallbladder, bile ducts, and duodenal mucosa, it also favors life in cold-water wells and estuaries and, notoriously, in the water supplies of Leningrad and elsewhere in the Soviet Union. In infected patients, the upper GI series may demonstrate spasm and thickening of duodenal folds (Fig. 3–4B) which disappear after treatment; biopsies may actually demonstrate tissue invasion. Their passage in feces is certain, but they are fragile and transparent. Thus, identification there is tentative and, as in any intestinal parasite, it can be further obscured by prior oral bismuth, kaolin, and, of course, barium sulfate. Endoscopic aspiration of cholecystokinin-stimulated duodenal bile may be necessary for specific diagnosis. Since treatment is simple (quinacrine or metronidazole), its use in well-water drinkers or tourists with diarrhea, nausea, weight loss, or low-grade fever should be considered. Unlike amoebae, they do not metastasize to liver or cause abscesses.

Strongyloidiasis is an acute form of nematode (threadworm) infiltration, particularly into the duodenum but into the large bowel as well. Symptoms include severe abdominal pain, nausea, and vomiting; intense eosinophilia is always seen. The upper GI series may be normal, or may also show effacement and sometimes polypoid thickening of duodenal folds, usually in the descending limb. Massive infestation in children or the immunosuppressed may end fatally.

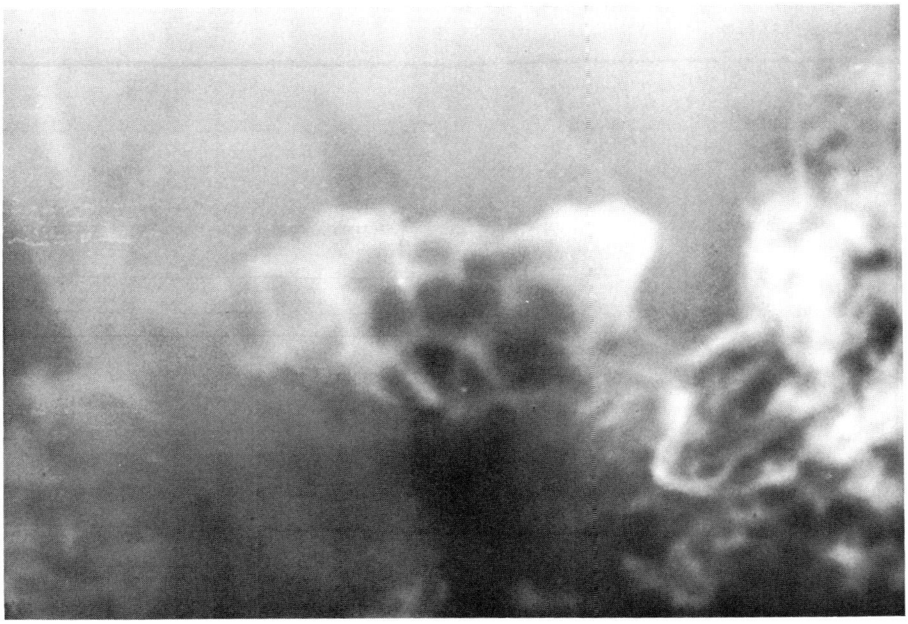

A

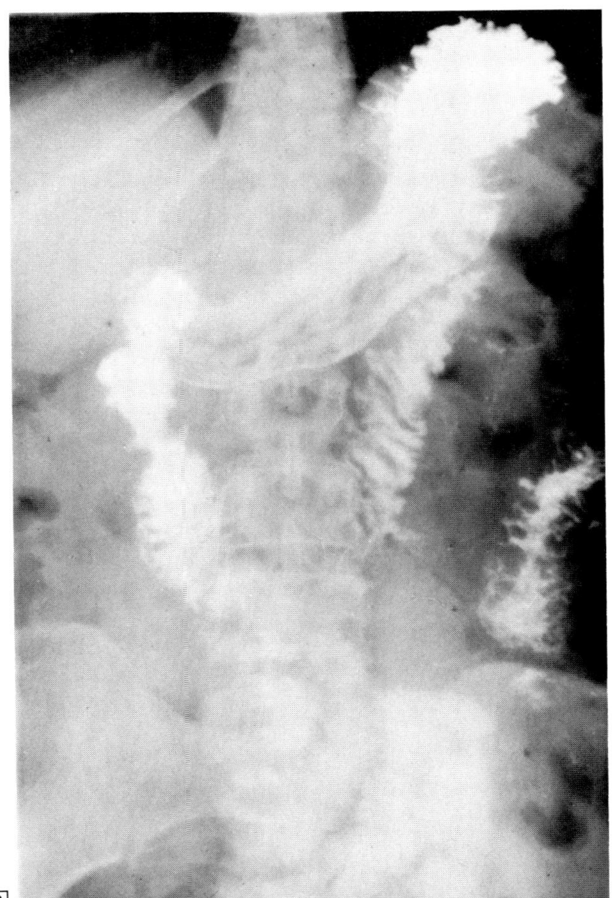

B

FIG. 3–4. A. Multiple, rounded radiolucencies of the duodenal bulb in cobblestone fashion, characteristic of Brunner's gland hyperplasia.
B. Giardiasis. Irregular stenosis and loss of small-bowel markings in upper second portion of the duodenum in a patient with nausea, weight loss, and diarrhea.

POSTBULBAR ULCER

Though only 1 or 2 cm distal, ulcers of the duodenum, beyond its bulb, often lack a typical, painful antecedent, instead usually appearing with hemorrhage. The bleeding is generally more rapid and voluminous than that emerging from bulbar ulcerations. These ulcers are usually associated with some mucosal deformity. Their healing generally occurs with stricture formation. Yet, their best demonstration (Fig. 3–5) is made radiologically, typically as an elliptic or ovoid, distal collection of barium. Because of the substantial accompanying mucosal irritability, postbulbar ulcers may be more easily identified on x ray by prior parenteral administration of atropine or glucagon, either of which is given to diminish gut motility.

If all the blood from a postbulbar ulcer is swept distally, and none is regurgitated back into the stomach, brisk bleeding may occur, understandably without nausea, hematemesis, or recoverable blood in a nasogastric aspirate. As with any atypically located disease, the illness can be missed visually, as well. The radiologist may terminate fluoroscopy when barium has filled the duodenal bulb, and the endoscopist, already finding a bloodless stomach and duodenal bulb, may not advance further. Though the majority of Zollinger-Ellison sydrome ulcers are bulbar, a postbulbar lesion should raise the possibility of hypergastrinemia.

Apart from careful attention to the patient's blood volume, medical treatment is identical to that of ordinary ulcers, including methods both proven and not yet proven effective in the acutely bleeding patient, e.g., H_2-receptor blockers, antacids, and mucosal protective (coating and prostaglandin-type) agents.

As in every upper gastrointestinal lesion that appears with bleeding, the risk of early rebleeding is high. When the diagnosis of postbulbar ulcer is made or at least attempted, a surgeon should be called, even if the patient has stopped bleeding or appears stable. Functioning in such a "what-if" mode is a courtesy to your consultant. After all, which of them might enjoy being called at the end of the day, or for that matter in the middle of the night, to see a patient who has been in the hospital for several days? Also, this form of anticipatory consultation provides the surgeon with a chance to consider operative strategy a little longer, also to the patient's benefit. Because postbulbar ulcerations are closer to the pancreas, gallbladder, and distal biliary ducts, they are less easily treatable by resection. In the face of active bleeding, many surgeons would be justifiably content with duodenotomy, oversewing the bleeding point, and, prior to closing, performing a quick truncal vagotomy.

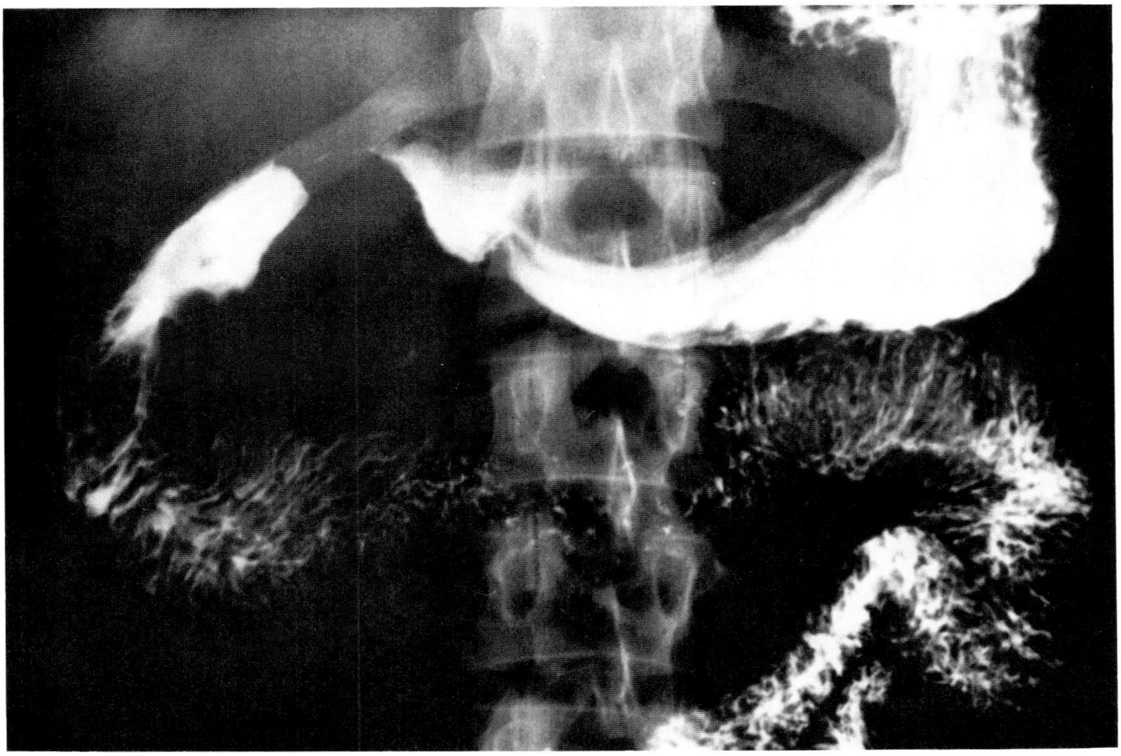

FIG. 3–5. Collection of barium (1½ in. in size) extends from the immediate post-bulbar region into the second portion of the duodenum. The well-outlined bulb, normal gastric rugae, and the unaffected proximal small bowel loops argue against a hypersecretory process.

CROHN'S DISEASE OF THE TERMINAL ILEUM

Though Crohn's "domain" was originally restricted to the distal small intestine ("terminal ileitis"), this disease can involve any portion of the alimentary canal and extraintestinal structures. Yet, the prececal ileum still remains the commonest initial target, with local fixed stenosis, loss or distortion of valvular markings, and visible ulcerations or nodular mucosal deformity seen here (Fig. 3–6) the most typical radiologic findings. Furthermore, thickening of the bowel wall and involvement or attachment of adjacent mesentery or omentum is often seen to displace contrast-filled, healthy small intestine out of the right lower quadrant, away from the deformed terminal ileum. This relatively barium-free area is usually ovoid or rectangular, often lies beneath a palpable mass pointing "northwest" out of the lower right abdomen, and is penetrated centrally by a trickle of contrast leading to the cecum. This narrowed segment often resembles frayed string, with multiple saw-tooth serrations, which sometimes extend as blind fistulae that occasionally perforate adjacent ascending colon (this is best) or, inappropriately, the bladder, vagina, rectum, or sigmoid, which may prematurely opacify on contrast x rays. Extraluminal collections of barium in the retrorectal space or right lower quadrant confirm an abscess.

Symptoms of ileitis often seem out of proportion to the extent of bowel involved, with fever, refractory diarrhea, and malaise, along with multiple protein, blood, and mineral deficiencies arising from only several diseased inches in an otherwise healthy 10- or 15-ft. small intestine.

Easy to understand when considering the fixed ileal stenosis, the precontrast plain film may show dilated, air-filled loops of bowel, suggesting the presence of obstruction, which is often the first stage in the appearance of illness. Other radiopaque, clinically important abnormalities seen in Crohn's disease can include ureterolithiasis, gallstones, skeletal underdevelopment in the young, and arthropathies, including sacroileitis and ankylosing spondylitis.

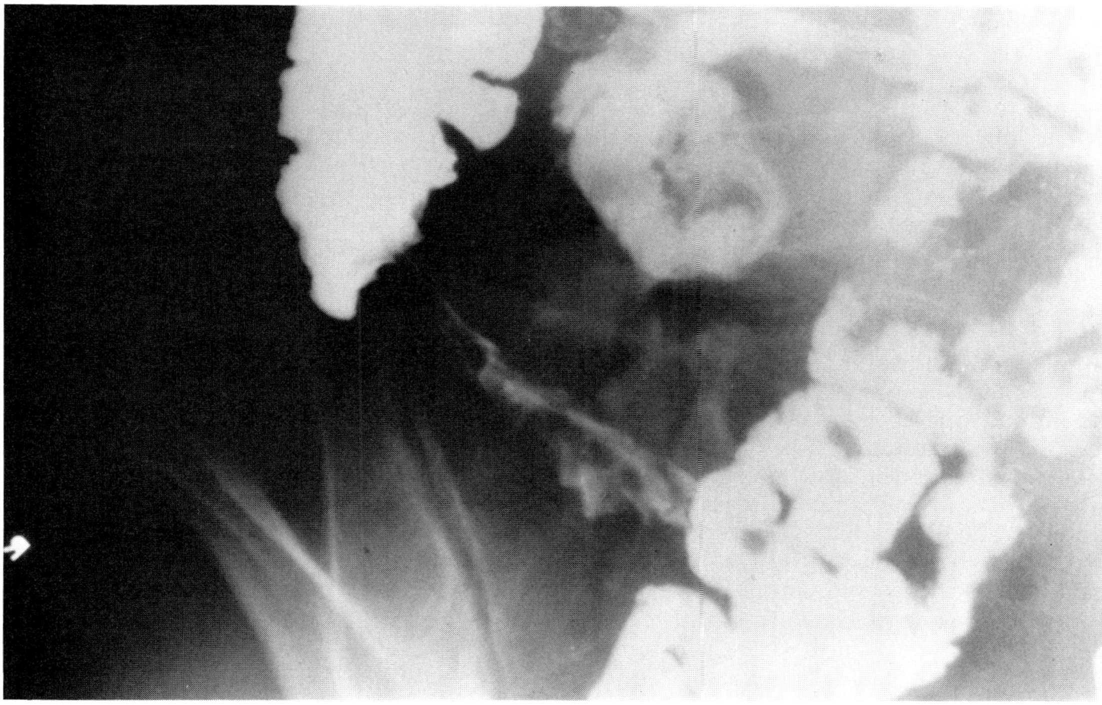

FIG. 3–6. A fixed, narrowed oblique loop of bowel is identified in the right lower quadrant, pointing at and eventually entering the ascending colon. Involvement of one loop of preterminal ileum in the pelvis is inferred.

RECURRENT CROHN'S DISEASE

Apart from a primary inoperability caused by extensive small-intestinal involvement, all the nutritional deficiencies, hormonal complications, and multiple organ-system involvement derive wholly or in part from Crohn's disease's most serious problem: recurrence after "curative" resection of presumably localized disease. One can assume that a clinically significant illness of unpredictable extent will develop again in half the patients undergoing operations for Crohn's disease. And this will happen in as few as 3 weeks to as late as 4 decades after surgery. Surgical decision-making in Crohn's disease is further influenced by the knowledge that one cannot "whittle" away indefinitely at recurrent small-bowel or colon inflammation without eventually encountering either life-threatening malabsorption or, at best, an ileostomy.

With progressively less bowel remaining after each operation, subsequent resections are more significant. The typical, unhappy result is a continued assault on the intestine's absorptive capacity, with reoperations followed by recurrences involving progressively less bowel. Each resection is of proportionately greater significance. One foot removed from a 10-ft small intestine constitutes a 10% reduction, whereas the same amount resected from an intestine already shortened to 4 ft will cost its owner 25% of the remainder. The nutritional consequences are obvious: these progressive intestinal resections resemble withdrawals from a bank account that gains no interest. To the patient, the social and economic results of chronic diarrhea and incontinence may be even more overwhelming.

Because the commonest initial location of Crohn's disease is the terminal ileum, the operation most frequently employed is local resection and an ileo-ascending colostomy. The amount of right colon resected is influenced by both the desirability of preserving the ileocecal sphincter and the distribution of the ileocolic vessels. Recurrences are characteristically at the new anastomotic site, at or near the hepatic flexure. All are seen in Figure 3–7A: the inflammatory stenosis approaching the right upper quadrant, involving at least 10 in. of fixed, thickened preanastomotic ileum. Healthy bowel loops seem pushed aside. A postoperative film following a second reoperation (Fig. 3–7B) shows recurrent stricture formation at a more distal anastomosis in the transverse colon, where fore and aft removal of eventually inflamed but previously healthy adjacent ileum and colon had been carefully performed. Even when "well," postiliectomy patients can have disabling diarrhea from their failure to resorb their own cathartic bile salts. Because of the occasional difficulty in distinguishing operative anastomotic deformity from recurrent disease, an early postoperative (6 weeks) small-bowel series is advisable.

No postoperative medical measures have been demonstrated to diminish either the frequency or activity of recurrences, but resection of floridly inflamed bowel in an actively ill patient is more likely to be followed by recurrence than is removal of a relatively quiescent stricture. The nature of recurrences tend to anatomically resemble the character of the primary disease (i.e., restenosis follows surgery for stenosis; fistulas seem to develop more often after fistulous bowel has been excised).

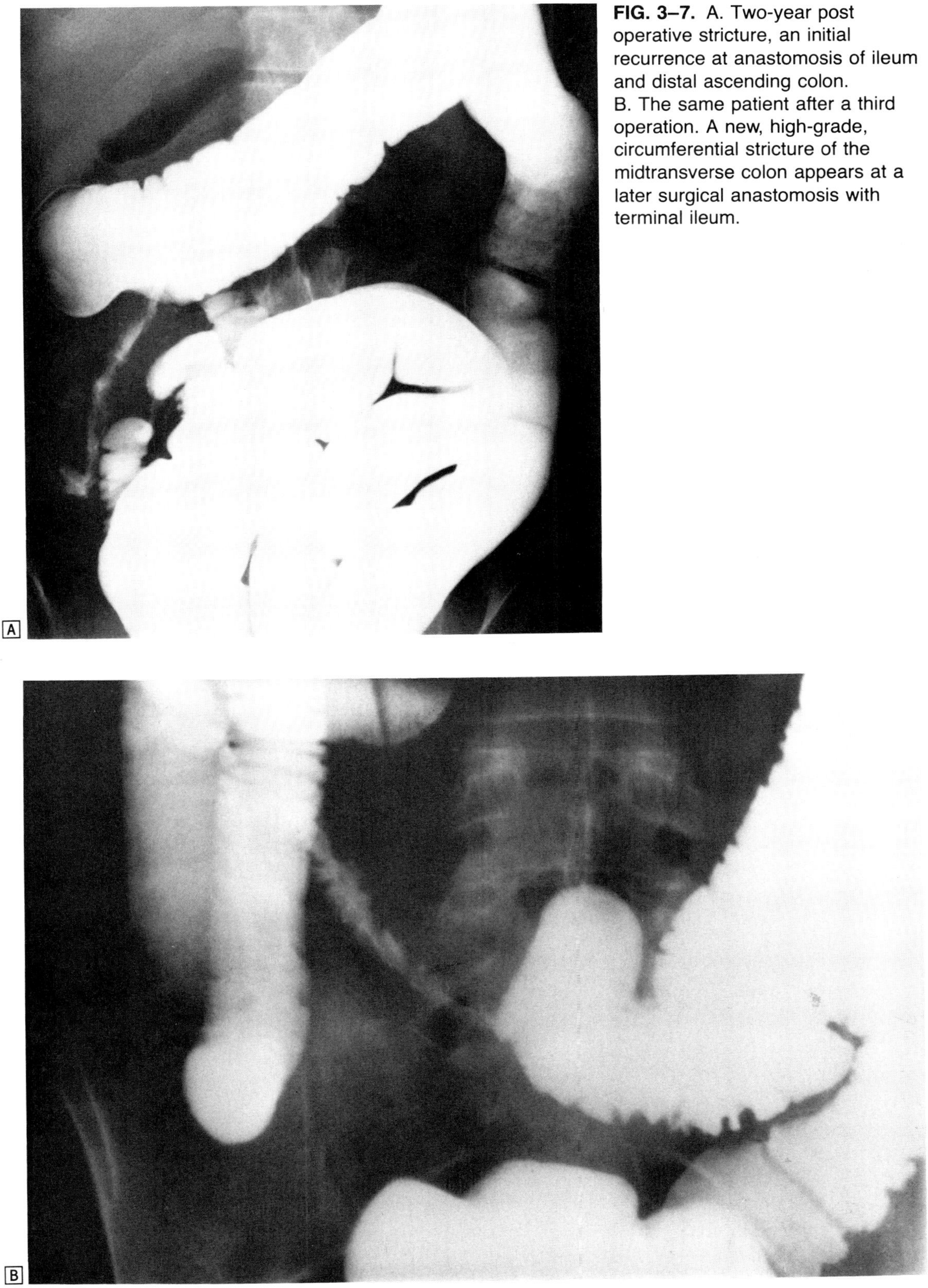

FIG. 3–7. A. Two-year post operative stricture, an initial recurrence at anastomosis of ileum and distal ascending colon.
B. The same patient after a third operation. A new, high-grade, circumferential stricture of the midtransverse colon appears at a later surgical anastomosis with terminal ileum.

JEJUNOILEITIS

Despite the position taken by some, Dr. Crohn included, that almost all patients with "his" disease needed at least one operation, there is a subselection of patients for whom surgery is almost always contraindicated, particularly those whose involvement appears to extend throughout the entire small intestine. Fortunately representing only a small percentage of the entire Crohn's population, patients with universal involvement also seem to have a more clinically indolent, corticosteroid-responsive disease, their course more of recurrent, episodic low-grade bowel obstructions, diarrhea, and perirectal infections. Despite apparent destruction of enormous amounts of their absorptive surface, most seem to enjoy surprisingly good nutrition.

The extent of the disease often comes as a shock; radiologic evidence of involvement includes multiple strictures, with intervening, dilated sacs of proximal and distal small intestine, often with communicating or blind intervening fistulas (Fig. 3–8). The valvular markings of the normal bowel are sparse. Fistulas to the rectum, bladder, vagina, abdominal wall, or buttocks may be evident. The distinction from extensive lymphoma, Whipple's disease, severe celiac sprue, or the rare ulcerative, nongranulomatous jejunoileitis may be difficult. Multinutrient malabsorption can take place, particularly of calcium, fat soluble vitamins, and B-12.

On physical examination, patients may demonstrate one or more masses overlying areas of thickened bowel or adjacent mesenteric reaction. Isolated distended loops of bowel may be felt or focal tympany heard.

Since there is rarely a single, resectable offending focus, decision-making is limited to choices of medical management. Apart from corticosteroid and the adjunctive use of antimetabolites (azathioprine and 6-mercaptopurine), the most promising choice appears to be long-term parenteral hyperalimentation. The fecal component of intramural and extramural infection is eliminated, as is the likelihood of luminal obstruction; nutrition is maintained. Occasional reports exist of significant clinical and radiographic regression of disease in patients with universal involvement treated this way. The financial burden of long-term hyperalimentation, however, could be staggering.

Treating recurrent obstruction by surgical division per serosa of only the muscular portion of lengthy small-bowel strictures has been reported. Local resections, absent any uninvolved areas, of course, mandates an anastomosis amidst diseased bowel, substantially increasing the risk of suture breakdown.

Bone loss from steroid-induced osteoporosis and calcium malabsorption are major complications of this form of disease and its treatment. The adjunctive use of calcium, vitamin D or its analogs, and possibly fluoride are mainstays of therapy.

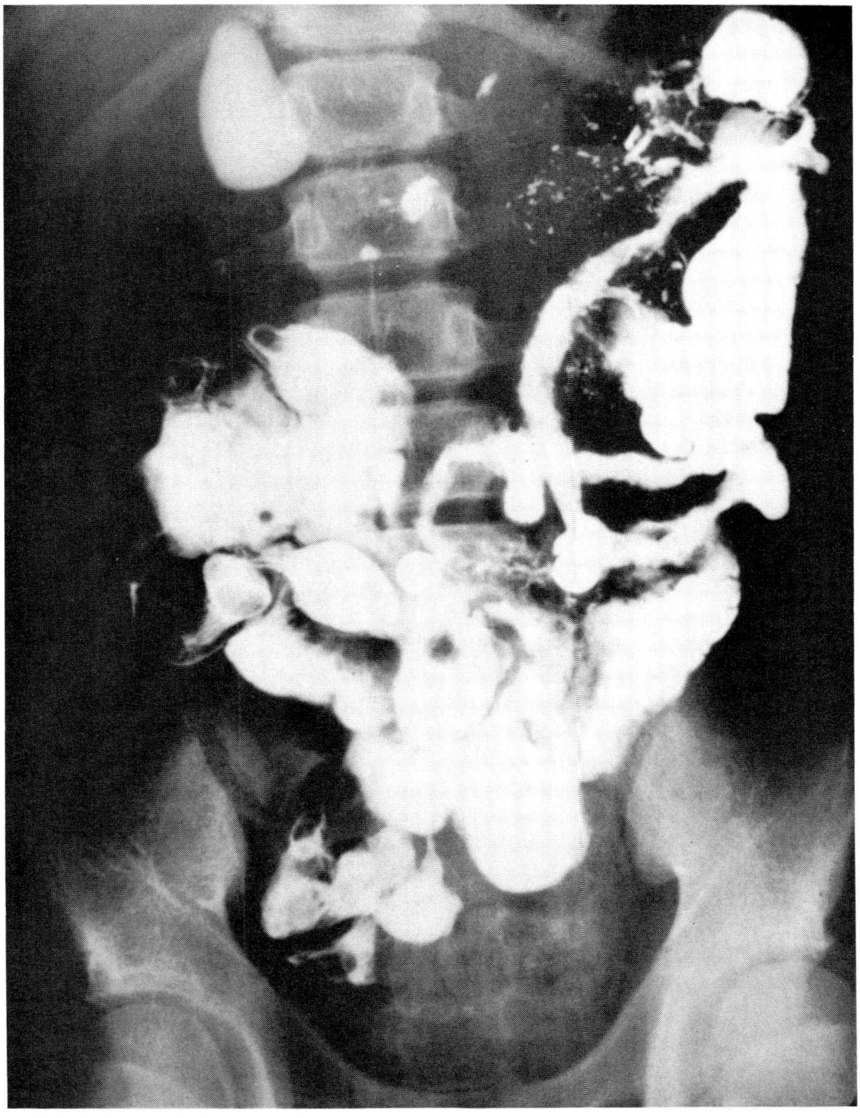

FIG. 3–8. Alternating multiple dilated and constricted loops of small intestine, with strictures and fistulae. The normal small bowel valvular pattern is absent throughout.

CELIAC SPRUE

This complex small-bowel disease can be thought of as the paradigmatic malabsorption syndrome. In it, small-bowel inflammation is typically initiated by a local, allergic-like contact reaction to the gluten contained in most cereal grains, resulting in decreased intestinal absorptive surface, striking loss of its villous height, and eventual atrophy. Mucosal cell loss also decreases available brush-border disaccharidases, further compounding the typical diarrhea, malnutrition, and fat-wasting of this disease. The extent of involvement varies among patients and clearly parallels the severity of the disease.

The commonest offenders are wheat, rye, or barley and the prepared foods containing them. Oats seem less toxic, and corn and rice are innocuous. The illness often appears in infancy, when cereals are added to the diet. In a larger number of cases, celiac sprue develops when the patients are middle-aged or elderly, occasionally discovered in "asymptomatic" form during a medical evaluation of weight loss, anemia, precocious bone fractures, or easy bleeding.

Patients typically present with frequent bulky, diarrheal stools and weight loss, the latter despite conscious, compensatory efforts at overeating. While an occasional patient recalls preferential selection of foods containing no gluten, the majority are unable to give a food-symptom link, yet most can associate their malnutrition with stool volume or frequency. Some celiac sprue patients relate a family history of diarrhea, "food allergy," or "colitis."

Stools of untreated patients contain a large amount of partially digested, malabsorbed fat, starch, and muscle. Peroral small-bowel biopsy reveals mucosal inflammation and flattening, which is characteristic, but not specific, for this illness. Similar biopsies can be seen in dermatitis herpetiformis, viral hepatitis, agammaglobulinemia, and Whipple's disease. X rays vary as widely as do symptoms. Plain films of the abdomen may show abdominal distention or soft-tissue wasting, or they may suggest ascites. Osteopenia may be evident, along with compression fractures, particularly in elderly females. Barium views of the small intestine can be normal in mild cases, but typically (Fig. 3–9) they show luminal dilation, thickening or effacement of jejunal and ileal folds, and intestinal hurry. The older description of segmentation and flocculation of small-bowel barium are noted less frequently with contemporary contrast suspensions.

The initial therapy is absolute restriction of gluten from the diet, an exercise made easier by consultation with a competent dietitian. The usual immediate responses are cessation of diarrhea, weight gain, and increased strength. Failure to improve usually follows the patient's incomplete adherence to their new diet, but is occasionally due to the inadvertent consumption of restaurant or prepared packaged foods containing wheat products such as starch fillers. Though intestinal sensitivity to gluten is usually lifelong, most patients, in time, understandably reintroduce some cereal grain into their diet, resulting in tolerable, continued diarrhea. Nutritional observation and vitamin supplementation may then be a lifetime requirement.

A small percentage of patients do not respond to even rigorous gluten restriction. Of those, most improve with orally administered corticosteroids. However, it should be recalled that a disease responsive to a drug may also impair its absorption, which is also the case with other unrelated, orally administered medicines, mandating increased doses or their parenteral administration. Some patients refractory to diet and steroids will be found to have small-bowel lymphoma, which may eventuate even in some responsive patients. A predisposition in sprue patients for gastric and esophageal carcinomas has also been reported.

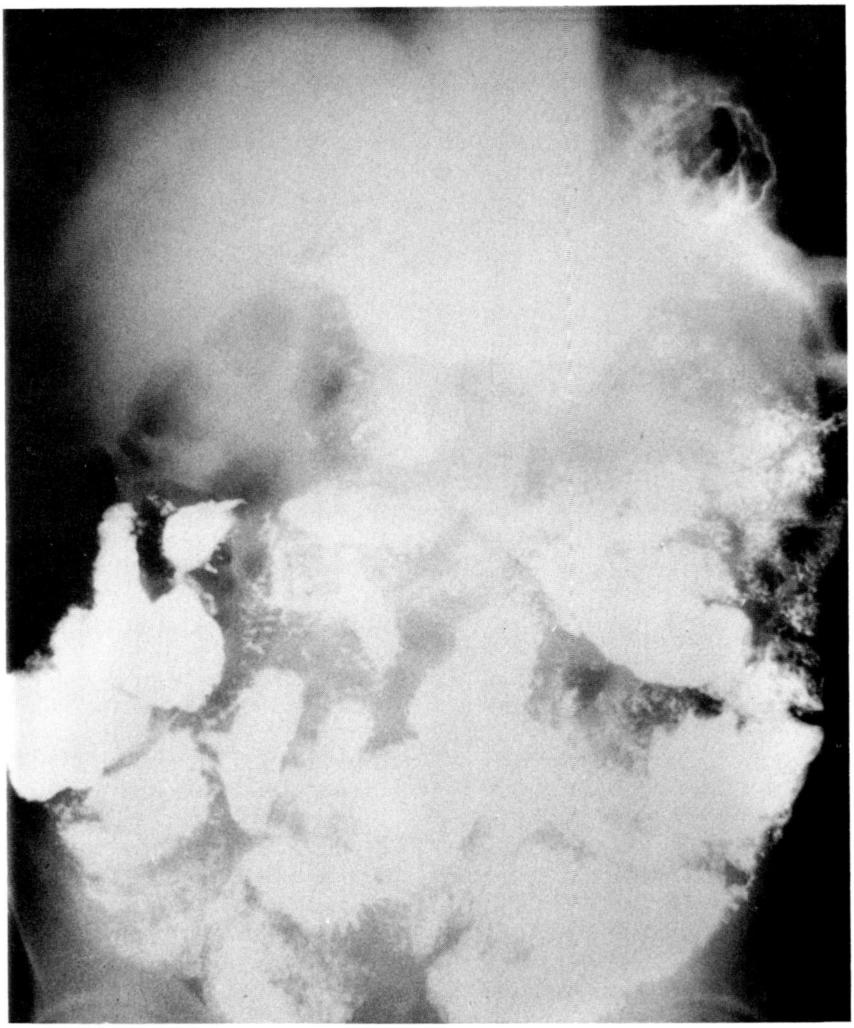

FIG. 3–9. Barium-filled midgut with conspicuous absence of normal valvular mucosal pattern and diffuse clumping or segmentation of contrast.

SMALL BOWEL LYMPHOMA

Because the small intestine hosts a sizable percentage of the body's lymphocytes, its potential as a focus for lymphoma is not surprising. These lymphomas are typically the non-Hodgkin's, large-cell type, and logically arise from the submucosal lymphoid follicles of the distal small bowel. They can be localized or diffuse, appear as a primary disorder or a satellite manifestation of generalized lymphomatous disease, and are observed increasingly in AIDS. The growth of the tumor, like the onset of symptoms, is usually indolent, with slowly progressive, refractory diarrhea and recurrent episodes of generally low-grade bowel obstruction. Ulceration into the lumen results in intestinal bleeding; perforation in untreated patients occurs rarely.

As the small-bowel x rays are nonspecific, exact radiologic diagnosis is not easy. When focal, lymphomas may appear as a circumferential, submucosal thickening with luminal encroachment (Fig. 3–10A), typically without evidence of significant proximal obstructive dilation. Extensive involvement (Fig. 3–10B) may suggest celiac sprue, another infiltrative thickened process (Whipple's disease, giardiasis, leukemia), or the intestinal edema of hypoalbuminemia. Crohn's disease or tuberculous enteritis can also resemble lymphoma. An extensive nodular pattern will resemble multifocal carcinoid tumor.

When large areas are involved, fixed, so-called aneurysmal dilatation (Fig. 3–10C) may be apparent; widened separation of loops is a manifestation of serosal thickening or intra-abdominal node involvement. Chronic diarrhea and malabsorption in lymphoma may be confused with, as well as preceded by, celiac sprue, particularly in Middle-Eastern males. The linkage between celiac sprue and lymphoma should be recalled, particularly when the former is unresponsive to gluten restriction or is followed by development of a mass. Peroral biopsy of the small bowel may be diagnostic or show a sprue-like mucosal atrophy. But if the radiologic lesion is distal and therapy (for example, corticosteroids) is ineffective, only direct examination and full-thickness biopsy are definitive and justified.

Because of the possibility for curative resection or the advantages of removing an ulcerated or obstructed segment, surgery should be considered at almost any stage of illness. Considering that much of the bowel wall is replaced by pharmacologically susceptible malignant cells, chemotherapy, while often dramatically effective, is not surprisingly followed by a formidable incidence of small-bowel perforation.

A diagnosis of secondary intestinal lymphoma is made easier by clinical and radiologic features of the primary disease, such as fever, weight loss, hepatosplenomegaly, and mediastinal and peripheral adenopathy. A decision favoring surgery in focal lymphoma is made easier by the understanding that between half and three-quarters of patients may be cured by local excision.

A
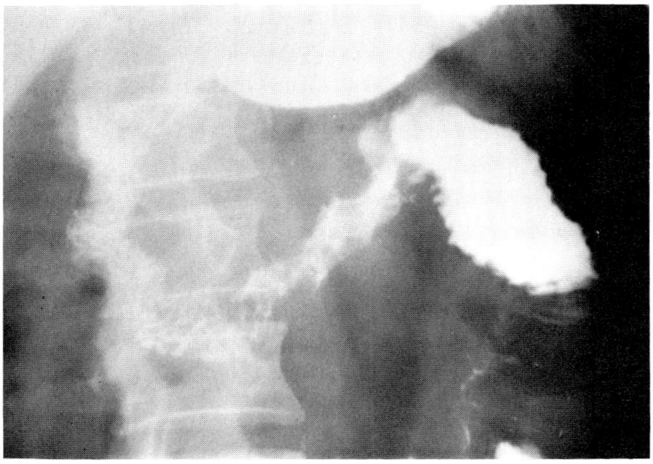

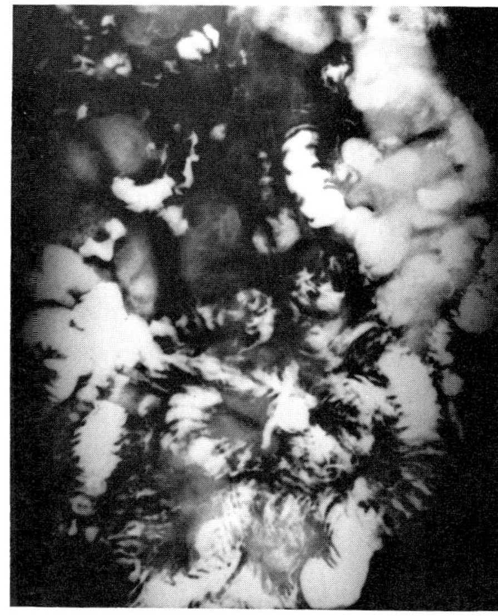
B

FIG. 3–10. A. Lengthy focal, but circumferential, thick irregular stenosis of the third portion of the duodenum.
B. Diffuse, extensive thickening of the distal small intestine in a poorly compliant, medically refractory celiac sprue patient. Persistence of radiologic abnormalities despite adequate therapy prompted laparotomy and full thickness biopsy, proving lymphoma.
C. Fusiform aneurysmal dilation of the ileum with intervening stricture formation in a medically treated lymphoma patient.

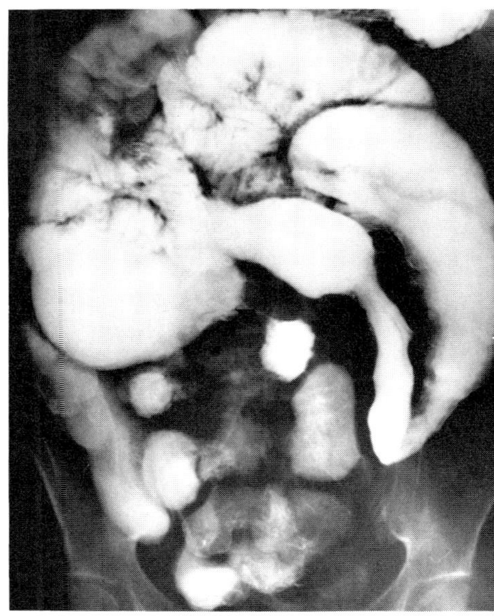
C

CARCINOMAS (PRIMARY AND METASTATIC) OF THE SMALL INTESTINE

Considering the frequency and the invariably benign nature of duodenal ulcers, it is sometimes difficult to realize that the commonest duodenal neoplasm is adenocarcinoma. Leiomyosarcomas, lymphomas, and metastatic tumors also occur and require consideration when dealing with atypical abdominal pain, bowel obstruction, or occult GI bleeding. Weight loss, early satiety, and abdominal distention relieved by vomiting suggest gastric-outlet obstruction. But endoscopy and upper GI series may be negative, particularly if the radiologist or endoscopist concludes the examination when the column of barium or the instrument's tip passes the duodenal bulb. Figure 3–11A shows a heaped-up tumor of the second and third portion of the duodenum that appeared first with brisk GI hemorrhage. Endoscopy revealed only blood regurgitating back from the duodenum, leading to the understandable mistaken conclusion that a duodenal ulcer was responsible. The lesion's similarity in both films implies its fixation.

Confirmation by biopsy is desirable, and if biochemical or CT-scan evaluation leads one to consider the disease confined, radical surgery should follow. In contrast to conventional pancreatic cancers, duodenal malignancies probably represent one rare justification for Whipple-type operations, which involve resecting the duodenum, the proximal two thirds of the pancreas, the distal stomach, and the spleen, while redirecting bile distally. Carcinoma of the ampulla of Vater is an entirely different, almost unique tumor, also potentially resectable, manifested by recurrent, often regressing biliary obstruction, chronic low-grade GI blood loss, and protracted, slow growth. Differential considerations of postbulbar duodenal lesions also include healed ulcers, focal duodenal Crohn's disease, and the circumferential entrapment of a pancreatic carcinoma.

While some studies show their frequency to be as high as ½ to 1% of all GI malignancies, nonlymphoid cancers of the distal small intestine (Fig. 3–11B) are rare. Few primary clinicians and general surgeons, and only a cluster of oncologists, encounter more than a case or two per decade, knowledge of them being like a bit of unforgettable stored computer data. Focal jejunoileal adenocarcinomas or leiomyosarcomas are cured infrequently by resection. Their clinical presentation is usually bleeding or bowel obstruction, but local or distant metastases may be evident first. An unquestioned predisposition for small bowel cancers occurs in celiac sprue and chronic Crohn's disease.

Metastatic tumors to the small intestine (Fig. 3–11C) are common, usually occurring as a late, postoperative bowel obstruction and, if identified, are best managed by decompressive bypass or exteriorizing surgery. Breast, pancreas, colon, lung, stomach, ovary, and melanoma are among the more common primary sources.

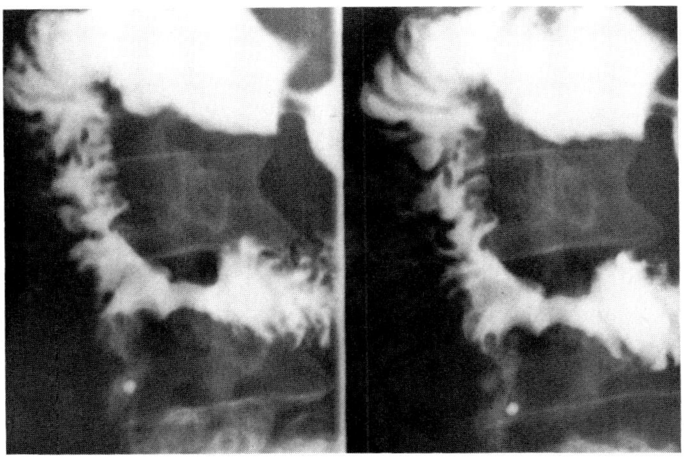

A

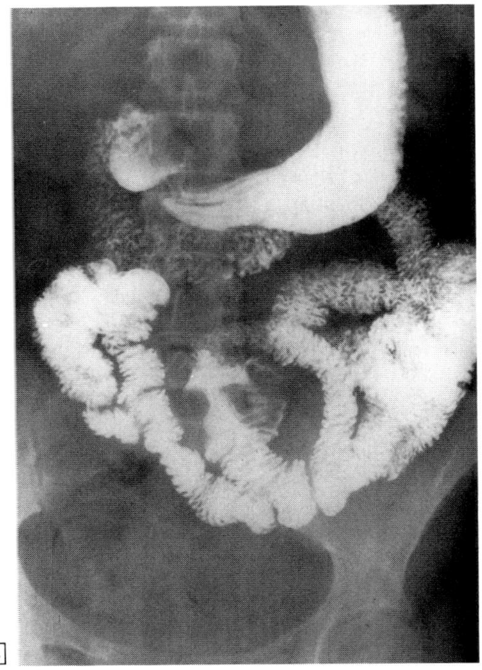

B

FIG. 3–11. A. Sequential films of rounded, asymmetrically constricting irregularity of third portion of duodenum.
B. Abrupt napkin-ring lesion in distal jejunum, indicating a circumferential adenocarcinoma. Absence of midgut dilatation suggests it is not yet obstructive.
C. Small-bowel metastases. Focal "fingerprint" nodular indentations on the small bowel. Fine sawtooth serrations on the opposite wall suggest lymphatic obstruction.

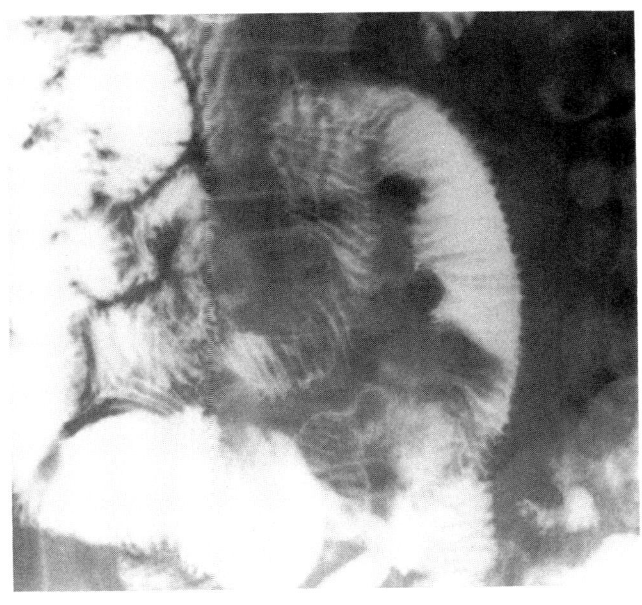

C

CARCINOID TUMORS AND THE CARCINOID SYNDROME

Arising from neuroendocrine (APUD) precursors, the benign carcinoid may be the commonest neoplasm of both the stomach and intestine. Almost half begin in the appendix, typically discovered incidentally following appendectomy. Rectal carcinoids are often found unexpectedly as yellowish submucosal nodules at proctoscopy. Nearly always benign, these carcinoids rarely, if ever, extend or expand. The syndome gets its notoriety from the unique, many-faceted behavior of biologically active, hormone-synthesizing metastatic carcinoids; these involve the liver and are usually of distal small-bowel origin. This fairly exemplary tumor-humor syndrome is typically characterized by watery diarrhea, which is accompanied by a characteristic purplish facial flushing, often with asthmatic wheezing.

The number of polypeptide-like hormones secreted by the tumors is high, including serotonin, histamine, and 5-hydroxytryptophane. The actual single cause of the syndrome is still debated, but the current leading nominee is kallikrein, which catalyzes conversion of kininogen to bradykinin. Serotonin's elaboration is probably responsible for the peritoneal fibrosis and retraction occurring in the carcinoid syndrome, and probably causes the pulmonary fibrosis and right ventricular enlargement seen in advanced illness. Urinary excretion of its metabolite, 5-hydroxyindole acetic acid, is elevated in almost all syndrome patients. The tumor's malignancy correlates with its size, and in the GI tract, these tend to collect around the terminal ileum and ascending colon.

When carried through the ileum and ascending colon, a small-bowel series is positive in almost all cases in which the syndrome is present. Careful attention will show that the tumors may be both extensive and, occasionally, multicentric. The lesions are predominantly submucosal, though ulceration may be present in advanced lesions. Cobblestone nodularity may be apparent (Fig. 3–12), often correlating with both a right lower (ileum) and upper (liver) quadrant mass. Plain films may reveal hepatic enlargement.

The use of H_2-receptor blockers is valuable when the tumor synthesizes histamine or originates in the stomach; cyproheptadine may antagonize endogenous serotonin. The best therapy of the carcinoid syndrome's diarrhea now appears to be somatostatin, which diminishes the satellite manifestations of the syndrome in almost 90% of patients with documented metastatic disease. Generally slow growing, the tumors are often discovered after metastases have developed; thus palliative hepatic resection should always be considered, particularly when drugs are ineffective. Antidiarrheals are a mainstay. Flushing from nonmetastatic, bronchial carcinoids may be more protracted; cure there may follow local excision.

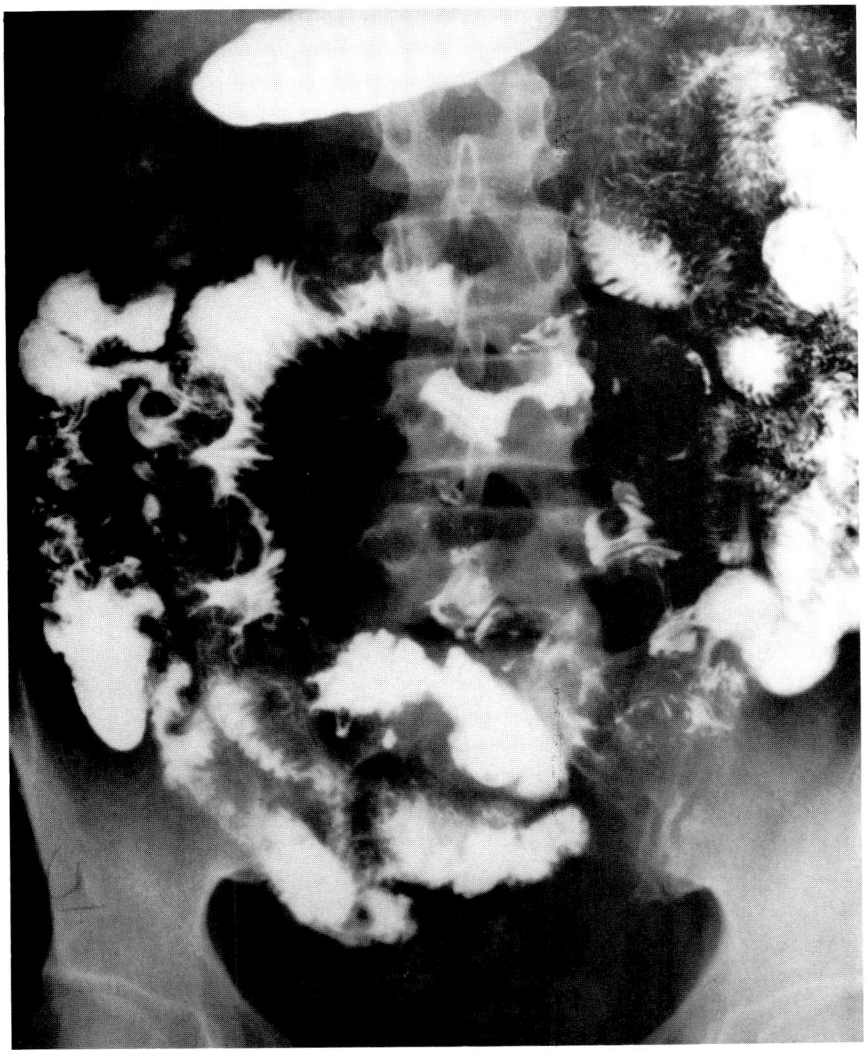

FIG. 3–12. Multiple, large rounded lucencies of mid and terminal ileum, with varying degrees of luminal narrowing.

DUODENAL DIVERTICULA AND COMMON BILE DUCT OBSTRUCTION

When multiple or associated with similar diverticula in the jejunum, these sacculations can cause intraluminal bacterial overgrowth and eventual malabsorption. But most duodenal diverticula are single, arising from the medial aspect of the second (descending) portion. They are generally unassociated with symptoms or signs of disease, and are manifested only as radiologic curiosities.

One interesting exception occurs when the common bile duct enters the duodenum through such a congenital diverticulum. Static, occasionally solidified intestinal contents can fill the diverticulum, occluding the ampulla of Vater and producing recurrent choledochal obstruction. Sometimes movement alone of the diverticulum may bend its junction with the distal common duct, resulting in acalculous cholangitis or nonalcoholic pancreatitis. The diagnosis should be suspected when recurrent cholangitis occurs in a patient without demonstrable gallstones, possessing only a typical duodenal diverticulum. Occasionally, swallowed barium itself will flow unobstructed via the diverticulum into the common bile duct (Fig. 3–13A). Operative cholangiography may also show a dilated, presumably occluded bile duct entering the mid duodenal diverticulum (Fig. 3–13B).

Bleeding correctly ascribed to duodenal diverticula is exceedingly rare and, unless endoscopically or arteriographically documented, is probably arising from another source. But diverticular bezoars (or enteroliths) do occur and are capable of including hemorragic or perforative mucosal erosions.

Small diverticula arising from the duodenal *bulb* mucosa may suggest peptic ulceration. Yet, the absolutely normal mucosa surrounding these tiny circular barium collections display no radiating folds, Brunner's-gland hyperplasia, or luminal deformities. In a patient with bleeding or pain, these benign, quiescent mucosal depressions, like postbulbar diverticula, argue for additional diagnostic studies.

Surgery of the complicated duodenal diverticulum producing jaundice, pancreatitis, or cholangitis must be exceedingly delicate, and is best limited to trimming diverticulum volume by partial excision, fixation to prevent kinking, and perhaps choledochoenterostomy. Unless enormous, solitary duodenal diverticula do not result in significant, upper intestinal bacterial overgrowth.

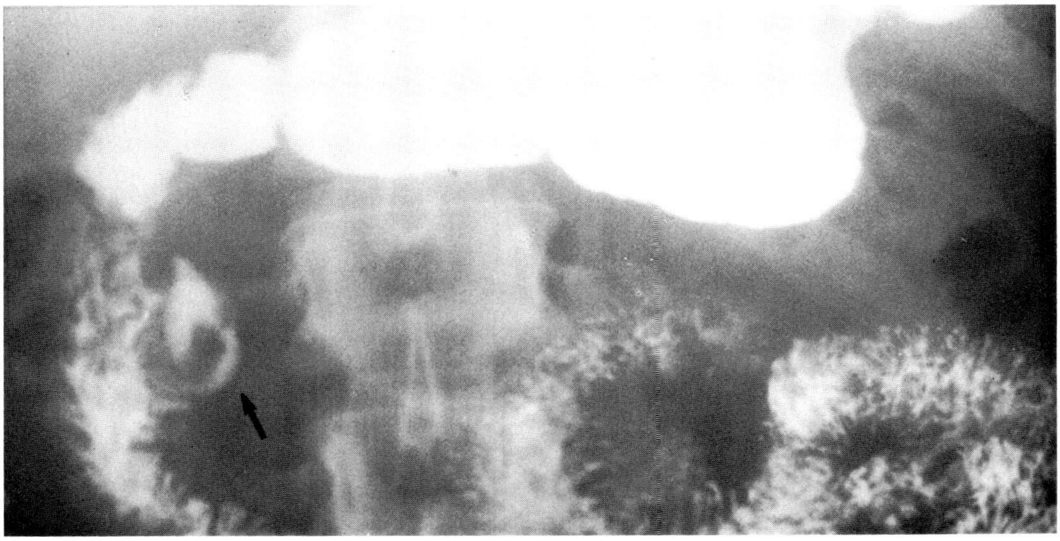

A

FIG. 3–13. A. Barium is seen traveling backwards ↑ up the common bile duct where it enters a midbulbar duodenal diverticulum. The normal choledocoal calibre argues against obstruction.
B. T-tube cholangiogram in a jaundiced patient showing distended common duct above entry into a diverticulum.

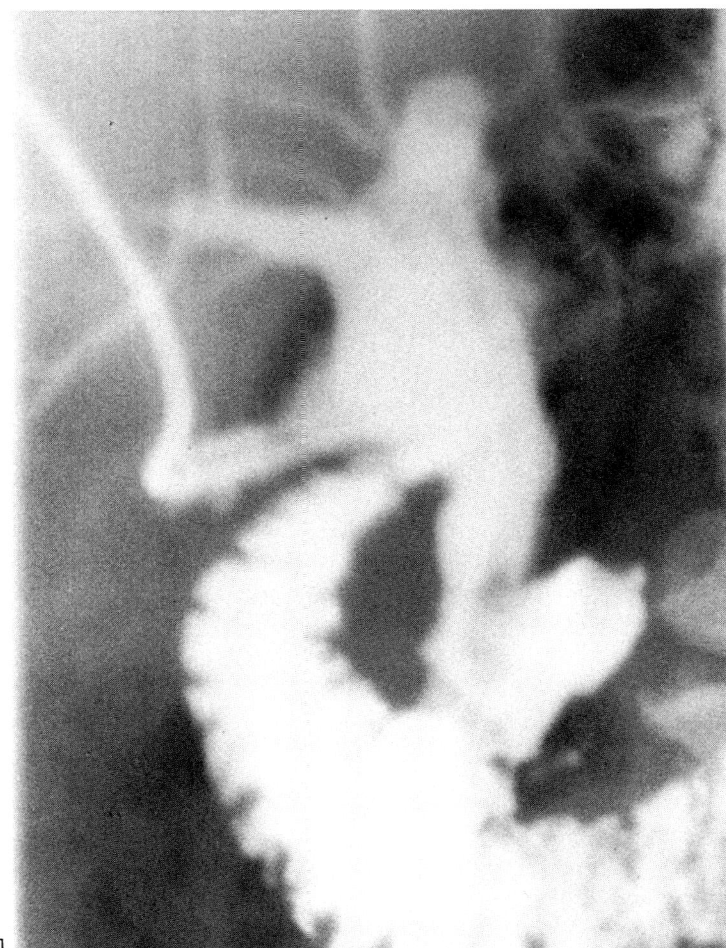

B

MECKEL'S DIVERTICULUM

Mostly a concern in pediatric medicine, this congenital abnormality is the intestinal (ileal) remnant of its fetal yolk-sac (vitelline) connection. Generally these abnormalities are asymptomatic, but on occasion contain heterotopic gastric mucosa which, when acid-secreting, can induce local ulceration. The typical lesion, though small, can appear with significant, painless GI bleeding, usually with maroon-colored stools. The diagnosis is often arrived at by exclusion, when recurrent hemorrhages are unassociated with retrievable blood by nasogastric tube or when one fails to locate a hemorrhagic focus at endoscopy, upper GI series, or the barium enema. However, if there is sufficient ileal reflux, the outpouching may be demonstrated (Fig. 3–14), generally arising between 6 and 15 in. proximal to the ileocecal valve.

Like most radionuclide studies done to localize GI bleeding, Meckel's scans are of only moderate, occasionally ambiguous value, unless the amount of responsible heterotopic mucosa is unduly large. Since identification of a gastric mucosa containing Meckel's diverticulum occurs because of its incorporation of technetium-99 pertechnetate, the clinician should recall that "hot spots" may also occur over certain enteric cysts, as well as in the gastric mucosa of a hiatal hernia or Barrett's esophagus. Absent the infrequent microvascular blush of a functioning diverticulum, angiography's value increases mostly with the identifiable extravasation of dye in the patient bleeding actively. It is sometimes also helpful to recall that these diverticula are always supplied by an individual branch of the superior mesenteric artery.

Unless this condition is asymptomatic, the treatment, of course, is small-bowel resection, which sometimes takes place when the Meckel's is found at a laparotomy performed for an unrelated condition. Occasionally, the diverticulum is large enough to wrap around and obstruct the small bowel or to induce this intraluminally through an ileocolic intussusception. These occur almost exclusively in children or adolescents. Rarely, hemorrhage will arise from ulceration due to functioning heterotopic pancreatic tissue.

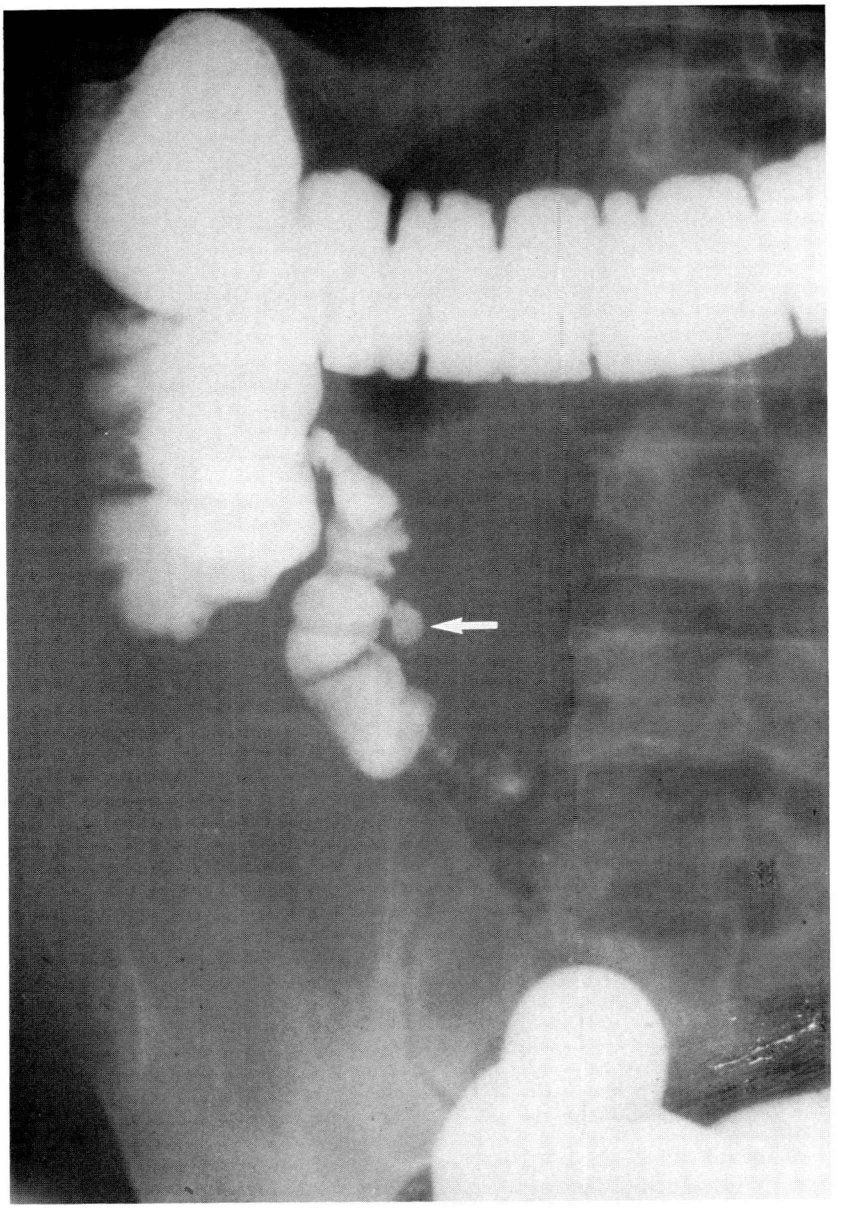

FIG. 3–14. Circular 1- to 2-cm outpouching from mesenteric border of ileum.

DUODENAL INTRAMURAL HEMATOMA

The penchant for submucosal hemorrhage in the duodenum derives from its retroperitoneal fixation, particularly where its third portion rides over the aorta, completing the last leg of its radiologic U-turn across the vertebral processes. Though midgut hematomas may occur spontaneously in anticoagulated or thrombocytopenic patients, the usual duodenal wall hemorrhage occurs where blunt midabdominal trauma is applied by an angry adversary's clenched fist. The duodenum cannot slither away from direct impact; hence, an intramural hemorrhage typically develops from extravasation of blood confined between submucosa and mucosa. Central abdominal pain, with occasional development of a midabdominal mass, and transitory rectal bleeding in an anticoagulated or recently intoxicated patient or an otherwise battered wife or child are added typical findings.

On this x ray (Fig. 3–15), the abnormality appears as an intrinsic, fusiform elevation of duodenal mucosa, with overlying nodular accentuation of intestinal markings, which are sometimes compared to a picket fence. If there is no significant tissue death, the mucosal changes gradually resolve, and the rectal bleeding is usually self-limited. Endoscopy is almost always negative, unless the instrument can be snaked distally enough to show blood regurgitating back from the postbulbar duodenum. A traumatic antecedent to a syndrome of central abdominal pain, mass, vomiting, or bleeding seems to argue against instrumentation or x rays. However, as anticoagulation can accentuate or disclose the bleeding of an otherwise asymptomatic cancer anywhere in the GI tract, and as trauma is often not the cause of an intestinal mass, followup films or endoscopic examination may be necessary to ensure both the resolution of the lesion and the absence of unrelated bleeding sites.

Duodenal hematomas rarely obstruct, become infected, continue to hemorrhage, or induce a perforative transmural necrosis, but these possibilities make surgical consultation necessary. Simultaneous traumatic pancreatitis may emerge to dominate the clinical stage.

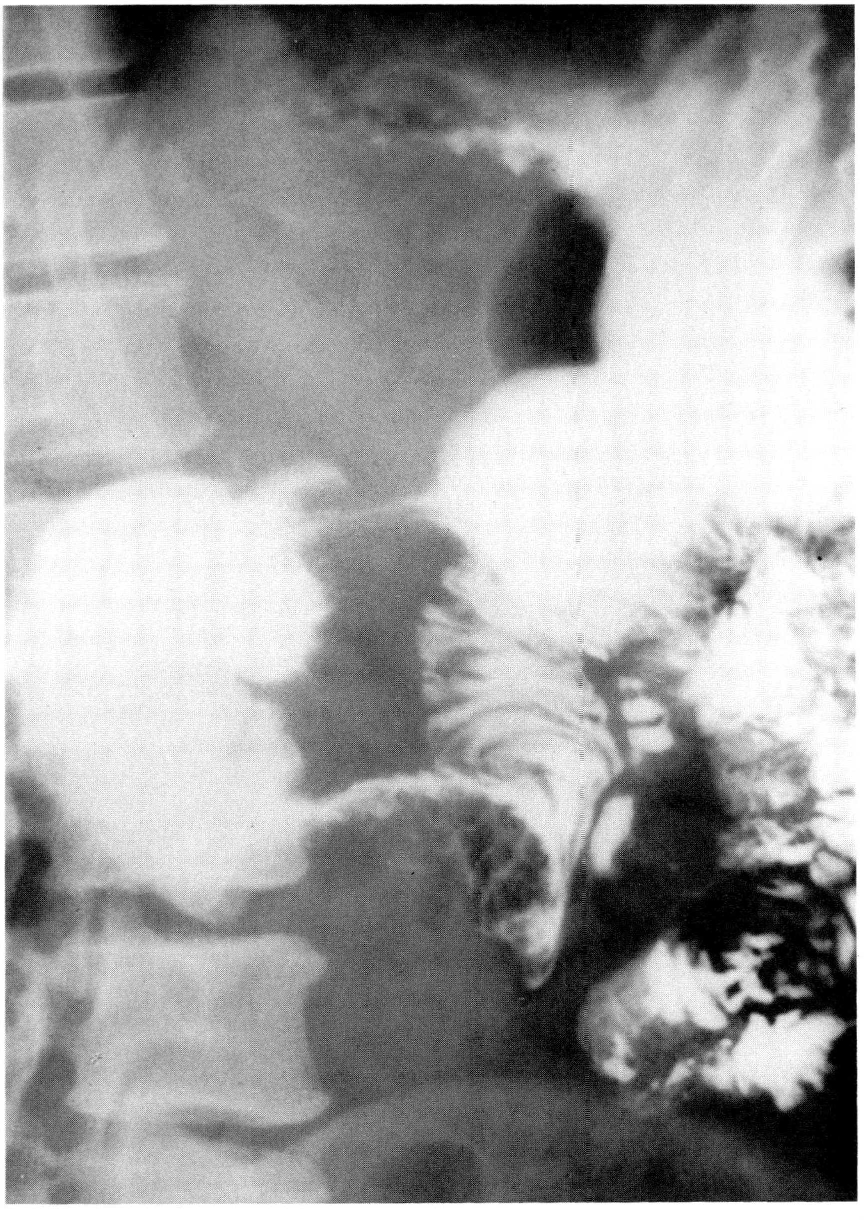

FIG. 3–15. Rounded and cobblestone textured elevations of distal third portion of duodenum, with partial obstruction to contrast flow. Followup x rays (6 weeks) are normal.

JEJUNAL DIVERTICULOSIS

Though rarely identified in childhood, this dramatic disorder must surely represent a congenital defect of connective tissue, favoring development of multiple, large, separate sacs protruding from the lumen into the wall of the upper small intestine or, less commonly, the ileum. Unlike their more common colonic cousins, they almost never bleed, perforate, or threaten peritoneal sterility, and likewise probably aren't extruded between hypertrophic muscle bands.

This typical x ray (Fig. 3–16) shows innumerable, ovoid, contrast-filled collections along the upper midgut. Because these diverticula are seen to empty barium poorly, their digestive contents also stagnate. This effects a massive, intraluminal microbial overgrowth, populating a normally near-sterile area with billions of organisms per ml of small intestinal juice; this overgrowth simulates the bacterial environment of the normal colon or static midgut in progressive systemic sclerosis, bowel amyloid, or the blind-loop syndrome. These bacteria dehydroxylate and deconjugate bile salts, lowering the amount available for digestion of dietary triglyceride. Accordingly, a painless, sprue-like diarrhea develops with steatorrhea, weight loss, and malnutrition, particularly with fat-soluble vitamin and calcium wastage.

As the bacteria metabolize away their host's intrinsic factor and dietary B-12 requirements, megaloblastic anemia, glossitis, and neuropathy may occur. Like the other absorptive manifestations of this disease, depressed B-12 absorption noted on the Schilling test normalizes only following administration of an oral antibiotic whose permanent, low-dose use will usually diminish small-bowel flora adequately to restore intestinal function. Further supplementation with calcium, vitamins (particularly A, D, K, and B-12), and dietary fat that is absorbable without bile-salt hydrolysis (such as medium- or short-chain triglycerides) seems logical.

Surgery is not required unless it is to resect a single exceedingly large or several proximate diverticula. Quantitative small-bowel culture, radionuclide breath tests for CO_2 and exhaled hydrogen, and measurement of serum bile salts or urinary bacterial metabolites are among the panoply of sophisticated (and costly) studies available to the clinician to diagnose intestinal overgrowth. The individual or aggregate superiority of these studies to the barium x ray and careful assessment of the patient's response to administration of a brief period of oral tetracycline therapy is doubtful.

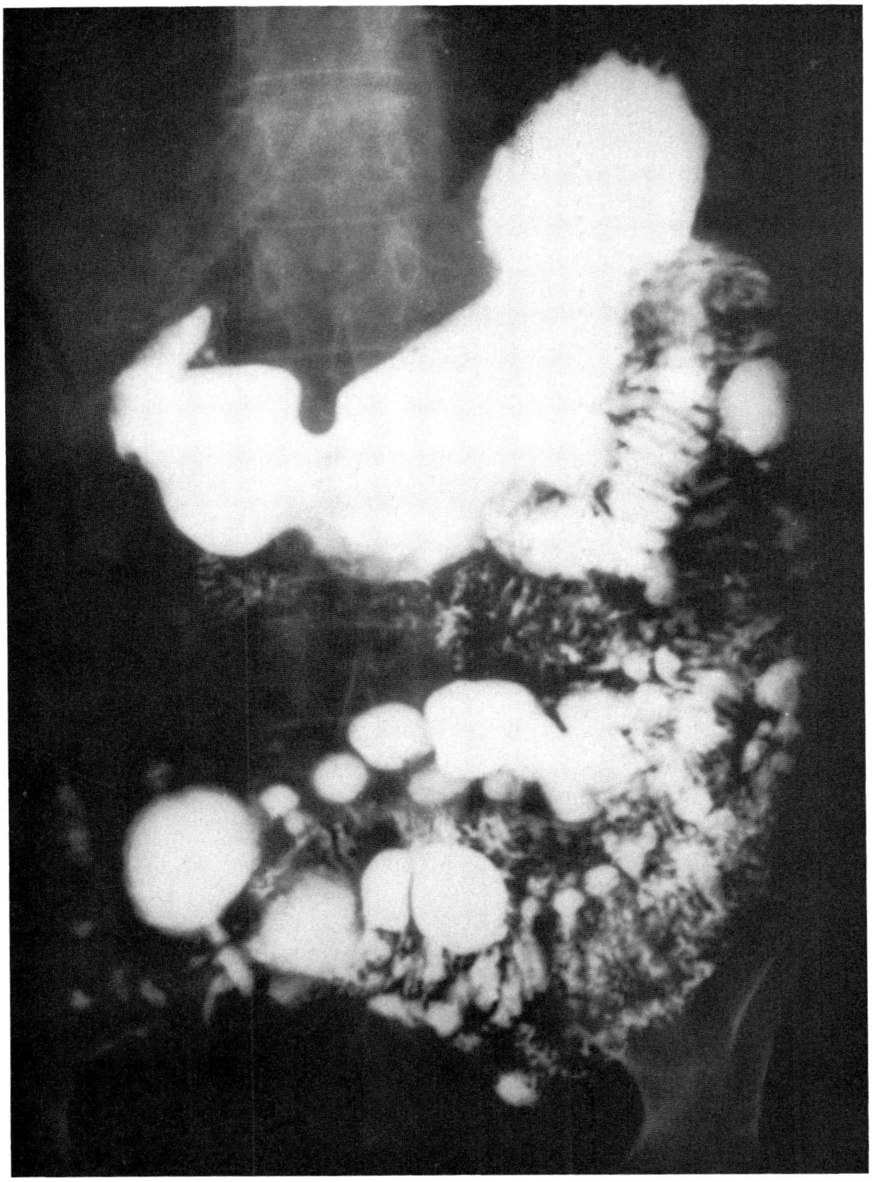

FIG. 3–16. Multiple, barium-filled outpouchings scattered throughout the small intestine, each sac assuming an almost colon-like calibre.

Exaggerated mobility of the small intestine may lead to a variety of acute and chronic, generally surgical disorders, the most serious of which is volvulus. Sometimes a consequence of congenital malrotations of the gut, these disorders generally develop following earlier abdominal surgery for acute, traumatic injury, such as stab wounds or auto accidents. Because their repair and the preceding intraperitoneal soilage or hemorrhage lead to significant peritoneal scarring, a focus is provided around which this critical, incarcerated twisting of small bowel, mesentery, and vasculature occurs.

The volvulus itself must be thought of as a discrete, often extensive obstruction, induced by focal rotation and sealed, sausage-like, at both ends; it is thus not decompressible by nasogastric suction, diarrhea, or vomiting. It is manifested by acute midabdominal pain and focal distension. Plain films (Fig. 3–17A) are likely to disclose a central collection of widely distended midgut, perhaps without air-fluid levels or gastric distention. The presence or absence of visible colonic gas contributes little. Bowel gangrene occurs rapidly, either from acute arterial insufficiency or venous obstruction with engorgement, and small-bowel resection is almost always required by the time of operation. The overriding issue is whether critical shortening of the midgut will result. "Second-look" procedures, 48 to 72 hours later, are often needed to ascertain the status of remaining bowel, particularly when the surgeon has allowed intestine of questionable viability to remain because of concern for the long-term nutritional complications of surgery.

Inguinal hernias, reducible or irreducible, are another form of visceral migration. They exist not around an adhesion, but through a weakened abdominal wall—in this case, at the inguinal canal leading to the scrotal sac. The hernia (Fig. 3–17B) is found filled with otherwise normal, though peripatetic, intestine.

Intussusception describes the bowel moving in upon itself, a slender loop usually prolapsing into a wider one, like a collapsing telescope. The commonest intussusceptions occur at the ileocolic junction, where the propulsive mobility of the large intestine seizes the valve and pulls the narrower ileum internally and distally. The herniated small intestine assumes an erratic, spiral outline, resembling a coiled spring. The majority can be reduced by the retrograde pressure imparted by barium enema, an attempt at which is seen in Figure 3–17C. Bowel obstruction occurs commonly; vascular infarction is a more serious complication of intussusception. Rare in adults, it is more commonly a concern of pediatricians and pediatric surgeons. The leading edge of an intussusception can be a polyp or cancer.

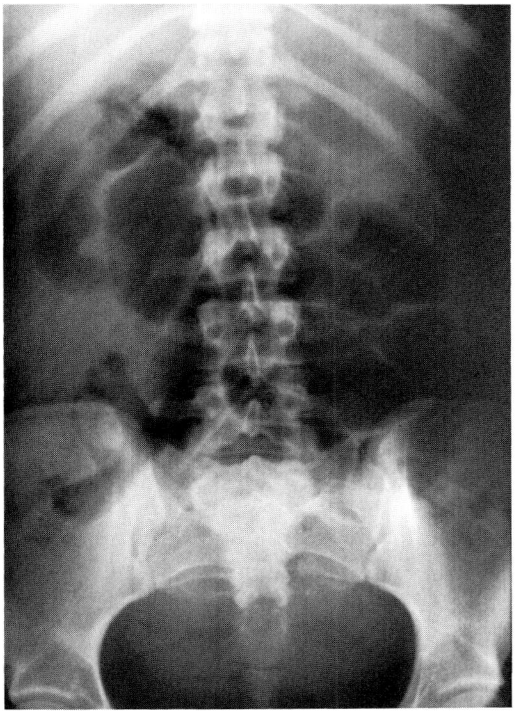

A

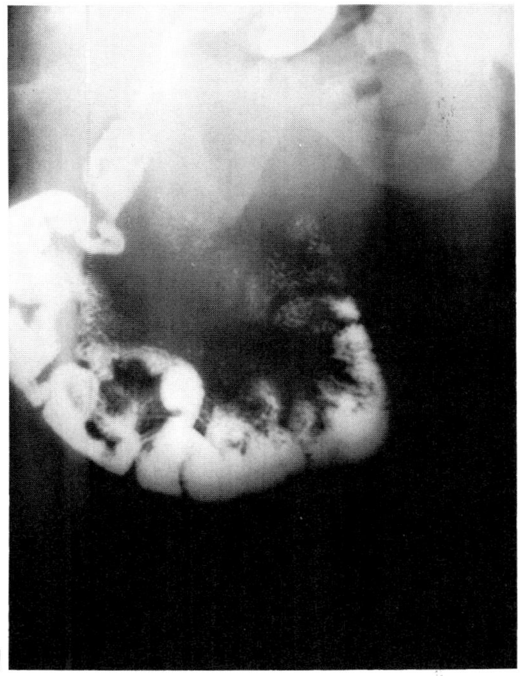

B

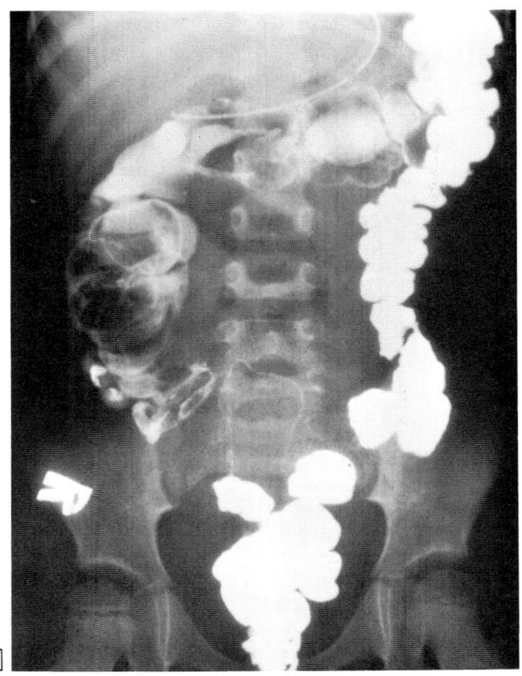

C

FIG. 3–17. A. Volvulus. Loculated, central cluster of widely distended small-bowel loops. Air is absent from colon.
B. Several feet of distal ileum noted well below the pelvis inside a massive, right inguinal hernia.
C. Intussusception. Coiled-spring appearance of ileum pulled into ascending colon, unrelieved by barium enemas.

SHORT BOWEL SYNDROME

The rapid entry of the shortened small intestine's contents into the colon or rectum constitutes one of the less remediable causes of maldigestion and malabsorption. Explaining the negative nutritional consequences by a fistula or the diminished length of bowel available for absorption seems simple. Yet, a variety of other factors are involved, whose understanding may afford some therapeutic opportunities for the clinician. These include poor mixing of foodstuffs with digestive juices, a peculiar form of gastric hypersecretion that sometimes follows massive small-bowel resection, a corresponding decrease in the brush-border enzymes (e.g., disaccharidases), and abbreviated physical contact of partially digested materials with luminal epithelium.

Causes of a shortened midgut are multiple; the more common include both multiple small-intestinal resections for recurrent or extensive Crohn's disease and surgery for massive intestinal infarction from adhesive bands, small-bowel volvulus, or physical trauma to the midgut or its vasculature. The best clue for identifying this disorder is not on the x ray, but on its requisition, which should describe prior surgery and its indications. The radiologic diagnosis is established by the paucity of otherwise normal, visualized small intestine (Fig. 3–18), recalling that a short circuit fistula will also speed rectal filling soon after barium is ingested. Since contrast may pass through the intestine in only minutes, the forewarned radiologist might choose to increase direct fluoroscopy time.

Treatment mandates full oral nutritional polypharmacy and, depending on the magnitude of the diarrhea and weight loss, adjunctive use of parenteral hyperalimentation.

Oddly enough, one additional operation may be useful. The resection, antiperistaltic reversal, and reanastomosis of a several-inch segment of distal small bowel can sometimes slow transit sufficiently to diminish stool frequency and nutrient loss. One must recall, however, that a too-lengthy reversed loop may induce obstruction; the required 180° turn on its axis can endanger the bowel's vasculature, while a tiny segment won't accomplish anything. H_2-receptor blockers to diminish gastric-acid hypersecretion and liberal doses of opiate and nonopiate antimotility agents are of undoubted value. Diarrhea may be improved by feeding glucose and isotonic electrolyte solutions. Supplemental pancreatic exocrine enzymes should be tried. On occasion, small-bowel absorptive function improves spontaneously, apparently through adaptive enhancement.

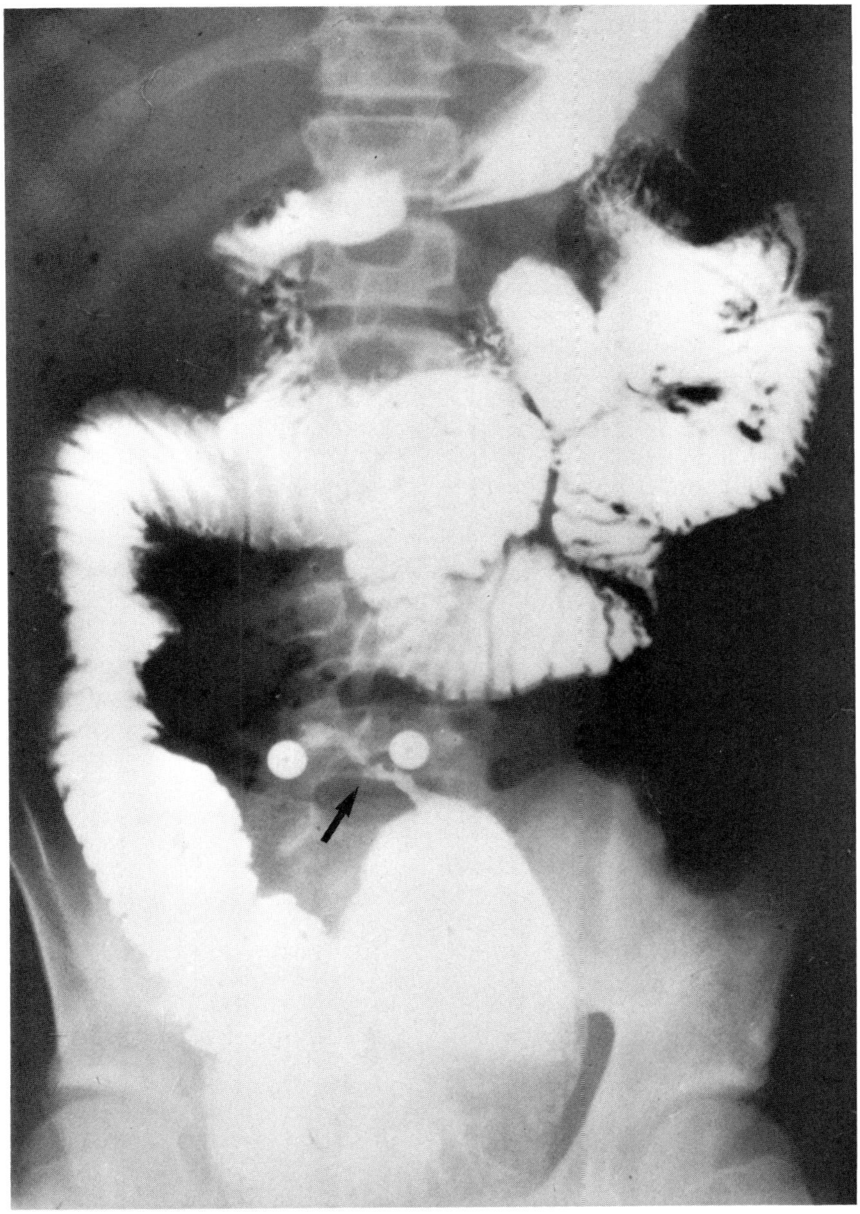

FIG. 3–18. Rapid filling of rectum in a previously unoperated patient. A jejunorectal fistula is seen entering the rectum.

SMALL BOWEL OBSTRUCTION

Speculations about small-bowel obstruction, complete or partial, are a persistent concern in gastroenterology, emergency medicine, and surgery, for which history complements both bedside and radiologic examinations. The pain pattern of obstructed patients is classically crampy, with a "sine-wave" distribution, in which pain gradually increases to its maximum while peristalsis becomes increasingly audible. Eventually generating enough pressure to overcome the obstruction, the distended bowel empties its trapped intestinal solid and fluid matter distally, giving temporary relief. If the obstruction is proximal, nausea will often exceed pain, and symptoms can be partially relieved by vomiting. Distal obstructive vomiting may be feculent and is less likely to decompress the obstructed segment.

Small-intestinal movements are continuous. Thus, standard x-ray films record only a static fraction of the bowel's activity and may not be capable of distinguishing between active obstruction and paralytic ileus. Examination of the flat and upright abdominal and chest films can ideally determine the degree and location of gaseous distension, the contour of bowel at a cutoff point, the presence of intraperitoneal air, and the progression or regression of the process.

The commonest cause of bowel obstruction is a previous intra-abdominal operation, resulting in one or more adhesive bands that entrap a pliable loop of small intestine. The second-commonest cause is carcinomatosis; hence, in either case the presence of and reason for an abdominal scar (or its absence) are valuable clues.

Acute small-bowel obstructions are generally associated with marked, air-filled distention of the small bowel (Fig. 3–19A) in which the valvulae conniventes are easily identifiable and the lumen is distended 4 or 5 cm in width. An acute cutoff point implies a high-magnitude obstruction, unlikely to be reversed by nasogastric-tube suction. A more common appearance includes the scattered low-grade air-fluid levels (Fig. 3–19B) seen in incomplete obstruction or as a nonspecific finding in patients with a nonobstructive disease such as postoperative ileus, acute pancreatitis, ulcerative colitis, or penetrating ulcer. Though often absent, air in the large intestine can occur even after complete proximal blockage.

A diagnosis of obstruction is suggested at the bedside, reinforced by plain abdominal films, and established by the instillation of contrast (Fig. 3–19C), which travels to a constant point, but no farther. Under these circumstances, treatment is surgical, preferably soon. The ongoing vasculature of a distended loop is problematic; at some point, bowel ischemia, gangrene, and eventual rupture await the indecisive physician and his patient.

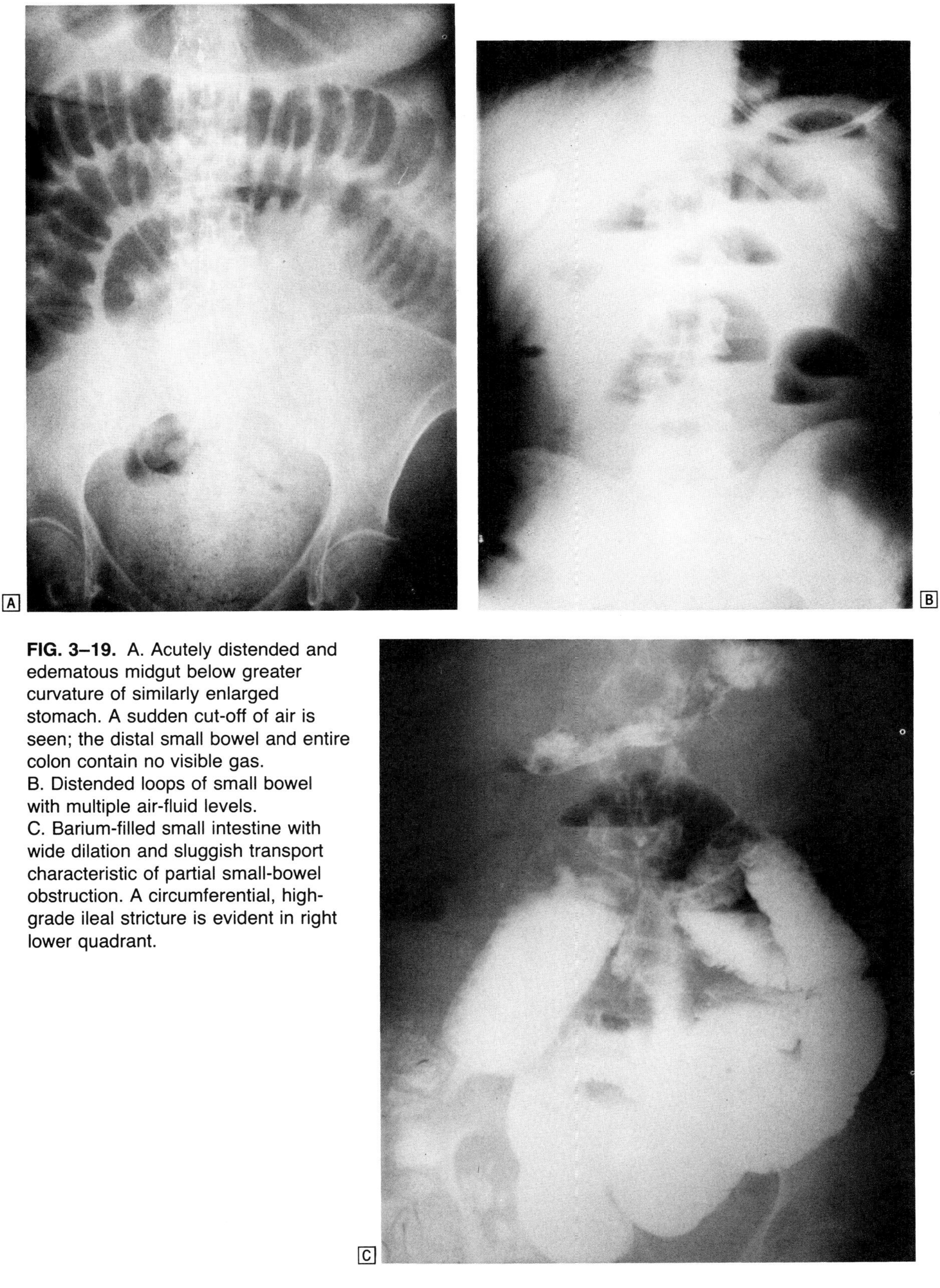

FIG. 3–19. A. Acutely distended and edematous midgut below greater curvature of similarly enlarged stomach. A sudden cut-off of air is seen; the distal small bowel and entire colon contain no visible gas.
B. Distended loops of small bowel with multiple air-fluid levels.
C. Barium-filled small intestine with wide dilation and sluggish transport characteristic of partial small-bowel obstruction. A circumferential, high-grade ileal stricture is evident in right lower quadrant.

SCLERODERMA OF THE SMALL INTESTINE

While the inexorable progression of systemic sclerosis usually parallels and is dominated by its pulmonary, vascular, or renal manifestations, its effect on the small intestine, like that on the esophagus, can be life-altering, though rarely life-shortening. Deriving from the identical smooth-muscle atrophy and fibrosis present in the scleroderma esophagus, the sluggish motility and secondary dilation of midgut involvement produces a stasis syndrome resembling that of patients with extensive jejunal diverticulosis. Because of its diminished motility, the small intestine becomes more like a storage organ, permitting its hypercolonization by aerobic and anaerobic bacteria. If aspirated, small-bowel fluid is found thick and fetid; quantitative cultures demonstrate billions of bacteria per ml. Through their deconjugation and dehydroxylation of bile salts, these organisms diminish dietary fat emulsification with malabsorption of fat and fat-soluble vitamins. As the bacteria are more successful competing for alimentary B-12, calcium loss and hyperprothrombinemia may also be compounded by megaloblastic anemia. The absorptive function of the small bowel villi is unaffected. This is really a maldigestive syndrome; the defect is intraluminal, as well as muscular.

On barium study, the intestinal muscle atrophy correlates well with agonizingly slow and sluggish transport and a particular, almost characteristic widening of the second and third portions of the duodenum (Fig. 3–20). Barium may remain in the intestine for days following ingestion. The colon may show large, wide-mouthed diverticula that are considered unique to scleroderma by some radiologists.

Never completely successful, treatment is constant, sometimes alternating administration of both absorbable and nonabsorbable antibiotics, which should lower the bacterial concentration sufficiently to improve absorption. Supplemental oral and injectable vitamins are also indicated, as is use of dietary medium-chain triglycerides, which do not require bile salt or pancreatic lipase for digestion. Promotility agents are probably indicated, but their value in improving digestion will be difficult to assess, particularly when diarrhea is present.

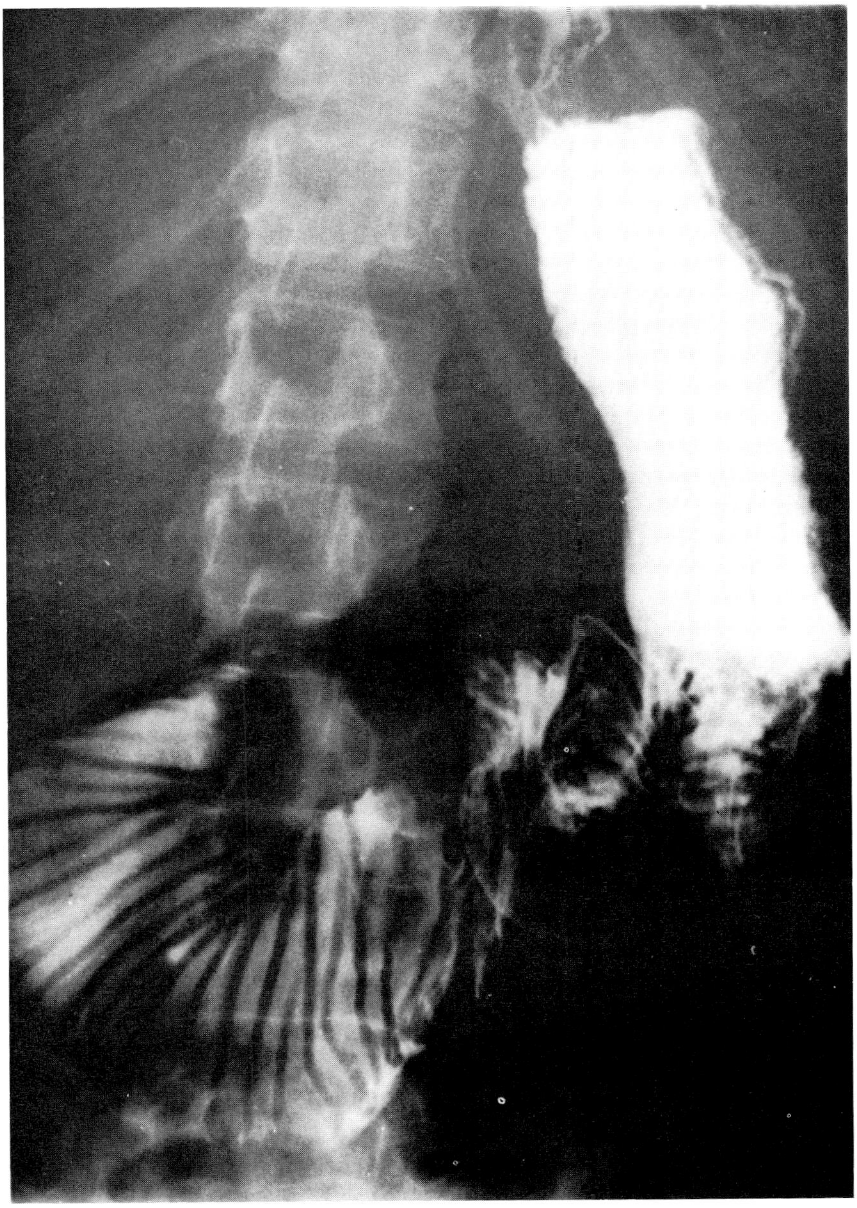

FIG. 3–20. Extraordinary widening of the duodenal sweep, with nonobstructive stasis in the stomach and small bowel. Note preservation of proximal small-bowel mucosal pattern.

PEUTZ-JEGHERS SYNDROME AND OTHERS LIKE IT

First described in this century, this uncommon disorder is manifested by multiple, hamartomatous tumors of the small intestine and, rarely, the stomach and colon. They are microscopically benign; instances of malignant degeneration have been reported. The syndrome derives from their familial incidence and associated multiple, mucocutaneous melanin deposits on oral mucous membranes, tongue, lips, nail beds, and fingers. Their commonest clinical manifestation is low-grade gastrointestinal bleeding. Since they typically occur in multiples (Fig. 3–21A), surgical treatment ought only follow an extensive intestinal survey and then, on some occasions, correspondingly thorough resection. Small-bowel and small-bowel-into-colon intussusceptions are frequent in Peutz-Jeghers syndrome.

A nonfamilial variant of intestinal hamartomas are so-called juvenile or retention polyps. These characteristically become apparent in the first decade of life and, apart from anal fissures, are probably the commonest cause of childhood rectal bleeding. Resembling typical adenomatous polyps or villous adenomas, the polyps are almost always pedunculated, spherical, and minimally lobulated. As retention polyps, they are filled with innumerable mucus-containing cysts, which are themselves lined with benign, glandular epithelium. They are highly vascular, almost always multiple, and never malignant. Accordingly, their colonoscopic removal can be completed in a single stage, meaning that the instrument does not have to be removed each time an individual polyp is transected, which is the usual case with potentially cancerous adenomatous polyps when it is critical to know the exact location of each lesion.

Nodular lymphoid hyperplasia may be seen in both children and adults, and commonly involves the Peyer's patches of ileal mucosa (Fig. 3–21B) or occasionally the large bowel; it is rarely significant. These lesions only faintly resemble true polyps and have been associated with deficiency of immunoglobulin A and, in those patients, vulnerability to parasite infestations, particularly Giardia.

Gartner's syndrome identifies the autosomal-dominant coexistence of premalignant colon polyps with cranial and long-bone osteomas, and a variety of cutaneous lesions, including fibromas and epidermoid cysts. Conspicuous mandibular enlargement is often the first clue. The skeletal and cutaneous lesions distinguish this syndrome from familial polyposis of the colon, as does development of dense, aggressive, postoperative intra-abdominal adhesions. Since total colectomy is usually required, these adhesions jeopardize ileostomy function and predispose the patient to recurrent small-bowel obstructions. Cancers in Gartner's have also been described in the ampulla of Vater, pancreas, and thyroid.

Cronkhite-Canada syndrome associates inflammatory polyps of the stomach and small intestine with decreased skin pigmentation, precocious hair loss, and dystrophic nails. Finally, some patients with thickened melanosis of skin folds (acanthosis nigricans) will be found harboring a gastric or colon cancer.

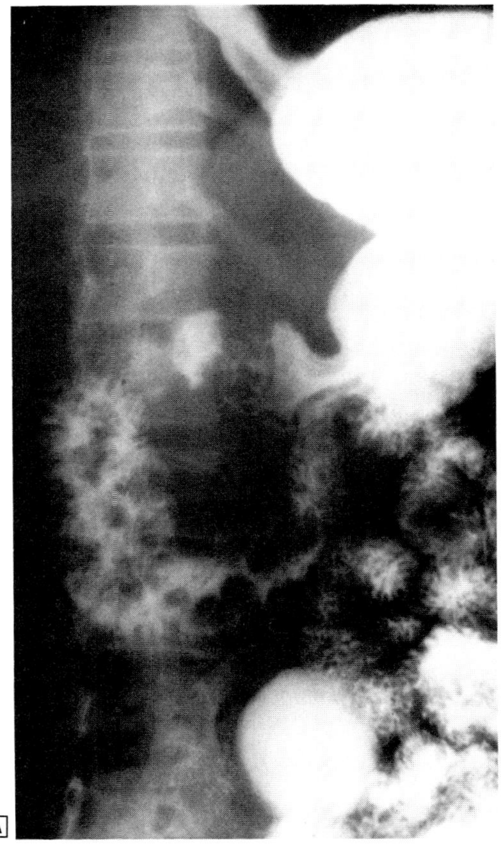

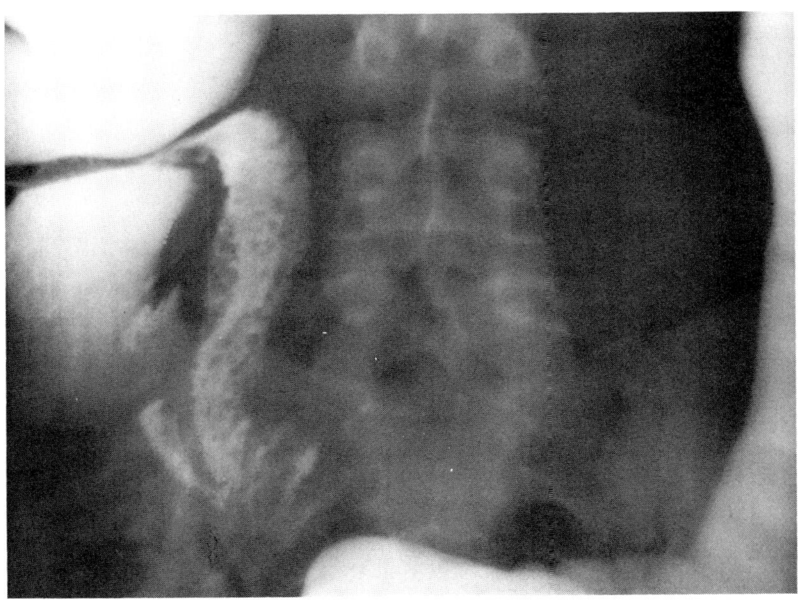

FIG. 3–21. A. Duodenal sweep, showing multiple rounded radiolucencies in a patient presenting with chronic GI bleeding. The valvular pattern is otherwise normal. Additional lesions are not evident in the remainder of the small bowel. B. Nodular lymphoid hyperplasia. Multiple tiny, circular radiolucent nodules of the terminal ileum, a generally benign finding.

EXTRINSIC DUODENAL COMPRESSION

Circumferential luminal compression by an annular pancreas is the commonest neonatal cause of duodenal obstruction and, when evident at birth, is seen commonly with other disorders, most conspicuously mongolism and, less often, focal bowel atresias. Unlike the heterotopic pancreatic tissue sometimes found in the duodenal or distal gastric wall (or a Meckel's diverticulum), the annular pancreas will rarely be found harboring a functioning insulin- or gastrin-producing adenoma. It reflects an embryonic failure of migration or fusion of dorsal and ventral anlage in forming the uncinate process; duodenal encirclement results. The usual annular gland produces no symptoms, but others may appear in adolescence or adulthood through a syndrome of recurrent, obstructive vomiting. Duodenal encroachment is inferred on x ray (Fig. 3–22A) as a circumferential, generally low-grade narrowing onto its descending limb, understandably associated with stomach and duodenal enlargement. In contrast with the more severe duodenal blockage occurring with primary mucosal or extrinsic tumors, pancreatitis, adhesions, or congenital bands, obstructive symptoms are neither severe nor progressive. A more indolent, chronic vomiting, sometimes lasting for years, often mistakenly ascribed to psychogenic factors, argues for this less serious, alternative consideration. The best "curative" treatment is a bypassing gastrojejunostomy.

In the compressive superior mesenteric artery syndrome, obstruction occurs more distally, at the third or transverse portion from focal compression by the superior mesenteric vessels. In Figure 3–22B, the stomach and most of the duodenal C-loop appear distended with barium. The intestine is abruptly blocked as it crosses the vertebral column right to left. Only a trickle of contrast escapes distally.

This syndrome is characteristically seen in asthenic females, whose contracted abdominal volume results from and may account for one remediable organic aspect of the autostarvation and vomiting in anorexia nervosa patients. The ideal treatment, of course, is to gain sufficient weight to allow the anterior abdominal wall to progress outward. If the patient is unwilling or the vomiting prohibitive, surgical division of the ligament of Treitz may drop the fourth portion of the duodenum inferiorly, releasing it from its compression between the superior mesenteric artery and vein anteriorly, and the aorta and vertebral prominences posteriorly. If this fails, gastrojejunostomy will be required.

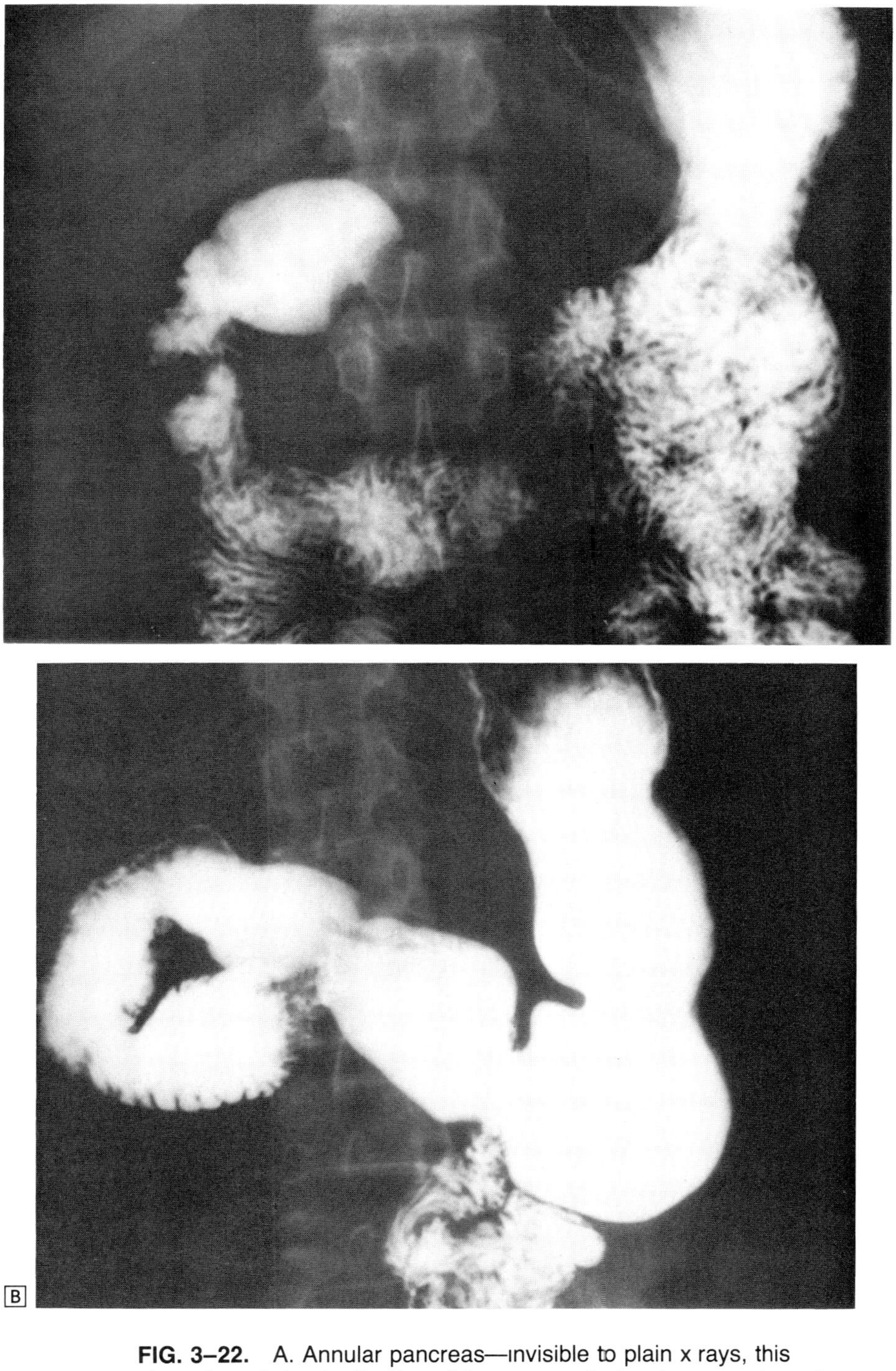

A

B

FIG. 3–22. A. Annular pancreas—invisible to plain x rays, this circumferential reduplication of the pancreatic head surrounds and constricts the obviously contracted, descending duodenal limb. B. Superior mesenteric artery syndrome—upper GI series with abrupt termination of barium flow at the junction of the third and fourth portions of duodenum.

GASTROINTESTINAL FOREIGN BODIES

Some are accidental, some intentional, others a feature of important organic or psychiatric disease, and whether "foreign" or domestic, macroscopic parasites are manifestations of defective hygiene and poverty. This brief, admittedly incomplete survey illustrates foreign bodies inhabiting esophagus, duodenal bulb, midgut, and rectosignoid.

The coin seen on end in the upper esophagus (Fig. 3–23A) is a common pediatric "crisis." Unlike quarters or half dollars, the smaller denominations are generally innocuous; they rarely obstruct or perforate, and respond to patience by their normal exit, typically a little shinier from exposure to gastric acid. Mid-esophageal impactions with coins are uncommon; blockages at the pylorus and ileocecal sphincter occur most frequently. Most endoscopes can be equipped with coin extractors, which, though imperfect, are an obvious improvement over laparotomy.

Acute esophageal obstructions in adults are usually caused by a large, poorly chewed meat bolus, trapped in a peptic stricture or a Schatzki's ring. Often coming for help to emergency rooms after their evening meal (when the culprit was swallowed), patients should be gently sedated and their mouths and throats kept clear by suction. Gentle pressure on a swallowed lubricated bougie will push most obstructions into the stomach. Endoscopic debulking by forceps often becomes an endless task and is rarely necessary. Secondary emetogenic tears of the esophagus may be induced through forceful, continuous retching, particularly when the distal esophageal mucosa is already inflamed.

Sharp-edged foreign bodies are quite another matter. A swallowed open safety pin or chicken bone will often perforate the upper esophagus. Cervical odynophagia or postprandial neck pain should prompt soft-tissue films, which may show the slenderest streak of retropharyngeal air (Fig. 3–23B) or subcutaneous or mediastinal emphysema. However, a suspected perforation can be precipitated or worsened by the air insufflation necessary for successful endoscopic visualization.

Figure 3–23C illustrates an obliquely placed cocktail toothpick, lodged in the duodenal bulb. Its immobility over a period encompassing three successive upper GI series argues that, absent manual extraction, it was there to stay. Like the more common impaction of a sharp-edged fruit pit, the risk of perforation and bleeding from a lesion with ends fixed on and into mucosa mandates duodenotomy and primary repair.

The tubular, straw-like radiolucencies in the midgut (Fig. 3–23D) represent a cluster of nematodes (Ascaris), generally appearing in the children of the poor, usually from the rural South. The organism's flamboyant lifestyle should be recalled: entry through the skin, travel via the vasculature, penetration into the lung, migration up the tracheobronchial tree and occasionally out the nasal passage, being coughed into saliva and, usually, eventually being swallowed into the intestinal tract. Their diet consists of human blood and tissue juices, and amidst all of this hospitality they enlarge and multiply, occasionally producing severe anemia or bowel obstruction.

Foreign bodies inserted intrarectally are those usually employed for their anticipated erotic potential. Figure 3–23E shows a battery-operated phallic vibrator, unfortunately manipulated above a point of easy extraction. Removal required general anesthesia and instrumental sphincter dilatation.

Gastric bezoars may follow regular ingestion of coagulable fruit pulp (pomegranate and persimmon), but they usually consist of retained food, following hemigastrectomy. Trichobezoars consist of the patient's own ingested, self-plucked hair, another explanation-defying habit; some psychotics will ingest anything, including table cutlery or hardware.

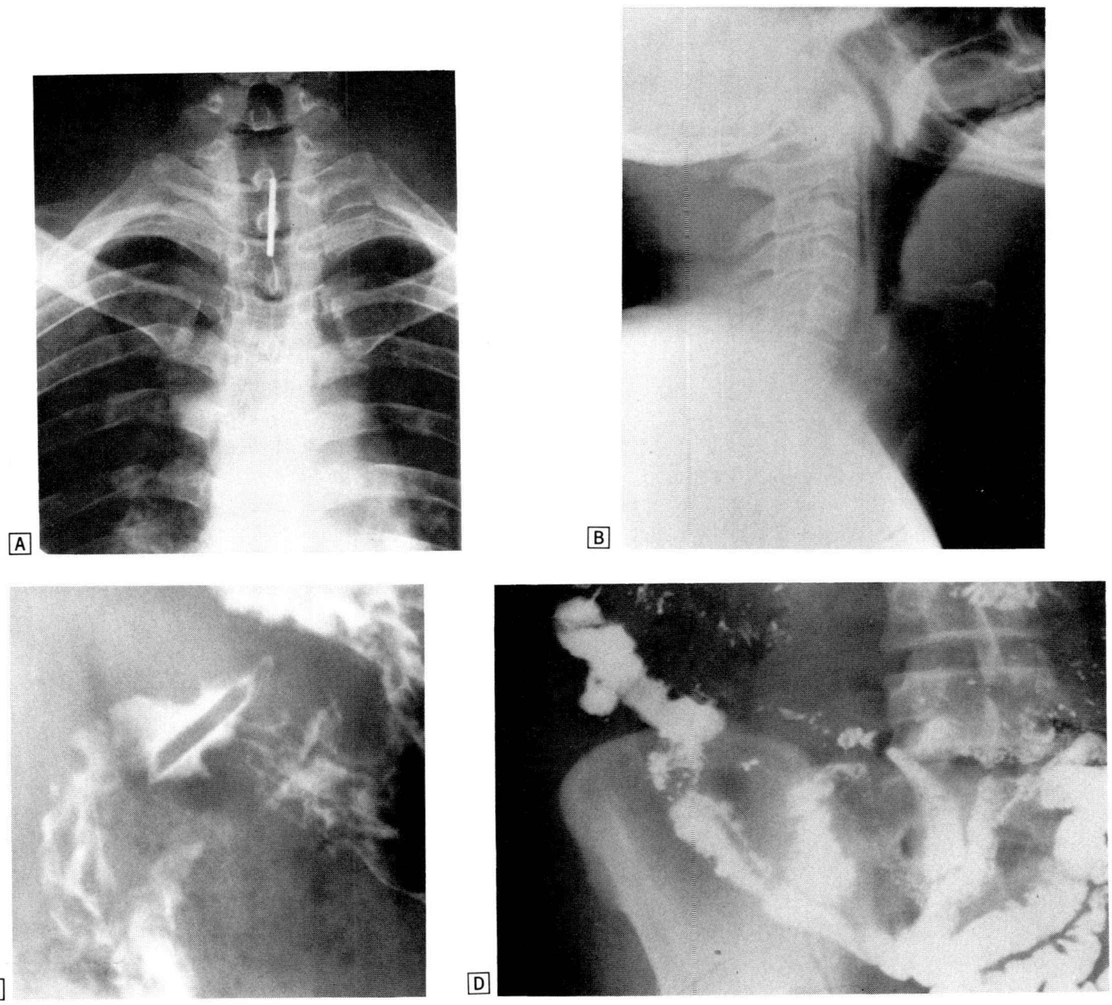

FIG. 3–23. A. Coin in upper esophagus, eventually retrieved by grasping forceps of a fiberscope.
B. Lateral view of neck of patient with perforated cervical esophagus. A dark streak of air is identified directly anterior to vertebrae and behind the pharynx.
C. Cocktail toothpick (minus olive) wedged obliquely in duodenal bulb.
D. Ascariasis—pencil-shaped radiolucencies amidst a barium filled ileum, one of dozens producing recurrent small-bowel obstruction in a malnourished, anemic tenant farmer.
E. Plain film of abdomen, showing upwardly pointing rectal vibrator in rectosigmoid. Surgical retrieval was required.

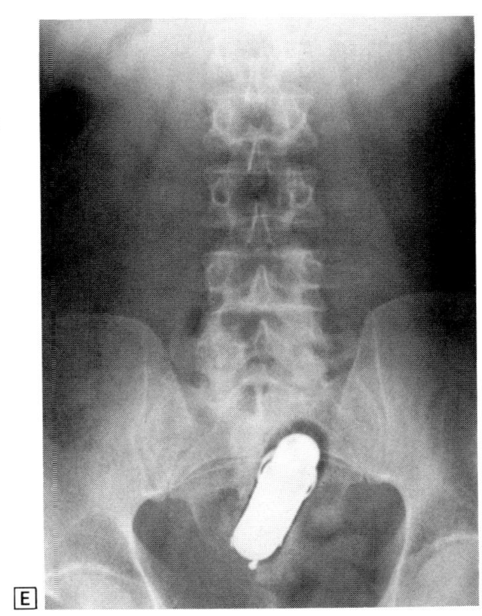

ILEOVESICAL FISTULA

One of the more visually striking and medically significant features of Crohn's disease is its capacity for fistula formation, which develops regularly from affected bowel to skin, perineum, and other hollow organs (normal bowel, bladder, vagina, renal pelvis). The transmural, including serosal, inflammation in Crohn's disease results in attachment to adjacent structures; thus, deep ulceration within the bowel makes these communications an understandable consequence. At first glance, this x ray (Fig. 3–24) looks like an otherwise uncomplicated small-bowel series but, while seeming to fill the rectum, the conspicuous absence of barium outlining the proximal colon argues against mere rapid transit through intact bowel. Indeed, the chestnut-shaped barium collection in the pelvis more closely resembles, and is, the urinary bladder with a prostatic shadow seen at its base. The tenting to its right is probably the distal end of an ileo- or jejunovesical fistula.

Such patients often present with pneumaturia, a dramatic symptom whose commonest alternative causes are diverticulitis and a cloacogenic pelvic or rectal cancer. Rarely healing spontaneously or with "medical" management, Crohn's fistulas involving other hollow organs typically require excision and resection of affected bowel, preceded by fecal-stream diversion through exteriorization of a proximal bowel loop or, to the extent possible, diminishing fistula flow through total parenteral hyperalimentation or an elemental diet. Primary Crohn's disease of the skin and enterocutaneous fistulas often respond favorably to systemic metronidazole, an agent whose antibacterial and anti-inflammatory capability make it comparable to salazopyrin's role in ulcerative colitis.

Patients undergoing fistula surgery should have preoperative computerized tomography, searching for an unsuspected abscess, either adjacent to the fistula or elsewhere in the abdomen. Though the bowel origin of an enterovesical, vaginal, or cutaneous fistula is usually evident, the circuitous path, if any, from a diseased ileum to a perirectal abscess is usually less clear and perhaps of only limited clinical interest. Much experience argues that Crohn's disease operated for fistulas recurs most frequently with fistulas; "like follows like" seems true also for resected bowel stenoses. Finally, though visually dramatic, intestinal fistulas, per se, do not mandate surgery, particularly if they are "internal" (bowel to bowel) or unassociated with sepsis, obstruction, or a malabsorptive short circuit.

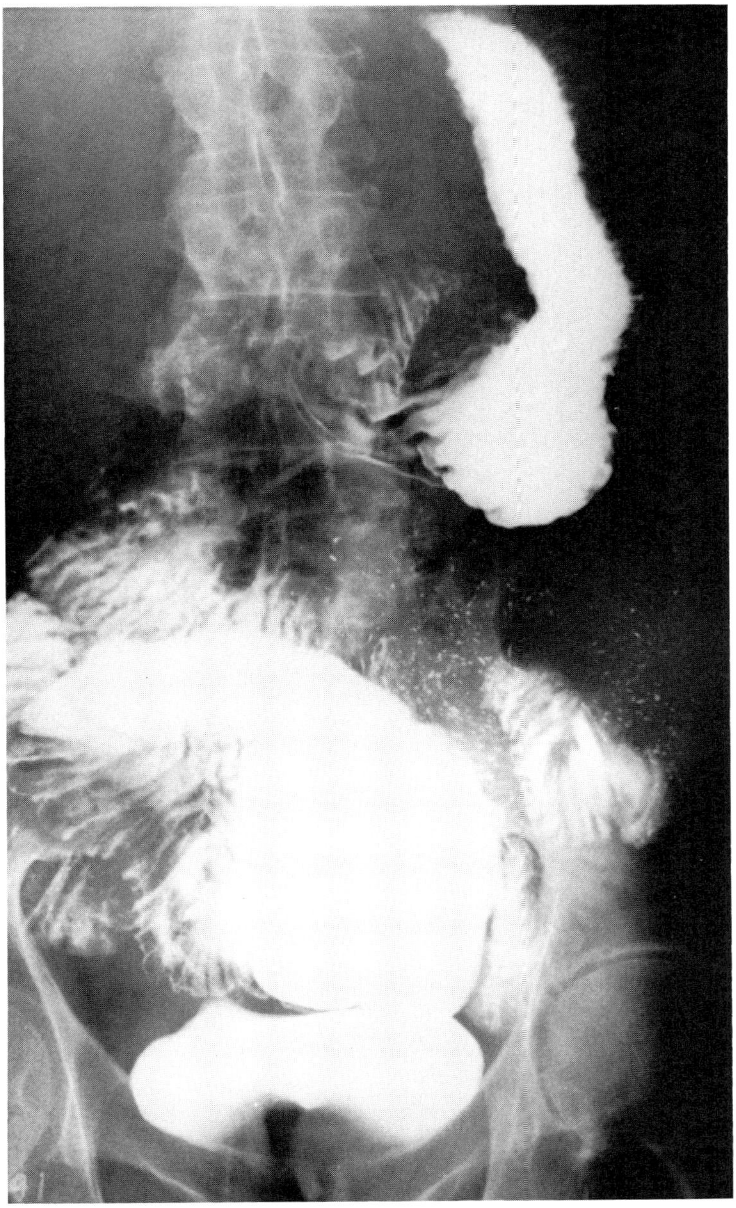

FIG. 3–24. Small-bowel series showing premature entry into pelvic reservoir, clearly the bladder. An impression of the prostate is visible at its base; upward tenting of contrast to the right of the bladder column is the probable site of the fistula's entry.

CHAPTER 4

THE PANCREAS AND BILIARY SYSTEM

GALLSTONES

Coming in many sizes, shapes, and specific gravities, floating, sinking, or dispersed in the gallbladder, and opaque or lucent to x rays, gallstones are typically composed of cholesterol precipitated from a bile with which it is supersaturated. When stones are multiple, small, or sludge-like, their extrusion into bile ducts is frequently associated with colic, jaundice, pancreatitis, or transiently deranged liver-function tests.

Though their diagnosis is now best made or confirmed by ultrasonography, the oral cholecystogram still has a place, particularly in the nonjaundiced patient, with a "normal" or equivocal sonogram, whose gallbladder incorporates or concentrates dye poorly or not at all. Occasionally, when stones are lucent and tiny, early films will appear normal; only after time are stones seen through a thinning fog of partially excreted or diluted gallbladder contrast (Fig. 4–1A). Because gallstones vary in specific gravity and content, recumbent x rays may fail to concentrate the gallbladder stones sufficiently to render them visible; hence, an upright film is indicated to show stones floating in a lucent band or falling into the most dependent portion of the gallbladder (Fig. 4–1B).

When there is a clinical or laboratory history suggesting cholangitis, or when gallstones are associated with pain, fever, or jaundice, surgery requires not only the removal of the gallbladder but x-ray, manual palpation, and visual (usually open) examination of the large bile ducts.

The major issue facing the clinician who diagnoses uncomplicated gallstones is how they are managed, whether through elective operative removal or masterful inaction. The typical syndrome of dietary-fat-induced right upper quadrant colicky pain radiating laterally or to the right shoulder helps erase indecision. Most physicians will withhold surgery from the nondiabetic patient with a single large stone and vague symptoms, while performing operations upon most diabetic patients (with questionable justification) whose stones are small or multiple, or those whose history suggests prior cholangitis or deranged liver function.

The prudent doctor needs to remind the patient with cholelithiasis that his abdominal pain may have another cause, and that surgery may purchase an oblique scar, medical bills, and some bad memories, but not relief. Likewise, there are instances when documented gallstones provide justification for surgical exploration, if the symptoms are worrisome and might or might not derive from stones, but cannot be attributed to any other disease. At surgery, cholecystectomy can be combined with palpation of the retroperitoneum and inspection of the abdominal contents.

The timing of cholecystectomy after acute cholecystitis is debated still. Surgical delay "to let things quiet down" jousts with the decision for early operation to prevent another attack, which could be complicated by sepsis, pancreatitis, or cholangitis. Until safe, painless, nonsurgical methods of stone dissolution are available, prompt operation seems both conservative and wise.

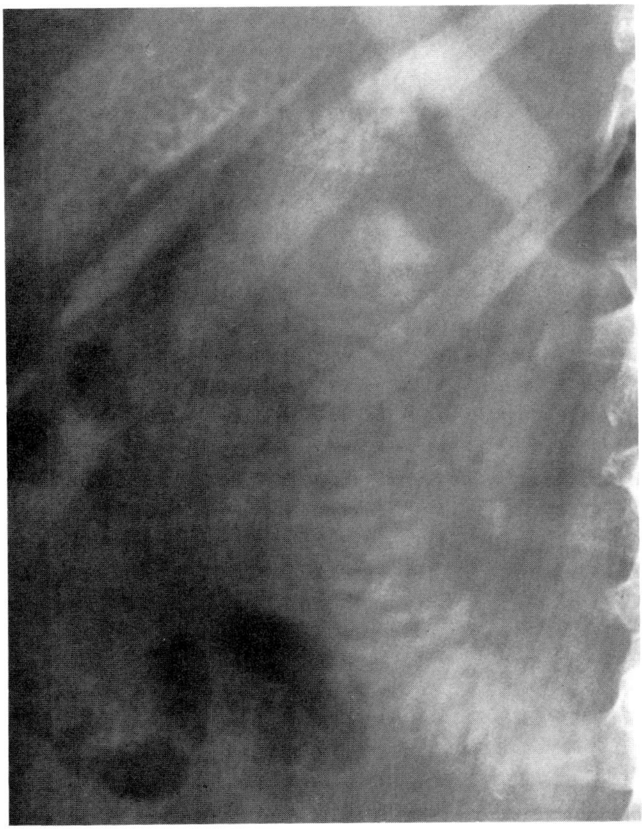

FIG. 4–1. A. Intravenous cholangiogram revealing hundreds of tiny radiolucent stones dispersed throughout the gallbladder. Dye enters a dilated common duct and partially into the duodenum.

B. A radiolucent layer of floating calculi whose specific gravity is somewhat below that of the dye-bile mixture. If this examination were done in the recumbent position, the stones might be sufficiently dispersed as to be "lost."

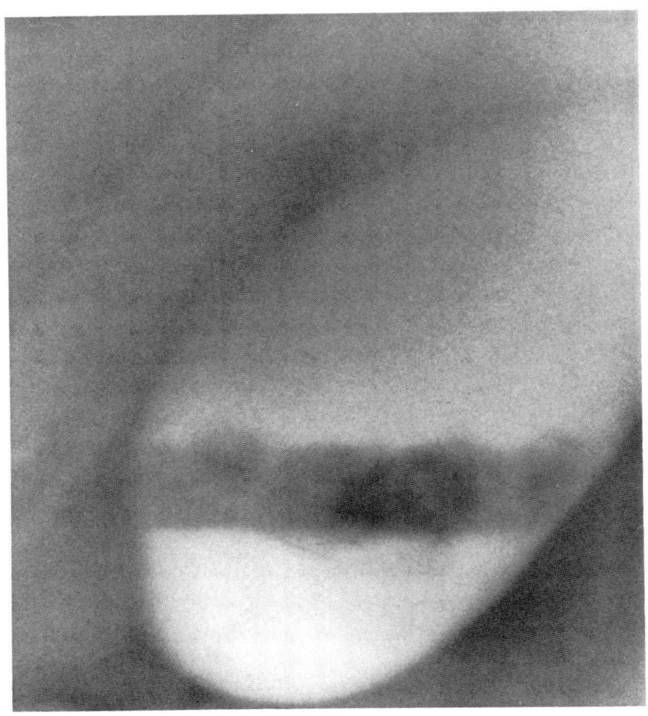

EMPHYSEMATOUS CHOLECYSTITIS

Most patients with acute cholecystitis respond well to initial nonoperative management that includes fasting, occasional nasogastric suctioning, or parenteral antibiotics. Some surgeons believe with justification that, absent evidence of common bile-duct obstruction, their patients will profit by a "rest period" that allows 4 to 6 weeks for the illness to become quiescent, reduce intraoperative inflammatory changes, enhance the identification of landmarks, and ease removal.

Emphysematous cholecystitis permits no such luxury. It constitutes an extraordinary surgical emergency, whose radiologic evidence mandates the same speed of action as that for proven peritonitis or a perforation threatening a pre-existing bowel obstruction. An occasional patient may seem deceptively well, but the majority are disturbingly labile, with severe right upper quadrant pain and tenderness arising from an infected, obstructed gallbladder.

The radiolucent, pear- or lightbulb-shaped abdominal lucency in the right upper quadrant on this plain film (Fig. 4–2) is a gas-filled gallbladder. It is always visible above the colon and lateral to the duodenum. Though not evident in this case, cystic duct and gallbladder stones are often present. It is also to be distinguished from the pneumatobilia accompanying a gallstone ileus. There, as in a biliary-enteric anastomosis, the gallbladder will be air-filled, but rarely distended, as it has been converted from a reservoir into a duct.

Absent any previous history of cholecystoenterostomy or the rare ulcer penetration into the common duct, emphysematous cholecystitis is an acute preperforative, often gangrenous, suppurative infection requiring immediate surgery.

As the risk of gram-negative septicemia is high, multiple antibiotics are necessary immediately, ideally employing those excreted in bile. Though rare, the chance of an anaerobic, gas-forming organism (e.g., Clostridia) cannot be ignored.

Postoperative fasting and resulting biliary stasis may induce severe cholecystitis in patients who undergo surgery for any reason. Once cholecystitis has been identified in this setting, treatment is drainage and resection, if possible. The abscessed gallbladder may distort anatomic landmarks sufficiently that the surgeon may have to be content with an exteriorizing cholecystostomy, which should provide adequate decompression.

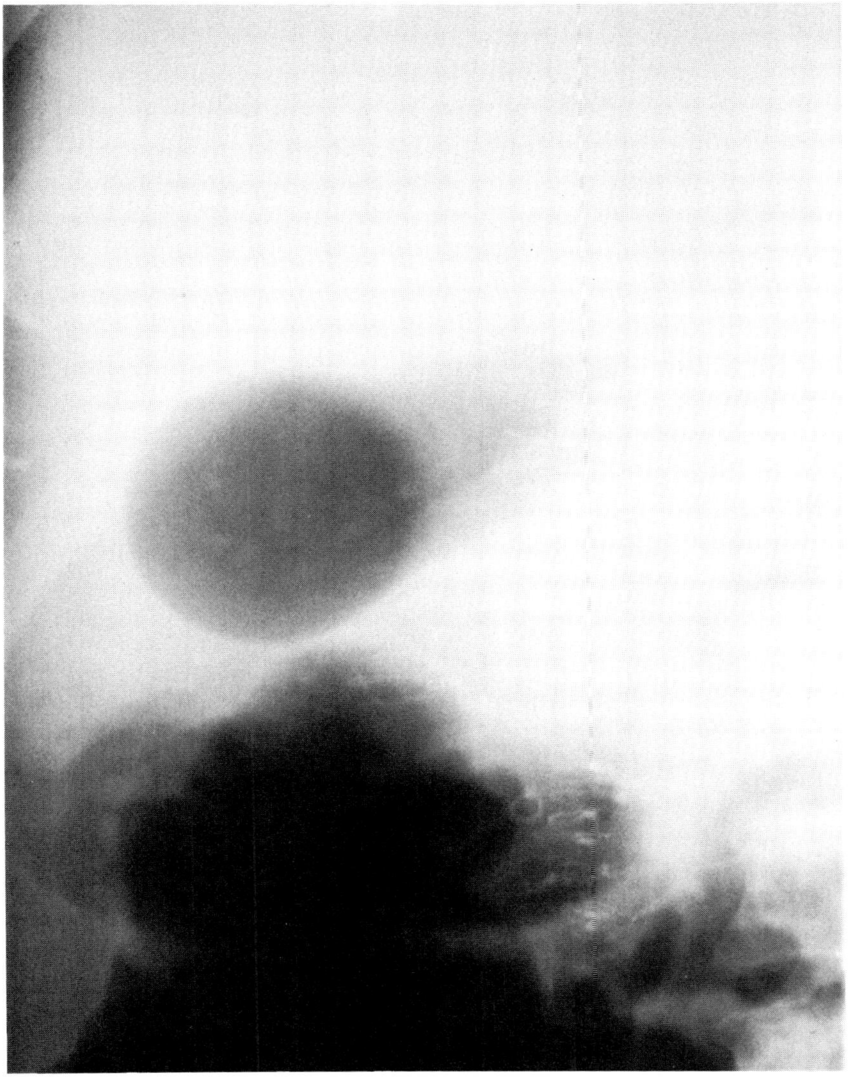

FIG. 4–2. The black pear-shaped lucency in the right upper quadrant, above the hepatic flexure, conforms perfectly with the outline of a gas-distended gallbladder.

GALLSTONE ILEUS

Not really a form of distal midgut paralysis, gallstone "ileus" describes the active small-bowel obstruction caused by a single large calculus eroding through the gallbladder wall into the intestine, to impact on and occlude the ileocecal sphincter. Three radiologic clues seen here (Fig. 4–3A and B) indicate its presence: (1) biliary air, unexplained by prior surgical biliary enterostomy; (2) small-bowel distension, suggesting obstruction; and (3) least common, a visible right lower quadrant calcified density, representing a gallstone. These patients may recall a background suggesting recurrent cholecystitis and typically have the acute onset of pain, nausea, and sometimes feculent vomiting of distal small-bowel blockage. Bedside and laboratory signs of cholangitis are usually absent, and pneumatobilia may be obscured by overlying loops of distended small bowel. Occasionally, swallowed barium will reflux from the perforated duodenum into the liver's ducts, outlining an intrahepatic system that resembles a set of deer antlers.

Biliary opacification following an upper GI series may also suggest duodenal-ulcer perforation into the choledochus, a previous sphincterotomy, or operative decompressive anastomosis between the biliary system and upper digestive tract. Though visually dramatic, barium in the biliary system is benign, not initiating the same inflammatory reaction it does in the peritoneal cavity.

Smaller stones may pass spontaneously through the bowel or, if they enter the stomach or duodenum, can be vomited up. Occasionally, they will be blocked at the pylorus, but then the x ray will show gastric as opposed to small-bowel distention. Of course, if the cystic duct is occluded, any fistula between the intestinal tract and the gallbladder will not result in air within the liver.

Management includes laparotomy, cholecystectomy, opening the ileum for stone removal, and, if found, the repair of the duodenal or jejunal site of gallstone penetration.

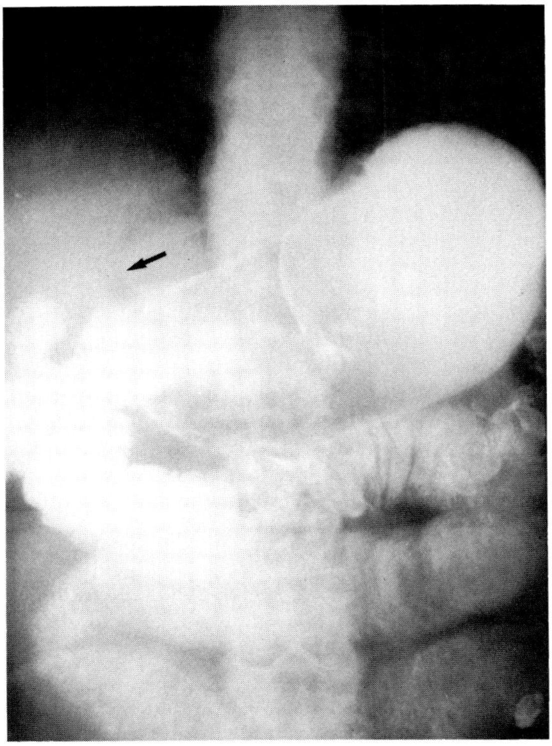

FIG. 4–3. A. Distended loops of barium-filled small bowel appearing simultaneously with air ↑ in the biliary system.

B. Plain film showing distended midgut, biliary air, and a calcified gallstone in right lower quadrant (at ileocecal sphincter).

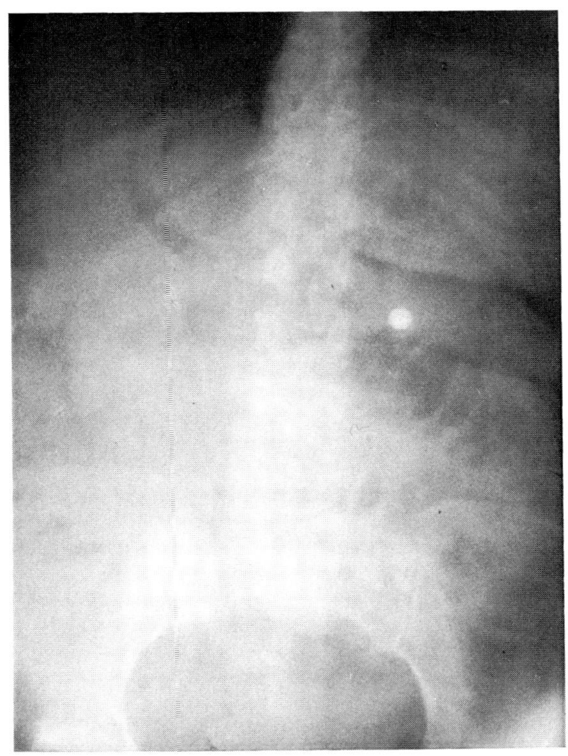

COMMON BILE DUCT STONE

However opacified, an inspected common bile duct must yield information on three issues: the caliber of the duct, the presence of any intraluminal defects, and the ease of entry of dye into the duodenum. The film opposite (Fig. 4–4) demonstrates the classic T-tube cholangiogram of a retained, obstructing common-bile-duct stone. The round intraductal radiolucent stone is obvious, permitting only a trickle of dye to enter the duodenum, opacifying its mucosa; a bit can be seen entering the main pancreatic duct. Proximal to the obstructing defect, the common bile duct is dilated, if not turgid. This examination is of a patient with recurrent fevers; it followed a cholecystectomy and common-bile-duct exploration, previously thought to have been curative. Reoperation is mandatory, as the likelihood of continued, significant difficulties in the unoperated patient approaches 100% within 2 years. The unhappy choices include sepsis from ascending cholangitis, bile-duct stricture, recurrent pancreatitis, and, less commonly, progressive hepatofibrosis (biliary cirrhosis).

Particularly reserved for the poor-risk patient, the "nonsurgical" options for managing this condition have increased. These options are now less diagnostic than therapeutic, including not only the use of cholesterol-solubilizing agents, but endoscopic sphincterotomy with stone removal by forceps and basket retrievers, choledochoscopy with similar "grabbers" and "crushers," and operative calculus dissolution by laser and sonographic lithotripsy. Greater experience argues for endoscopic retrieval, with the understanding that its employment per duodenum can introduce unsterile intestinal contents into an obstructed biliary system. Thus, if stone retrieval is unsuccessful, the risk of cholangitis is substantial, and open surgical repair should proceed directly. In truth, endoscopic stone removal and cholangiopancreatography are almost specialties in themselves and should be attempted only by the most skilled and experienced operators.

During the initial surgery of choledocholithiasis, careful operative cholangiography should be considered the minimum diagnostic procedure, probably supplemented by examination of the opened common bile duct, its irrigation and sludge removal, and passage of dilators across the ampulla into the duodenum, all of which are to precede a second, confirmatory T-tube dye study.

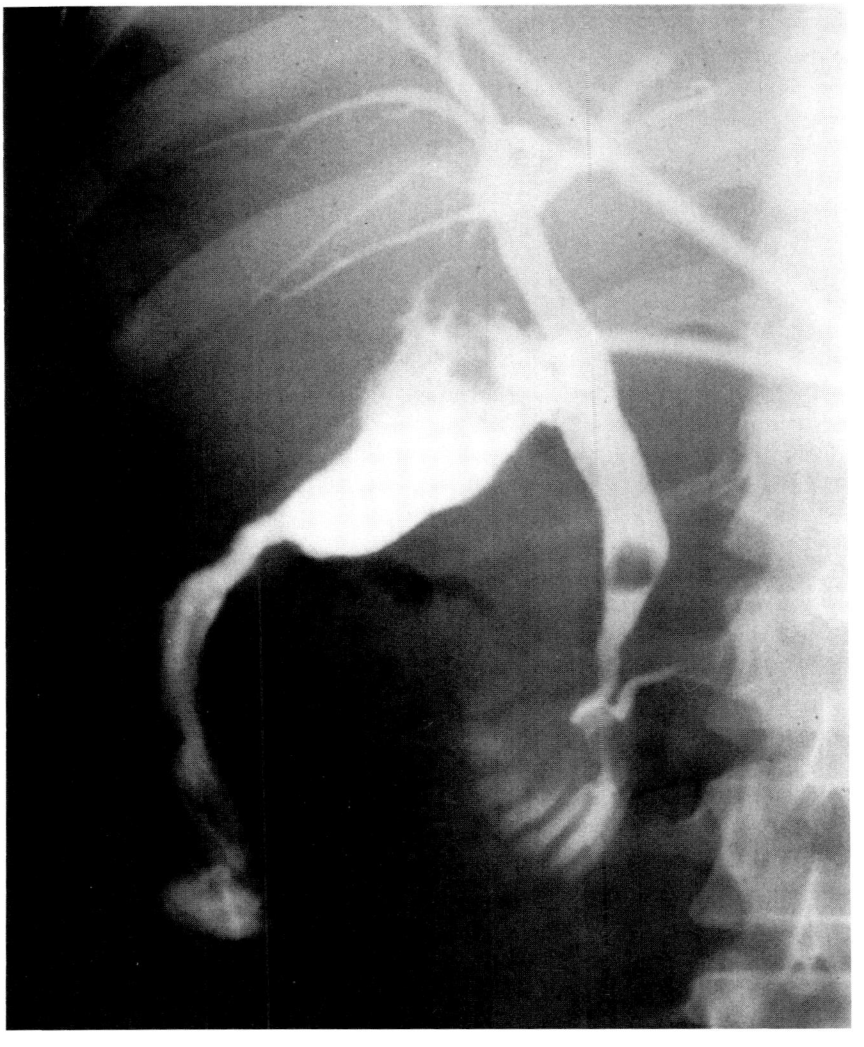

FIG. 4–4. T-tube cholangiogram illustrating spherical radiolucency in the distal common duct, with proximal dilation and minimal passage of dye into the duodenum.

BILIARY STRICTURE

Focal, non-neoplastic stenoses of the common bile duct are usually traumatic, occurring either from the localized injury of an impacted gallstone or during a difficult or complicated cholecystectomy, particularly if common bile duct exploration is performed. The site of T-tube placement is at particular risk for stricture. Post-inflammatory stenoses are extremely serious, since they are difficult to repair or reverse and almost always result in some form of continuing cholestasis. They present an immediate risk for suppurative cholangitis and, in the long term, chronic jaundice and cirrhosis. Biliary infestation by Clonorchis sinenses is a less common cause, but it should be considered in a jaundiced patient from the Far East or Southeast Asia.

The biliary stricture syndrome includes recurrent fever, altered liver-function tests, and typically faint jaundice following gallbladder surgery. An obstruction is best found via T-tube opacification, as in Figure 4–5. Typical strictures are unifocal and smoothly tapering, with some element of proximal ectasia. Their multifocal location raises the possibility of sclerosing cholangitis or, less commonly, local extension of a cholangiocarcinoma. The delicacy of the reparative surgery cannot be overemphasized. Direct repair of the stricture itself, when successful, is the most rewarding, but this generally risks restenosis following healing. Most surgeons think that the conservative approach is stricture bypass through a proximal choledochoenterostomy.

Because the majority of biliary strictures begin after operation, some can be traced to inadvertent ligation, incision, or division of the common bile duct. Complete ductal obstruction will then be followed by rapidly increasing jaundice, but rarely to a point at which the value of surgical repair has been lost. Biliary strictures should always be thought of as treatable; a passive approach will almost always result in cirrhosis or death from septicemia or multiple hepatic abscesses. Even when previous attempts at operation have been unsuccessful in experienced hands, there may be an opportunity for transhepatic stricture dilation or hepaticojejunostomy. If portal hypertension has already developed, an operation is certain to be bloody, and if anything therapeutic then is to be done for a recalcitrant stricture, portal decompression, perhaps using a distal splenorenal shunt, may be required initially.

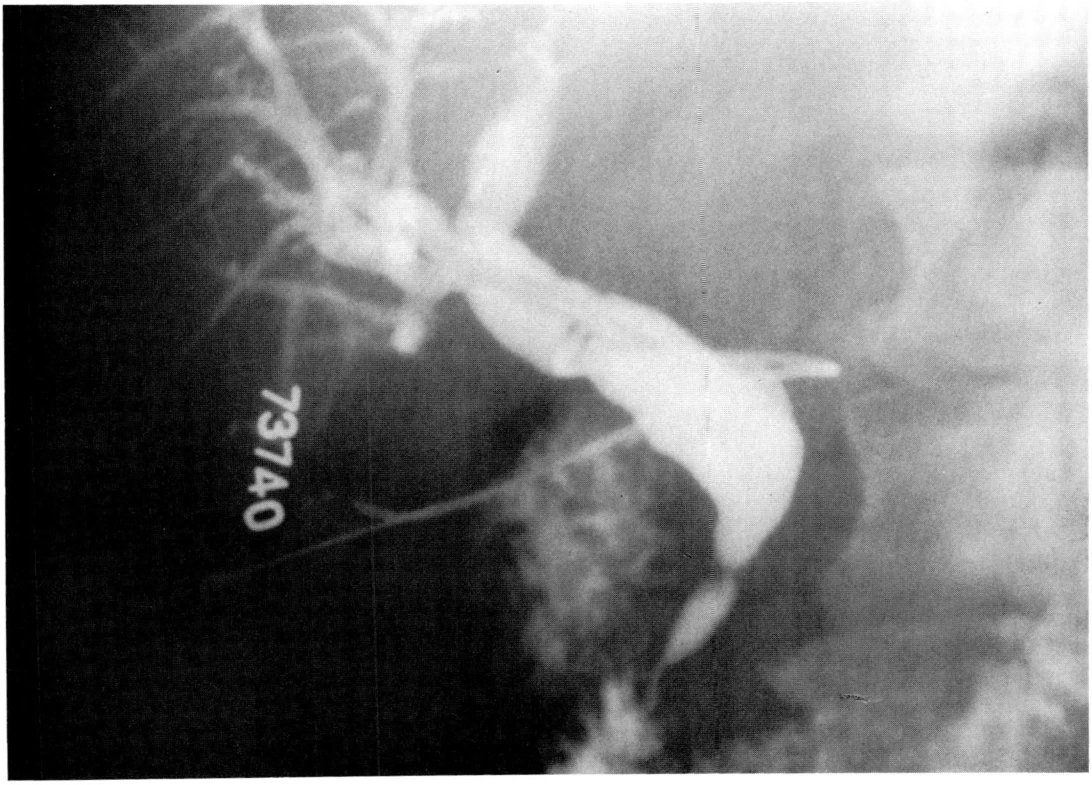

FIG. 4–5. Operative T-tube cholangiogram showing swollen intrahepatic and common bile ducts divided abruptly by a slender, radiolucent compression defect, representing old surgical injury or a scar from a previous stone or drainage tube.

ACUTE PANCREATITIS

Whether acute or chronic, pancreatitis is a curious manifestation of the body's capacity for self-destruction. Though the exact cause is unknown, the sudden release into tissue of pancreatic enzymes, ordinarily confined in cytoplasmic granules in inactive form, results in a multimechanism liquefactive digestion of the very gland that produced the once-innocuous, now responsible enzymes.

The majority of affected patients are alcoholic, and most attacks occur following binge drinking; a smaller abstemious percentage have gallbladder or common-bile-duct stones or sludge, and those remaining demonstrate a variety of ascribed etiologies, including hypertriglyceridemia, a locally penetrating ulcer, chronic renal failure, hypercalcemia, vasculitis, and metastatic or primary pancreatic cancer. The characteristic clinical feature is abdominal pain, generally central and unremitting and typically radiating posteriorly into the back, probably because of the pancreas's retroperitoneal location. As the inflamed gland begins to swell, the duodenal C-loop may widen, where, later, an inflamed pancreatic head may actually envelop the descending limb of the duodenum or obstruct the common bile duct.

In Figure 4–6A, several of these conditions are inferred: Separation of the first and third portions of the duodenum, impingement on its descending limb, and, in the midst of the pancreas, tiny speckles of calcification suggesting one or more earlier attacks. Another radiologic manifestation, poorly explained but considered characteristic of acute pancreatitis, is the so-called "colon cutoff sign": a characteristic, transverse colon air-fluid level on upright film (Fig. 4–6B) that is probably a focal ileus, reflecting involvement of the distal transverse or proximal descending colon by an adjacent inflamed pancreatic tail. Typically localized, the necrotizing inflammatory process sometimes "extends" anatomically and physiologically to life-threatening proportions.

In severe acute pancreatitis, calcifications may be seen throughout the abdomen and occasionally in bone marrow or adipose tissue as circulating activated lipases catalyze the digestion of tissue triglycerides into fatty acids, which then combine with calcium to form radiopaque "soaps." Blood and fluid loss into the peritoneum is common.

Treatment, while nonspecific, is directed first at repairing the metabolic and volume implications, particularly fluid loss, hypocalcemia, and anemia. Psychosis, adult respiratory distress syndrome, pleural effusions, tense ascites, abdominal wall or perineal hemorrhage, severe hypocalcemia, or a major fall (or rise) in hematocrit are poor prognostic signs. Gastric-acid production, which stimulates pancreatic secretion, must be decreased; therefore, nasogastric suction, H_2-receptor blockers, and antacids probably all play some modestly helpful role. Multiple-site surgical drainage of the necrotic peripancreatic detritus is occasionally lifesaving. Most pancreatitis is probably never diagnosed, but simply noted as just another somatic complaint in an incorrigible alcoholic.

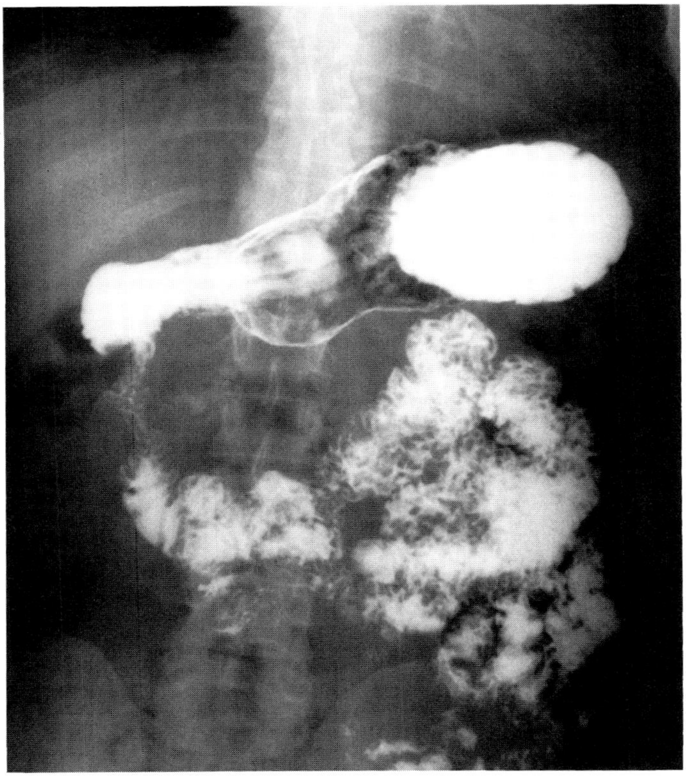

FIG. 4–6. A. Widening of the duodenal C-loop with constriction of the second (descending) portion implies pancreatic swelling. Flecks of calcification suggest previous inflammation in the pancreatic head.

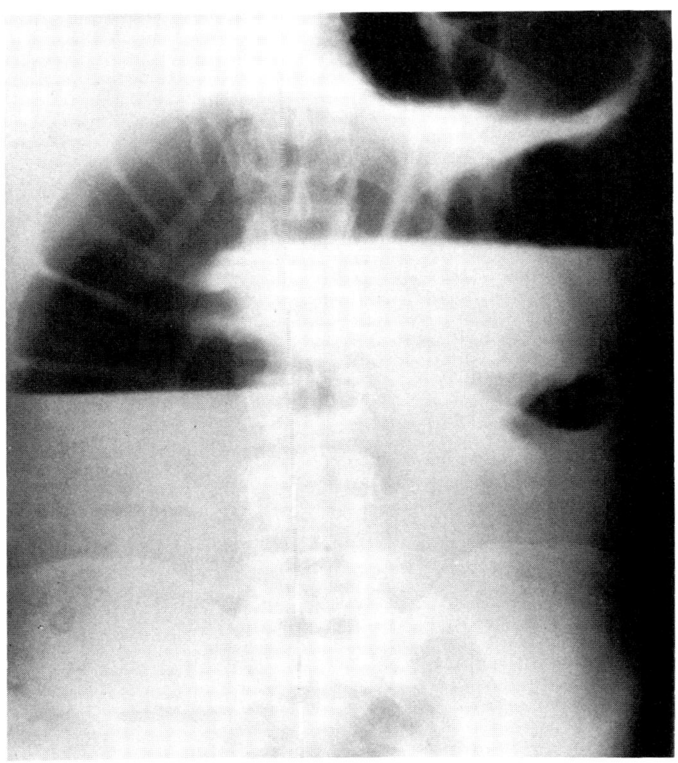

B. Colon cutoff sign. Segmental ileus with air-fluid levels in transverse and proximal descending colon, a rare but characteristic sign in acute pancreatitis.

PANCREATIC PSEUDOCYST

Reflecting the incomplete resolution of a severe acute pancreatitis, pseudocysts represent the confined, unlined collection of unresorbed necrotic, liquified adjacent fat, muscle, and pancreatic acinar and ductal tissue. Considering the digestive potency of the exocrine enzymes unleashed during inflammation, a centrifugal liquefactive result is not surprising. Their clinical significance derives from their potential for pain, dissection, mass effect, and infection. One of these features is clearly illustrated on the film opposite, where an enormous cystic pancreatic phlegmon occupies most of the left upper quadrant, essentially negating the stomach's reservoir capacity. A tiny rim of barium flows along the greater curvature; the body and lesser curvature are compressed leftward and anteriorly.

Some pseudocysts continue to expand. Because their leading edge can solubilize tissue, they may drain spontaneously by perforating into the descending colon, stomach, and rarely, small bowel. Entry into a hollow organ may produce sudden intestinal bleeding, occasionally along with diarrheal stools, which, if analyzed, will be found rich in amylase, trypsin, and lipase.

Apart from chronic pain, the commonest clinical impact of pseudoycsts is infection, even without penetration into the bowel. It should be emphasized that nearly all undrained pancreatic abscesses are fatal. Parenterally administered antibiotics will not penetrate them adequately, and fever or other signs of septicemia, developing in the course of pancreatitis, is likely to mean serious abdominal infection. CT scan of the cyst may show bubbles in an heterogeneous retroperitoneal fluid collection.

Drainage of pseudocysts can often be left to the capable interventional radiologist; the percutaneously placed drainage tube, even when placed acutely, may accomplish nearly adequate evacuation. When surgically exposed, pseudocysts are best treated by evacuation and anastomosis of an ideally mature cyst wall with jejunum or stomach. When emptied, the cyst's infection risk disappears and it usually closes, replaced by a fibrotic and calcified scar. Most pancreatic pseudocysts probably resorb spontaneously and, like episodes of acute pancreatitis, are often misdiagnosed as an alcoholic's bellyache. Unfortunately, many sufferers will continue drinking for analgesic purposes, worsening the underlying disorder.

Pseudocyst formation may occur in any form of severe pancreatitis, and though nonalcoholic causes remain a clear minority, associated gallstones, hyperlipidemia, or penetrating ulcers must be considered, particularly given their therapeutic potential. As pancreatic pseudocysts represent the undrained residue of an autopancreatectomy, they are likely to be followed by exocrine and endocrine insufficiencies which, while serious, are trivial when compared with the burden of chronic pain.

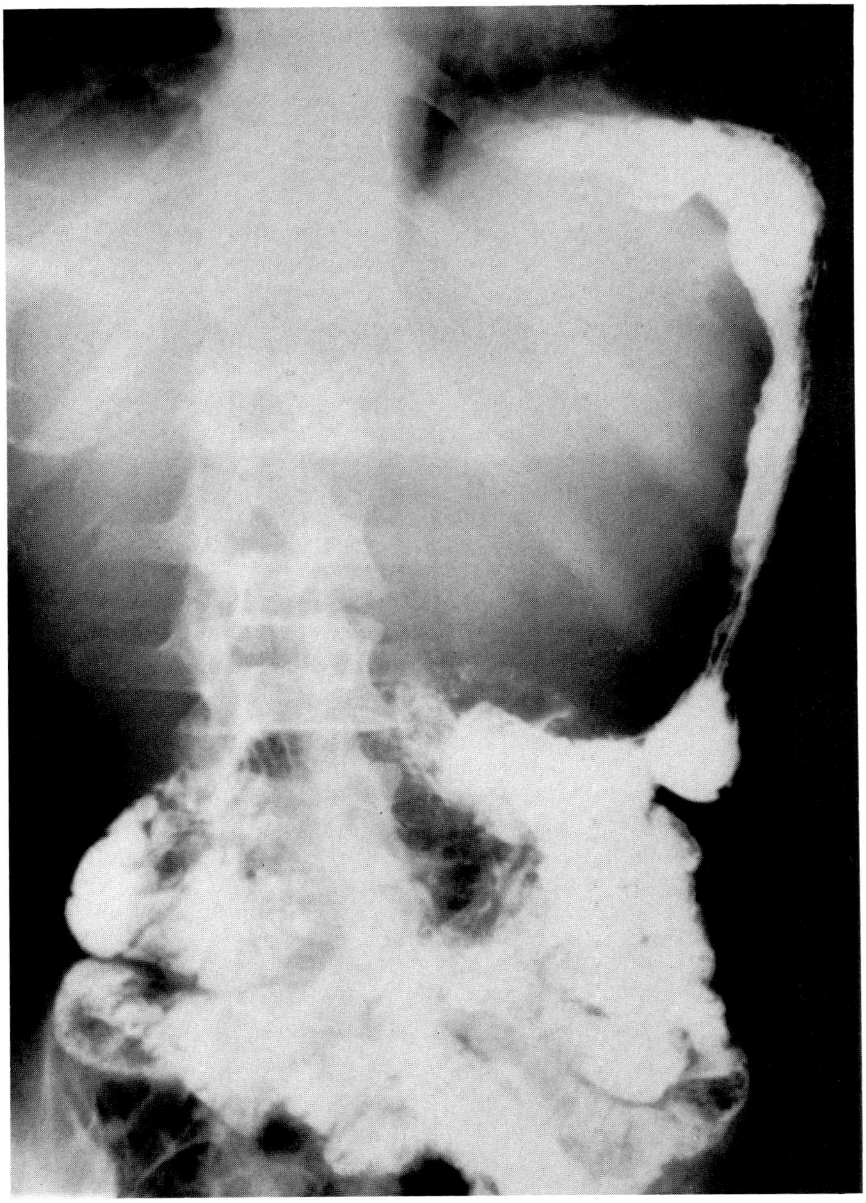

FIG. 4–7. Swallowed barium displaced down and leftward, representing extrinsic pressure on stomach by an enormous pancreatic cyst. Haziness in the upper central abdomen reflects its liquidified center. Small bowel and transverse colon also are pressed into the lower half of the abdomen.

CHRONIC (CALCIFIC) PANCREATITIS

Chronic calcific pancreatitis is the often visible reminder of earlier, usually multiple attacks of acute pancreatitis, particularly in alcoholic patients. On abdominal plain films, some radiopaque punctate-mottling is evident, typically at or around the pancreatic head or uncinate process. This mottling sometimes extends to a diffuse, almost plaster-cast outline of the gland itself (Fig. 4–8), defining head, body, and tail. Though glandular reserves are substantial, varying degrees of endocrine and exocrine insufficiency are understandably associated; these tend to be a late manifestation of calcinosis. While the diagnosis of calcific pancreatitis is extremely easy, management of pancreatic maldigestion and diabetes is more difficult, requiring pancreatic supplements (particularly lipase) in large doses, along with attempts at gastric alkalinization; the enzyme's maximum effectiveness is usually at a pH of 5 or higher.

The most perplexing therapeutic issue in these patients is chronic pain. The regular use of analgesic will almost certainly eventuate in addiction, particularly in patients with a history of substance abuse. While finding a focal cyst or stone at CT or sonogram is seductive, operative drainage or duct-stone removal is difficult, delicate, and hazardous. Most clinicians feel that when dealing with a largely nonfunctioning gland in a pain-debilitated patient, total pancreatectomy is probably best. Celiac-axis blockage is rarely successful, and spinal-cord pain surgery (rhizotomy) is difficult and risks paraparesis.

Pancreatectomy, however, makes the need for enzyme and nutrient supplements a certainty, and the diabetes of postpancreatectomy patients tends to be extremely brittle. The worst risk of surgery, apart from its mortality, is that pain may not be relieved, usually raising speculations about any residual glandular stump usually at the head. Surgeons who perform only an occasional pancreatectomy often overestimate or exaggerate the amount resected; the phrase "95% pancreatectomy" is generally employed. The preoperative problems are difficult enough, but operation, once decided upon, is probably best done as a radical procedure, as though performed for cancer of the duodenum or ampulla of Vater, including duodenectomy to ensure complete eradication of the pancreas. Unoperated chronic pancreatitis is a frequent precursor of pancreatic adenocarcinoma; partial or complete radiologic disappearance of established pancreatic calcifications may suggest this.

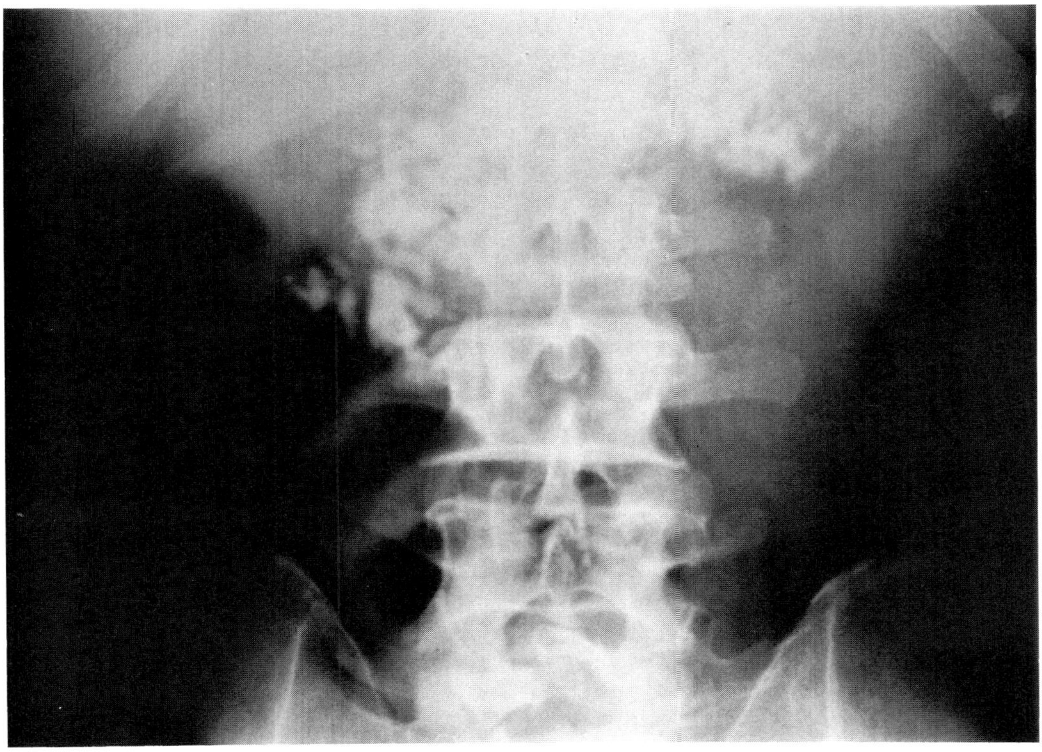

FIG. 4–8. Patchy pancreatic opacifications involving uncinate process, head, body, and tail, indicating near-total glandular destruction.

CARCINOMA OF THE HEAD OF THE PANCREAS

Most pancreatic and biliary malignancies are now diagnosed and histologically confirmed through sonography or CT-scanning guidance. Yet the first investigation of abdominal pain using barium x rays may suggest pancreatic cancer, particularly through the mass-effect widening of the C-loop, its duodenal perimeter. Beginning as subtle, centrifugal intestinal pad effects, pancreatic tumors widen by circular distortion (and entrapment), spreading the pylorus, antrum, and greater curvature of the stomach away from the transverse duodenum, seen dramatically in Figure 4–9A. Midabdominal or back pain is the presenting symptom in more than 90% of patients with pancreatic cancer, while in a smaller number, tumorous ablation of pancreatic exocrine and endocrine function causes malabsorption or diabetes first. When the common bile duct is involved, pruritus and deepening double-digit hyperbilirubinemia follow, rare in uncomplicated calculous disease.

Distal biliary obstruction can also be inferred when gallbladder enlargement is evident on an upper GI series. In Figure 4–9B, the descending portion of the duodenum is concave, pushed leftward by a faintly outlined, pear-shaped, and bile-distended gallbladder. Though this x ray will associate with sonographic or CT evidence of a huge gallbladder, pancreatic mass, or bile-duct ectasia, the film alone tells much.

Courvoisier's pertinent but imperfect axiom is that only undiseased gallbladders are capable of distention; hence, a palpable gallbladder implies pancreatic cancer, not cholecystitis or cholelithiasis. However, many patients with malignant obstructive jaundice do not have enlarged gallbladders, and a palpable gallbladder may not derive from a malignancy (e.g., obstructing cystic duct stones). Courvoisier's law amended is that a palpable gallbladder indicates only that its owner requires operation to relieve a benign or malignant blockage at the cystic, common-bile-duct, ampullary, or pancreatic levels.

Because adenocarcinoma of the pancreas is always fatal, logic argues for only palliative surgery, particularly since the radical regional pancreatectomy and Whipple procedures have a formidable operative mortality and almost no chance for cure or prolongation of life. Those rare long-term survivals wistfully recalled by some surgeons probably involved wide removal of an aggressive, obstructing pancreatitis or a less virulent duodenal or ampullary cancer.

Therefore, the surgical implications of pancreatic cancer are relief of actual (or anticipated) biliary and gastric-outlet obstruction. Despite the newer endoscopic or radiologic biliary drainage, operative cholecystoenterostomy or choledochoenterostomy diminishes jaundice best, with fewest postoperative complications. The frequency of eventual extrinsic malignant pyloric obstruction argues for simultaneous, prophylactic gastroenterostomy.

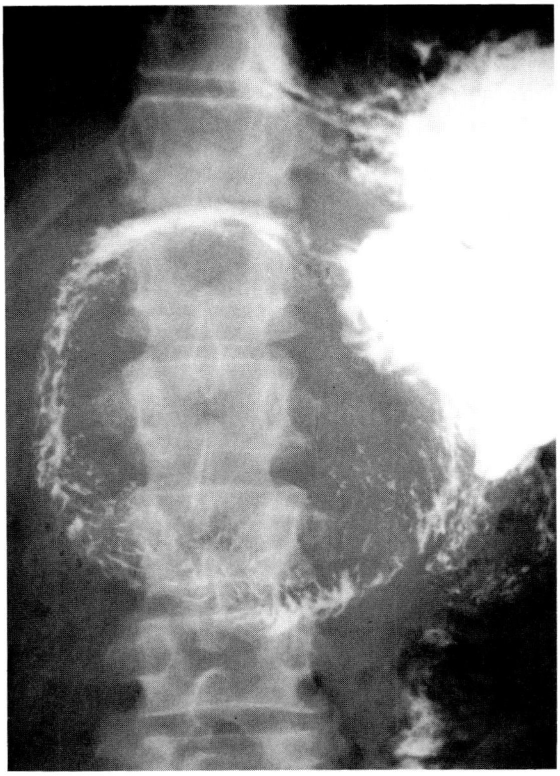

FIG. 4–9. A. Spherical stretching of the duodenum around the pancreatic head, and near-total blockade of the gastric antrum.

B. Biliary obstruction. Note leftward impression on descending limb of the duodenum, conforming to the faint outline of a distended, bile-filled, undoubtedly palpable gallbladder.

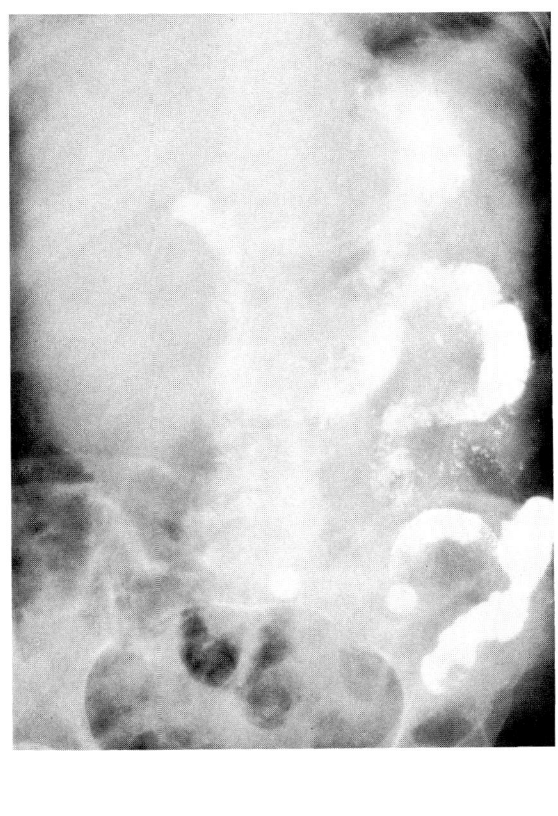

CARCINOMA OF THE BODY AND TAIL OF THE PANCREAS

As their U.S. incidences rise and fall respectively, carcinoma of the pancreas seems to be supplanting that of the stomach in frequency. When cancer begins in the midportion of the pancreas, its symptom is most often midabdominal pain, generally continuous and worsening, typically with radiation into the midback. Though pancreatic replacement by tumor rarely causes exocrine and endocrine insufficiency, this sequence deserves consideration when unexplained, chronic diarrhea or unexpected diabetes occurs in an adult with (or without) an unresolved bellyache.

Because the pancreas does not opacify with oral or rectal barium, the symptomatic tumor is often misdiagnosed as hypochondriasis, "irritable bowel," or "ulcer disease," particularly when chronic abdominal pain fails to correlate with a routine biochemical or radiologic abnormality. For conventional films to be of value, the tumors must have grown sufficiently to displace the stomach, small bowel, or colon.

In carcinoma of the *body* of the pancreas, duodenal C-loop widening (Fig. 4–10A) extends more leftward, separating the third portion from the greater curvature of the stomach. Its retrogastric location may cause indenting of the posterior wall of the filled stomach, as viewed from the side. When the lesion involves the tail of the pancreas, a small-bowel series may display a barium-free area in the left upper quadrant (Fig. 4–10B). Because much of the splenic vasculature is intrapancreatic, unexplained, painless splenomegaly may derive from tumorous thrombosis of the splenic vein.

Chronic pancreatitis and cancer can furthermore be confused; some pancreatic cancers are very desmoplastic, and a single biopsy of a malignant tumor may not yield convincing diagnostic tissue. Similarly, pancreatitis may be locally aggressive, producing obstruction of the choledochus, duodenum, transverse colon, and even encasement of the stomach. While the early diagnosis of pancreatic cancer or chronic pancreatitis may not extend a patient's life, extreme caution must be exercised in mislabeling either. As invasive radiologists routinely perform "skinny-needle" pancreatic biopsies safely under CT scan or sonographic guidance, the reluctance of some surgeons to biopsy the pancreas adequately for fear of inducing pancreatitis or a nonhealing fistula seems exaggerated. Despite pancreatic carcinoma's essential incurability, early, elective gastrojejunostomy may prevent or delay gastric-outlet obstruction from aggressive local invasion by adjacent tumor.

It should be recalled that pancreatic carcinoma is substantially more common in alcoholics, particularly those with a history of pancreatitis, and that unexplained disappearance of established pancreatic calcinosis may indicate cancerous degeneration.

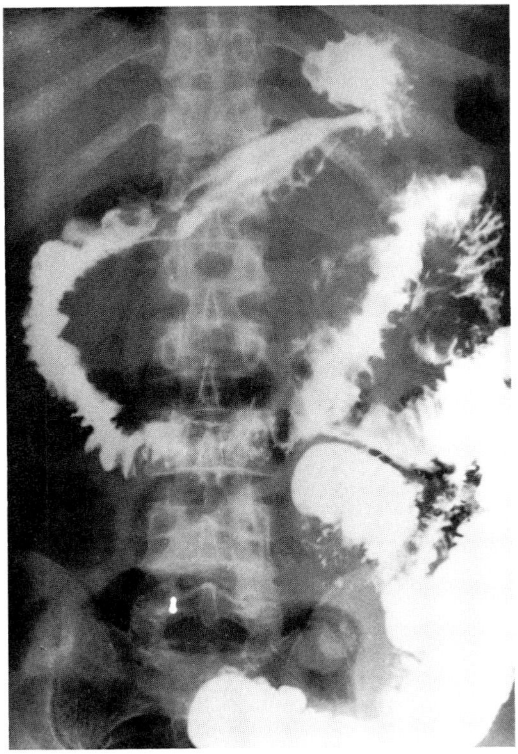

FIG. 4–10. A. Diffusely widened duodenal sweep, with serration of its mucosa and upward displacement of gastric body.

B. Left upper quadrant, barium-free area, outlining a tumor of the tail of the pancreas. There is no widening of the C-loop.

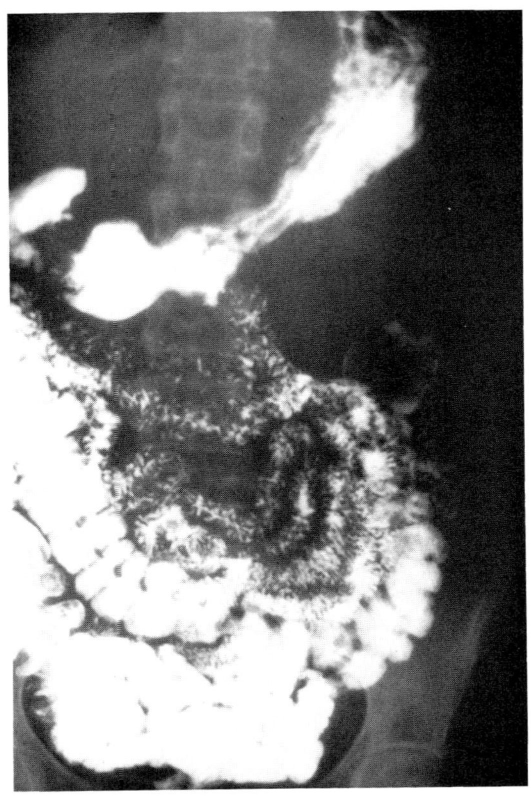

SCLEROSING CHOLANGITIS

This is usually a "secondary" disease, as approximately 80% are associated with ulcerative colitis or Crohn's disease of the colon, and fewer with inflammatory vasculitis or idiopathic retroperitoneal fibrosis. Pathogenesis aside, the disease derives from chronic inflammation in large and middle-sized bile ducts, progressing to multiple discrete high-grade fibrotic stenoses of both intrahepatic and extrahepatic channels with progressive jaundice and cirrhosis. Because the disease is multifocal, no single surgical management method is uniformly effective, although some attempt at decompressive stent placement or exteriorization of bile from a dilated lake seems logical. Apart from infrequent and incomplete responses to steroids, pharmacologic therapy is generally ineffective. When ulcerative colitis is associated with this disease, colectomy is occasionally advocated, but its effect on the cholangitis is unpredictable.

Important for the clinician are its distinctions from hepatitis, the occasionally severe pericholangitis associated with ulcerative colitis, primary biliary cirrhosis, and cholangiocarcinoma. Rarely extensive, biliary cancer tends to be unifocal, though typically seen with progressive, rarely remitting cholestasis. Hence, visualization of intrahepatic and extrahepatic ducts, though risky, is unfortunately necessary. This is accomplished by an operative cholangiogram (surgery), endoscopic retrograde cholangiopancreatography (with the danger of inducing enteric organisms into an obstructed choledochus), or percutaneous "skinny-needle" cholangiography. While safest, the latter is often least satisfactory because of the understandably high failure rate in trying to penetrate mostly narrowed, as opposed to dilated, intrahepatic ducts.

The cholangiogram of Figure 4–11 reveals a diffuse beaded stenosis whose alternatingly narrowed and dilated ducts involve the entire intrahepatic and extrahepatic biliary system, including the gallbladder. Progression to biliary cirrhosis is typical; to cholangiocarcinoma, rare. Therapies with bile-salt chelating agents or antimetabolites have their advocates. Liver biopsy distinguishes this form of cholangitis from primary biliary stenosis, in which the inflammatory process obliterates the tiniest bile ducts within portal areas and the process is strongly associated with the antimitochondrial antibody and hypergammaglobulinemia M.

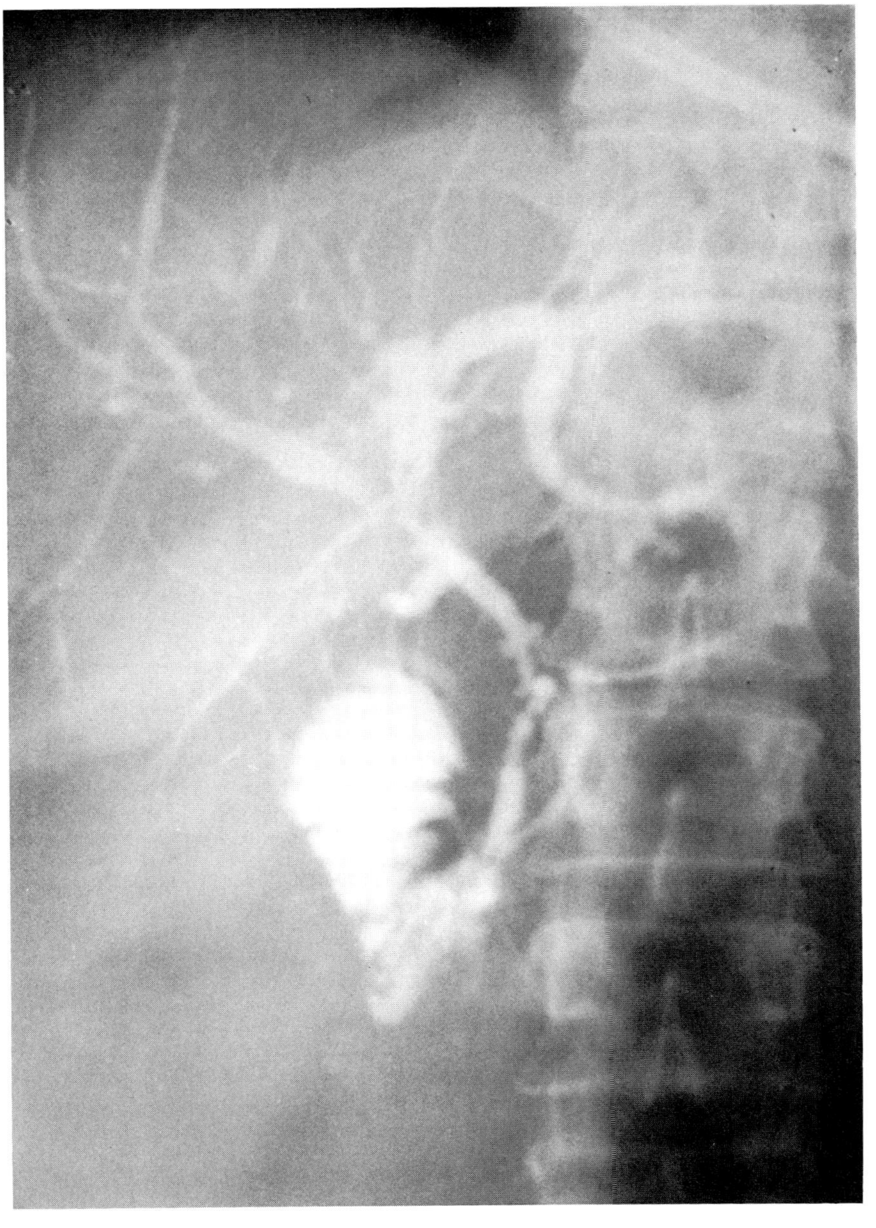

FIG. 4–11. Cholangiogram showing beaded narrowing and sacculation of common bile duct; irregular dilation of proximal intrahepatic tributaries is apparent.

CHOLEDOCHAL CYST

This focal, occasionally diffuse, sometimes congenital cystic dilation of the common bile duct is an intrinsic cause of recurrent jaundice and cholangitis. Occasionally appearing in early childhood, the choledochal cyst produces acute attacks that may seem like cholecystitis but in fact reflect inflammation only within the proximal intrahepatic channels, which may demonstrate further cystic change. Like gastric cancer, it is far more common in the Far East, perhaps induced by endemic biliary parasites such as Clonorchis sinensis.

A junction between the pancreatic and common bile duct often coexists with these cysts, suggesting that choledochal reflux of pancreatic juice may be playing a pathogenic role, though some element of congenital thinning or weakness almost certainly must be present, as well. Sonography provides the best clue to diagnosis of the cyst, which may contain multiple calculi. Endoscopic retrograde cholangiography can also identify the lesion but carries an infectious hazard, as introduction of dye via duodenum will always transfer intestinal bacteria into this largely stagnant bile lake.

Whether choledochal cysts are the cause or the result of recurrent attacks of obstructive jaundice does not alter their obligation for surgical excision, leaving only a cuff of cyst anastomosed to an opened loop of small intestine. Excision and drainage should probably always be accompanied by a cholecystectomy.

Figure 4–12 discloses an enormous, saccular, stone-free cyst, which was dye-filled at an operation preceded by recurrent attacks of fever and jaundice in a patient whose gallbladder opacified normally on oral cholecystogram.

Advocates of total cyst excision and biliary-tract reconstruction point to the low but ineradicable incidence of carcinoma in choledochal-cyst remnants, as well as to the need for reoperation for stenosis after simple cystenterostomy. In truth, exact procedural decisions are almost never arrived at preoperatively; the precise anatomy and surgeon's capabilities or enthusiasm can be resolved only with the abdomen opened. Congenital cysts occasionally rupture spontaneously and, when present in the young, are usually associated with an epigastric or right upper quadrant mass. When the cyst involves the duodenal wall, recurrent pancreatitis is an understandable consequence.

Dilatation of only the intrahepatic bile ducts is another disorder, occasionally associated with progressive hepatic fibrosis (Caroli's disease).

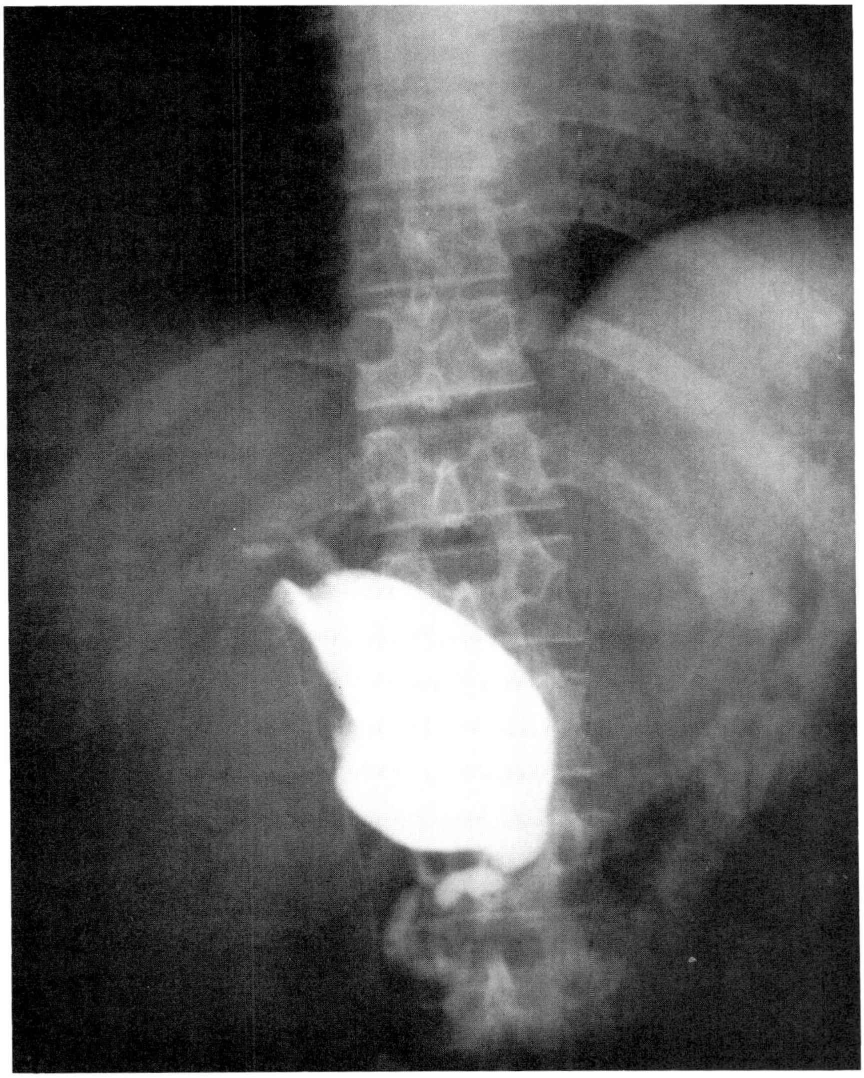

FIG. 4–12. Operative cholangiogram showing ovoid dye collection adjacent to and emanating from common bile duct.

CHOLANGIOCARCINOMA

Biliary epithelium rarely undergoes carcinomatous degeneration. But a syndrome deriving from tumor located at the critical junction of the right and left hepatic ducts deserves mention. It includes progressive obstructive jaundice without evidence of any of its more typical causes, such as biliary stricture, the common-bile-duct stone, pancreatic tumor, aggressive pancreatitis, or carcinoma of the ampulla of Vater. At exploration, biliary dilators drop easily from the common duct into the duodenum. The explanation for this "negative" exploration is that the lesion, though obstructive, was largely intrahepatic. The diagnosis can be made with cholangiography, best done by the percutaneous, transhepatic route. The classic tumor is identified in Figure 4–13, showing a smooth, diffuse stenosis of the major distal ducts of the intrahepatic lobes. Pre-existing ulcerative colitis with pericholangitis may predispose the patient to cholangiocarcinoma, including tumors of the gallbladder; certainly this is true with antecedent sclerosing cholangitis.

When the gallbladder does not opacify on x ray, films should be searched first for evidence that dye has been ingested; tablets taken as directed the night before x ray are typically seen in the right lower quadrant the following morning. Nonopacification may result from dye retained in an obstructed stomach, the tablets having been vomited, severe diarrhea, disturbed liver function, or a diseased gallbladder's failure to concentrate.

Most patients with primary gallbladder cancer are jaundiced at the time of presentation; the initially asymptomatic tumor generally progresses upward by local extension into the common bile and hepatic ducts. Accordingly, cholecystography is rarely employable in the setting of gallbladder carcinoma. Some carcinomas of the gallbladder are said to associate with pre-existing gallstones; this is debatable and none usually are evident at surgery. The gallbladder-cancer-prevention argument for cholecystectomy in asymptomatic patients with gallstones seems statistically insupportable.

One benign radiolucency seen with oral cholecystography is a mucosal polyp. Such polyps consist of well-differentiated glandular tissue and are devoid of malignant potential; when seen with "biliary" symptoms, mucosal polyps are probably not their cause. They are nearly always benign, and adherent to the wall from which they arise. In contrast with most calculi, polyps will not shift with changes in the patient's position.

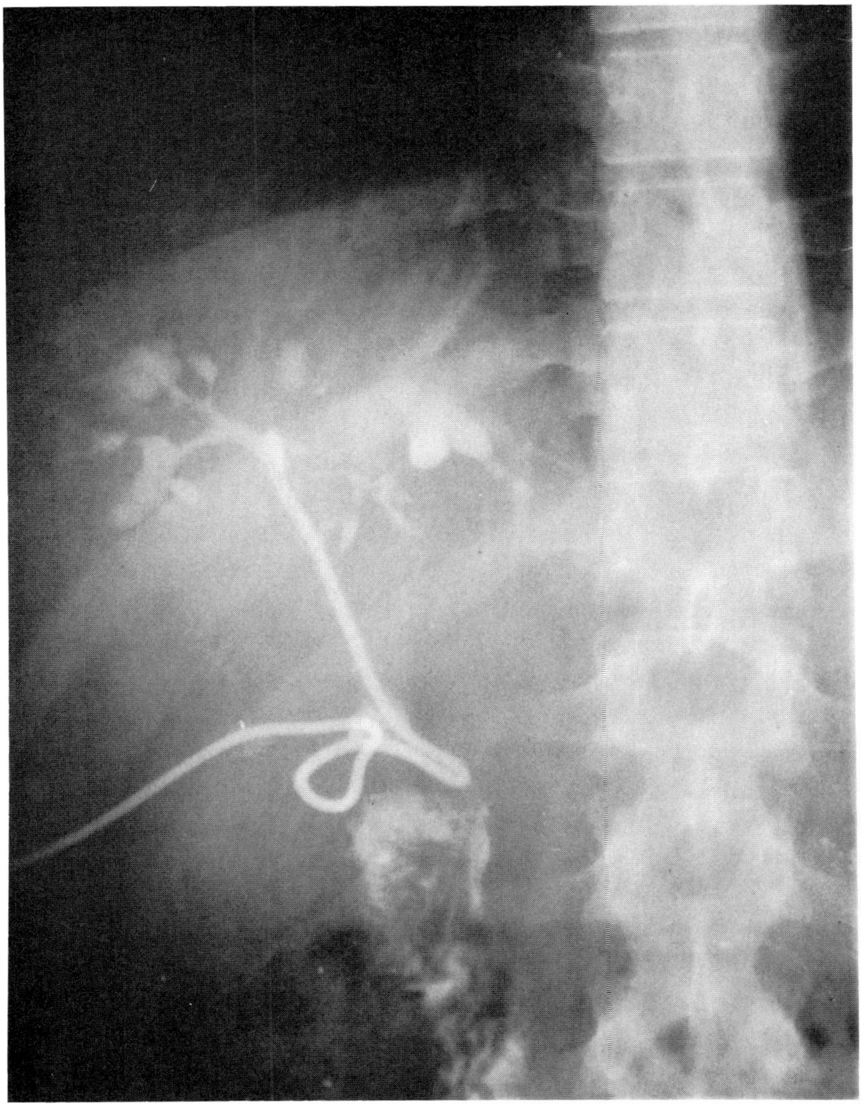

FIG. 4–13. Operative cholangiogram showing smooth extensive constriction of right and left hepatic ducts with proximal dilation into bile lakes, implying a largely inoperable cholangiocarcinoma.

ADENOMYOSIS

Taken after a fatty meal, Figure 4–14 demonstrates a persistent, variably prominent, horizontal radiolucent web of hyperplastic mucosa and musculature of the lower third of an hourglass-shaped, dye-filled gallbladder. Distinguished from the less-prominent "Phrygian cap"of a sharply angulated gallbladder and not diagnosable by sonography or CT scanning, adenomyosis is a form of acalculous cholecystitis, becoming symptomatic (postprandial, right upper quadrant pain) when this clamp-like septum occludes the lower segment of a contracting gallbladder from the rest of the biliary system. The tiny flecks of dye around the teardrop-shaped inferior portion are Rokitansky-Aschoff sinuses. Cholecystectomy is curative.

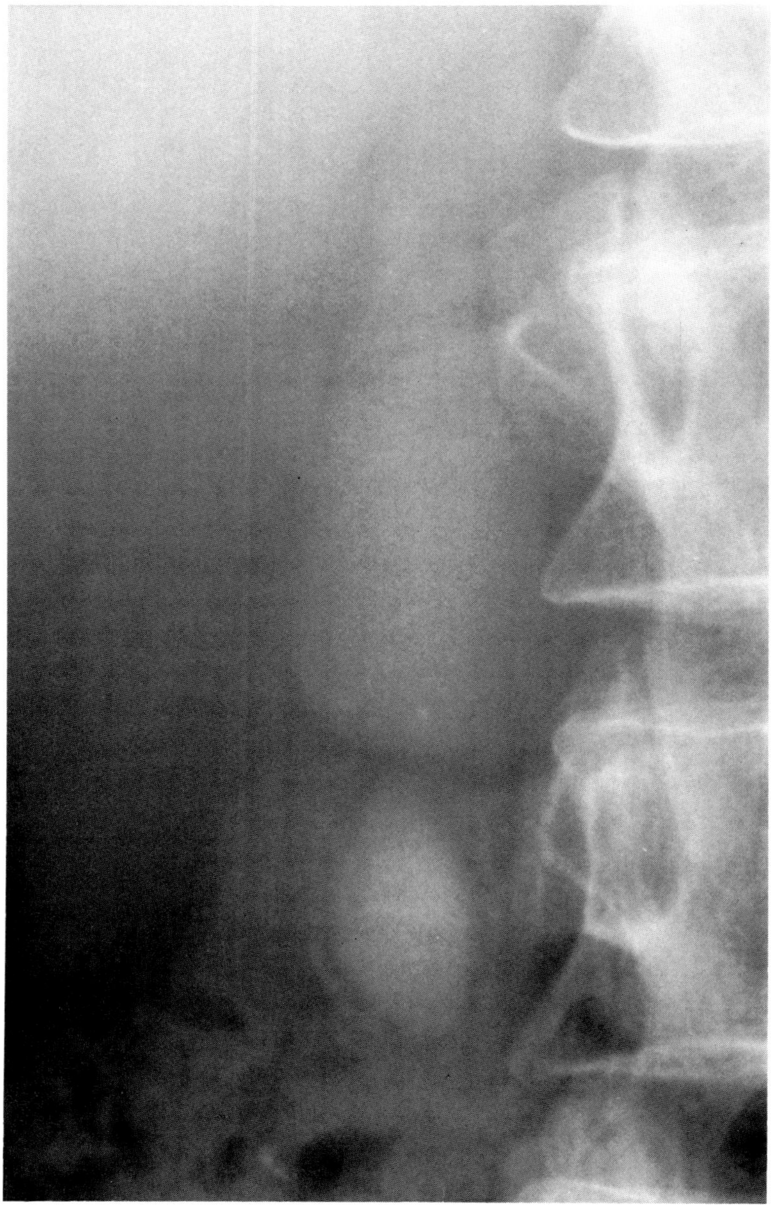

FIG. 4–14. Cholecystographic dye fills the gallbladder, lobulated by a horizontal radiolucent ellipse of adenomyosis. The narrowed lower portion is surrounded by intramural collections of dye (Rokitansky-Aschoff sinuses) in a thickened wall.

ROKITANSKY-ASCHOFF SINUSES

More microsopic than radiologic, these mucosal and submucosal ulcerations of the lower gallbladder wall (Fig. 4–14) are indicative of cholecystitis. They are small and difficult to see, particularly since the gallbladders they inhabit concentrate dye poorly. One of the rarer cholecystographic signs mandating surgery (or at least a diagnosis of an inflamed gallbladder), they are to be distinguished from cholesterolosis ("strawberry gallbladder"), a benign, noninflammatory deposition of cholesterol along the normally functioning gallbladder mucosa (Fig. 4–15). Because of difficulty in distinguishing cholesterolosis from cholecystitis or gallbladder cancer in a nonjaundiced patient, cholecystectomy is sometimes reasonable.

A small, irregularly outlined gallbladder (microgallbladder) suggests progressive circumferential encroachment into the gallbladder bed from a tumor-filled liver or the occasional small, intrahepatic gallbladder.

EXTERNAL BILIARY FISTULA

Opaque material in any lower quadrant seen draining from an intrahepatic radicle of an obviously enlarged liver argues for a traumatic fistula. Painful and dangerous, bile peritonitis must be treated quickly by laparotomy and decompression drainage. Contrasted with illnesses or operations in which bile is diverted into the stomach or small intestine, intraperitoneal biliary fistulae are almost always iatrogenic, resulting from complicated surgery or from a percutaneous liver biopsy done in the presence of an extrahepatic biliary obstruction. While the frequency of this disease has decreased from early identification of dilated biliary radicles by sonography and CT scanning, the popularity of percutaneous or transendoscopic biliary stents will probably prompt the disease's resurgence.

Parasitic cysts rarely, if ever, rupture spontaneously; however, single or multiple bile-containing nonparasitic cysts can hemorrhage internally. Spontaneous *hemo*peritoneum occurs in 20% of patients with hepatoma.

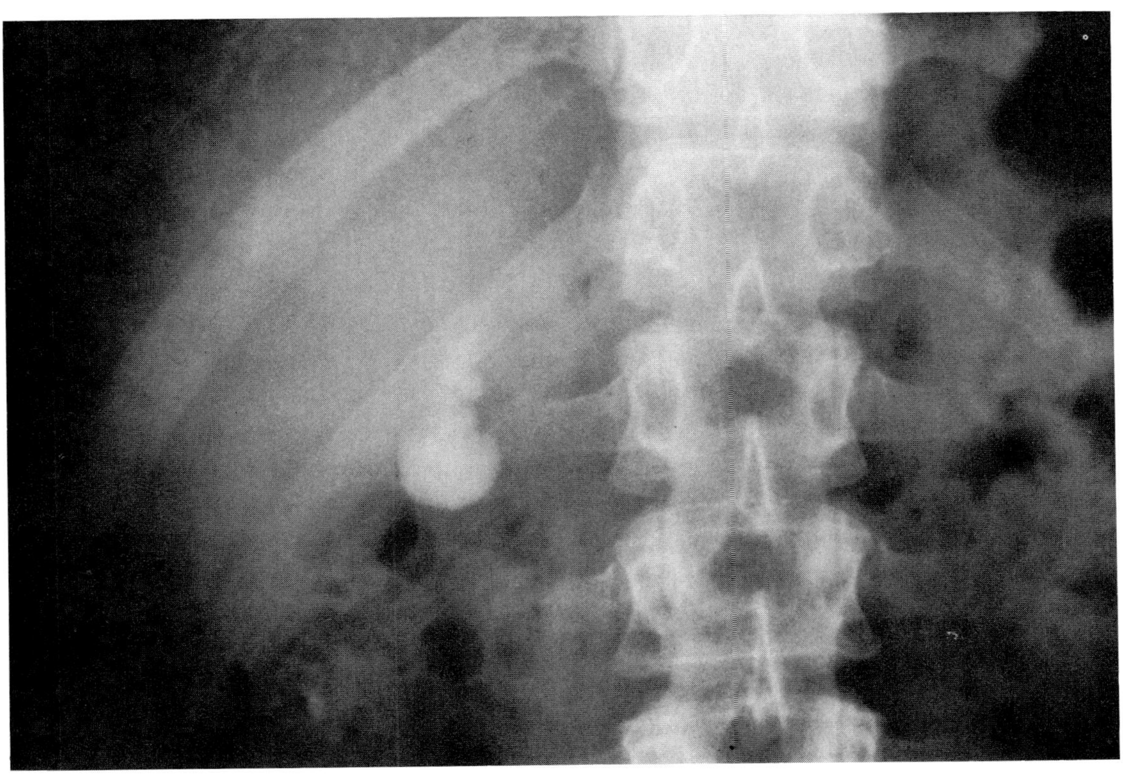

FIG. 4–15. Cholesterolosis. Diffuse irregularity in the wall of a gallbladder, with normal concentrating function.

VARIOUS ABDOMINAL CALCIFICATIONS

In both the acute and chronic clinical settings, plain abdominal films may disclose unexplained though important opacities, reflecting a variety of problems of medical and surgical implications. The commonest, of course, are single or multiple gallstones, generally seen where expected, within the gallbladder itself. Rarely varying in shape or mobility, they may remain unchanged for years. Attitudes about asymptomatic stones vary from decade to decade, with surgery historically advocated for the young diabetic with multiple small stones.

Also in the right upper quadrant, a large, often spherical, but occasionally pear-shaped opacity reflects smooth calcification of the entire gallbladder wall, the "porcelain gallbladder" (Fig. 4–16A). Like Rokitansky-Aschoff sinuses, this condition indicates chronic though presumably inactive cholecystitis. Its removal for cancer prophylaxis may have a statistically supportable rationale, as more than a few reports exist of gallbladder malignancy supervening in these patients.

Calcifications within the liver may include aneurysms, metastases, and parasitic cysts, most notably Echinococcal, which are generally large and irregular (Fig. 4–16B), appearing in patients of Levantine extraction with protracted exposure to sheep and dogs, the parasite's intermediate hosts. Occasionally visible in the spleen, brain, or lung, the cyst's clinical or serologic diagnosis is not usually difficult. However, the need for resection or drainage of expanding cysts in the liver is unpredictable and occasionally critical, given their penchant for intraperitoneal rupture. Cysts of the adrenal gland and mesentery may calcify in either upper quadrant. The multiple particulate calcifications of splenic histoplasmosis (Fig. 4–16C) are common. Splenic artery calcifications are more medial and often of a corkscrew or tubular configuration. If the calcifications are saccular, an aneurysm is inferred, and as they are fragile, they probably should be resected when identified.

Noncalcific masses in any quadrant are suggested by their displacement of organs from their area of enlargement. Chronic massive splenomegaly argues for myeloproliferative or lymphoproliferative disease or, when acute, for traumatic or spontaneous rupture of the spleen (Fig. 4–16D). Calcifications within the abdominal aorta, pancreas, ovary, renal pelvis, and parenchyma are self evident.

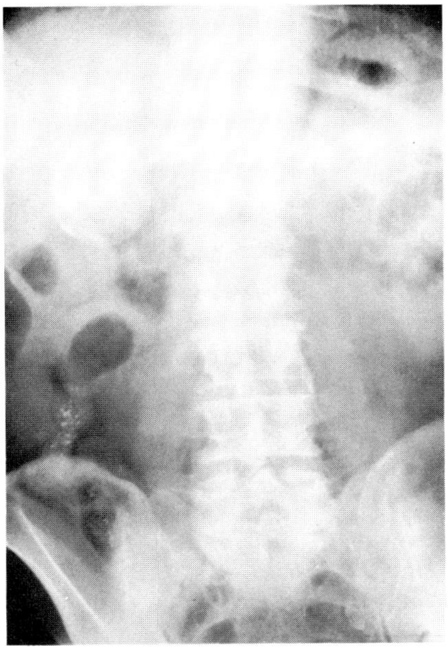

A

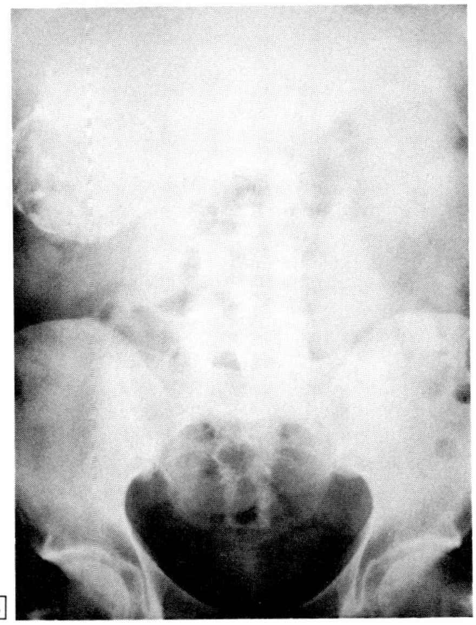

B

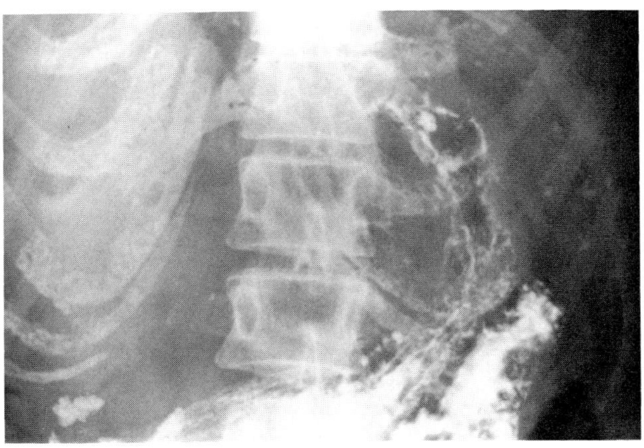

C

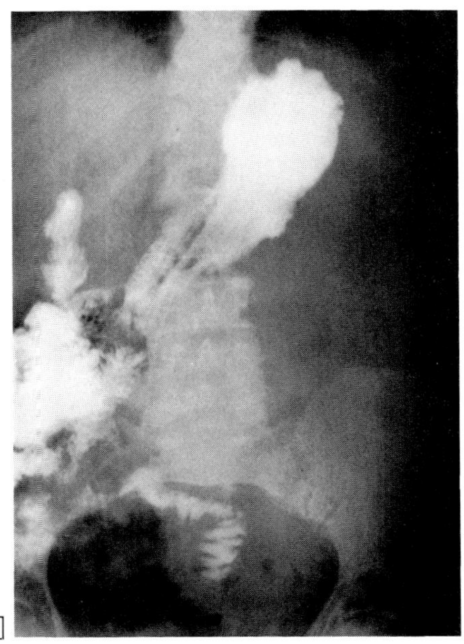

D

FIG. 4–16. A. A smooth, sharply demarcated, rounded calcification outlining the perimeter of a universally calcified gallbladder. No cholecystographic dye has been administered, and no calcifications are noted elsewhere.
B. The second calcification is more extensive, with indistinct superior edges and a shaggy, mottled outline, classic for an echinococcal cyst.
C. Late film following completion of upper GI series showing mottled calcification in left upper quadrant, representing healed, inactive splenic histoplasmosis. The costochondral cartilages are also calcified, an unrelated finding.
D. Massive splenomegaly on upper GI series in a patient with left upper quadrant mass developing following an auto injury. Displacement of the stomach medially suggests splenomegaly, in this case, an enormous subcapsular hematoma.

CHAPTER 5

THE COLON

ACUTE ULCERATIVE COLITIS

Ulcerative colitis rarely ulcerates, per se; indeed, it is a more typically infiltrative, diffusely necrotizing process, while isolated, discrete, punched-out ulcerations are more common to the Crohn's variant. Though it is emphasized repeatedly that the patient acutely ill with rectal bleeding and diarrhea should be spared the preparation for and instillation of a barium enema, we are sometimes fooled. The symptoms of even severe colitis may be deceptively less dramatic than the extent of disease disclosed on x-ray examination. An instance in which the x ray does hold unhappy surprises is the bowel loop seen in Figure 5–1. In this closeup of the splenic flexure, the penetrating nature of the severest inflammatory process is apparent. The barium appears to filter out of the lumen, intertwining through a lacy bowel wall rendered porous or spongy. Any mucosal barrier to the flow of contrast from the luminal side to the still-intact serosa seems to be lacking.

Obstinate reliance on medical therapy in the face of this degree of colon injury risks catastrophe. The absence of haustrations and the tubular quality of the colon outline suggest chronic disease, but this degree of mural necrosis is not uncommonly seen in first attacks of acute ulcerative colitis.

Concurrent, sometimes polymicrobial portal and systemic bacteremia should be anticipated, and patients so obviously ill should be managed with multiple parenteral antibiotics in generous doses, which may reduce the risk of septic shock and eventual peripheral (usually liver) abscess formation. The immediate distinction between Crohn's disease and ulcerative colitis is unimportant, but determining whether or not the colonic inflammatory process is infectious (i.e., medically curable) is vital.

Though a steroid's prejudicial effect on healing is well known, a brief, intensive course of corticosteroid management is usually rational. But if agreed upon, it must be combined with repetitive, scrupulous bedside examinations. Severe acute colon damage predisposes a patient to toxic megacolon, so regular x rays of chest and abdomen are needed, also to assess for the presence of intraperitoneal air. Failure of this degree of colitis to respond to medical therapy in 48 hours mandates surgery. Once made, a decision for colectomy does not eliminate the risk of death. Ulcerated to this extent, colonic tissue will often tear intraoperatively with the slightest manipulations. A live patient remains the pre-eminent goal.

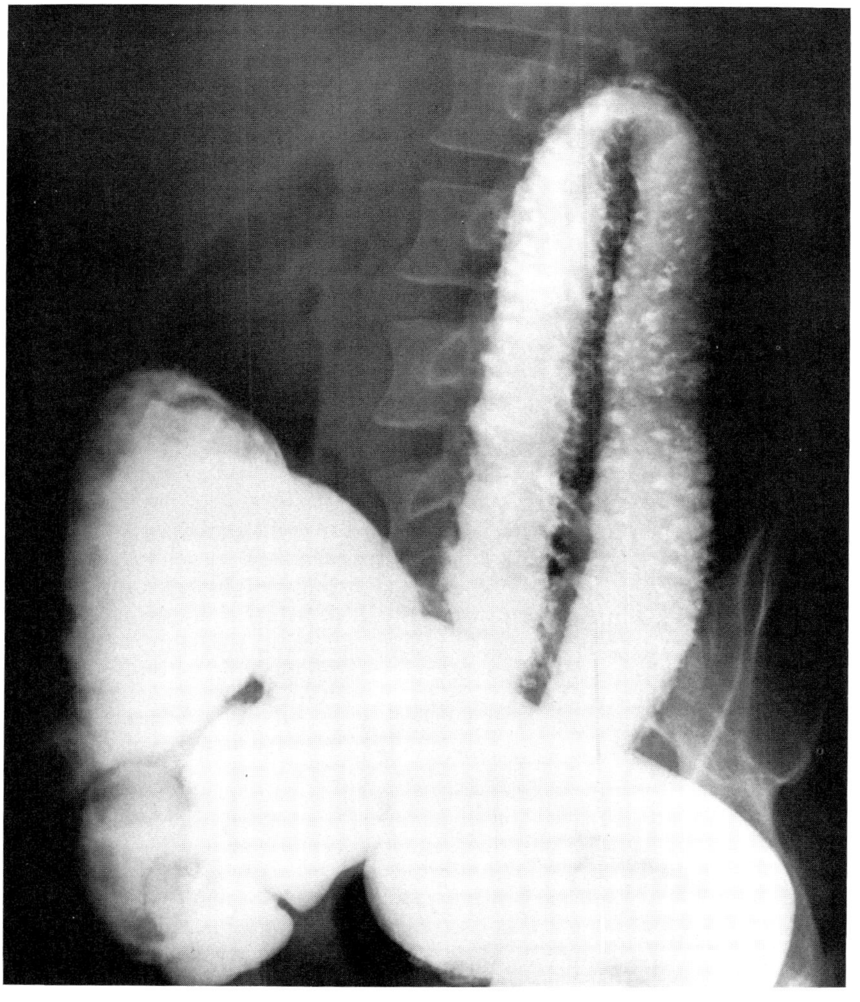

FIG. 5–1. Multiple intramural ulcerations noted in splenic flexure with parallel submucosal tracking in the descending colon.

TOXIC MEGACOLON

A nightmarish manifestation of fulminating inflammatory bowel disease, particularly ulcerative colitis, toxic megacolon must be dreaded as a life-threatening, segmental paralysis of a bowel about to perforate. This condition is associated with deep and generally diffuse mucosal necrosis; although some patients may continue to defecate, the colon is apparently so damaged that it ceases effective emptying, and it will distend to the point of rupture. Plain films of chest and abdomen show a gas-filled, often nonhaustral segment of widely dilated transverse colon across the upper abdomen (Fig. 5–2), with deep ulcerations occasionally visible on mesenteric and antimesenteric borders of the dilated loop. Sometimes precipitated by excessive use of antimotility agents, a premature barium enema or its preparation, or hypokalemia, the condition can also develop in severe amebic dysentery, Shigellosis, or Crohn's disease. Megacolon should be considered whenever an unstable colitis patient develops distention, signs of peritoneal irritation, or a sudden rise in temperature or white count, or when bowel sounds decrease. Of almost equal importance is megacolon's distinction from a more benign ileus or a "sentinel loop" of any origin, such as pancreatitis, ischemic colitis, or fecal impaction.

Because of the risk of colon necrosis, immediate surgery should be considered unless a reversible, precipitating factor is identified, the patient can be examined hourly, effectiveness of therapy is assessed, and a surgical consultant is alerted. Standby medical treatment should include antibiotics in rational multiples; suction by long tube; high-dose corticosteroids; blood, protein, and electrolyte replenishment; the withholding of antimotility agents; and ordering enough followup chest and abdominal films to make an x-ray technician feel abused.

Some advocate immediate decompressive surgery by temporary tube cecostomy and ileostomy until the patient is stable; others prefer a one- or two-stage proctocolectomy. The possibility that the colon may tear when manipulated should be made clear to the surgeon, who, wishing to avoid the horrendous prospect of peritoneal contamination, might well wrap the colon in a moistened towel while removing it. The risk of inducing toxic megacolon is a major reason to defer barium enemas in the patient acutely ill with fever, diarrhea, and rectal bleeding.

Recalling that toxic megacolon could be precipitated by a *second* bowel disease in a previously stable patient, a wise clinician will consider (and perhaps treat empirically for) a superimposed amebic or pseudomembraneous colitis.

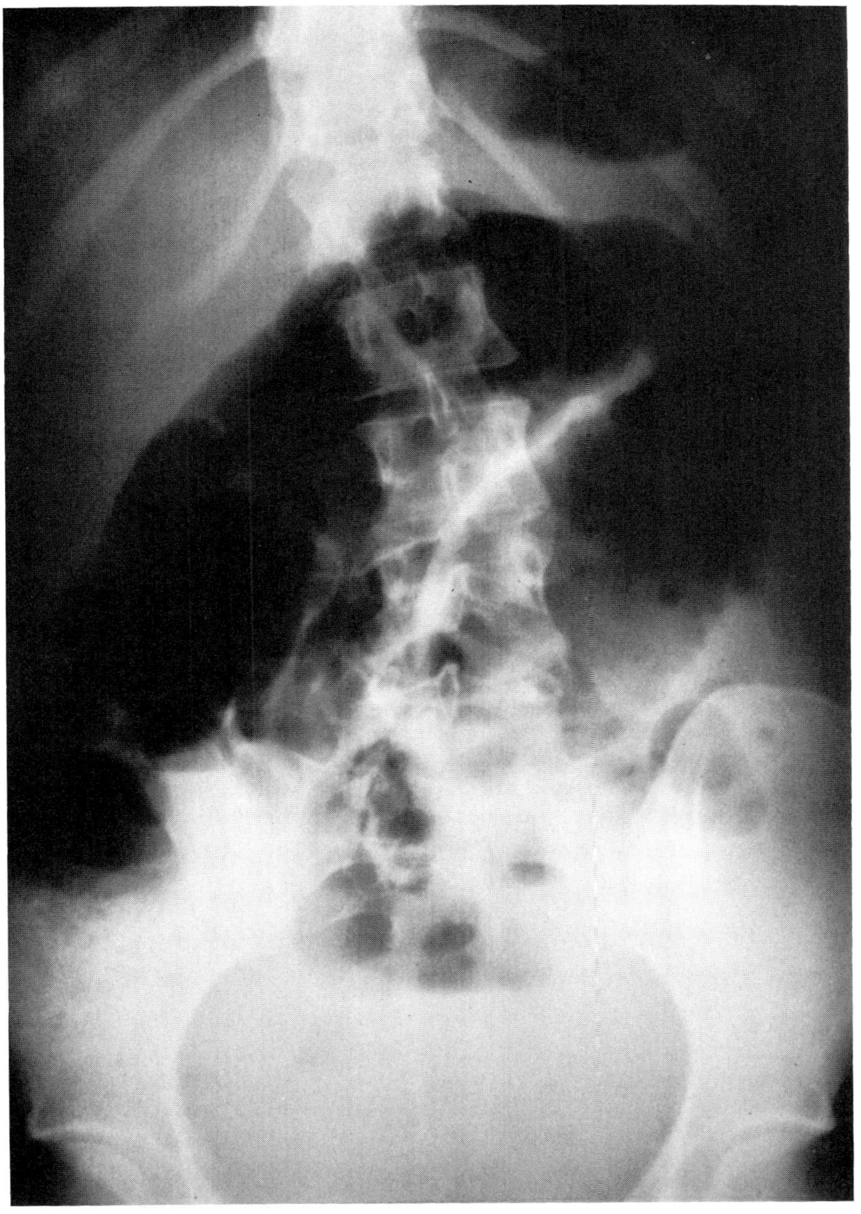

FIG. 5–2. Widely dilated, preperforative transverse colon, demonstrating irregular, nonhaustral, ulcerated mucosa.

CHRONIC ULCERATIVE COLITIS

Several more classic features of chronic ulcerative colitis are well represented by Figure 5–3, and their clinical implications are easily inferable. The initial distal colonic locus of illness and its subsequent retrograde progression are evident in Figure 5–3A, a film of a 16-year-old male who had been growth-retarded from 10 years of chronic illness or its steroid therapy. The last two thirds of the colon are cylindrical and featureless, appearing much like a garden hose, while haustrations and ability for dilation seem preserved in the ascending colon. Circumferential stenosis typically follows chronic inflammation anywhere in the alimentary tract through infiltration of fibrous tissue leading to fixation with luminal narrowing. This frequent colonic "cylindrization" (Fig. 5–3B and C) has understandable clinical implications: a severely reduced storage capacity in which muscular contractions anywhere in the bowel transmit quickly to a contracted rectum, producing an irresistible defecation reflex.

The life-altering curses of urgency and tenesmus are serious enough in adults but tragic in this teenager with a refractory stool frequency of 20 to 30 movements per day. The added feature of fecal incontinence is unbearable. Protocolectomy and conventional ileostomy was followed by an understandable growth spurt, and the patient's happy disappearance from the physician's roll of regular visitors.

In the patient with established chronic illness, the conventional anti-inflammatory therapies are usually incompletely successful. While the traditional criteria for operation (hemorrhage, perforation risk, malignant degeneration) may not be satisfied, the burden of chronic illness to the patient may be overwhelming. All too often, the physician, not the patient, needs convincing of the benefits of surgery.

Contending with an ileostomy is not entirely blissful, but is usually preferred to battling with chronic ulcerative colitis of the kind seen here. Postoperative patients may be an increased risk for bowel obstruction and nephrolithiasis, but the hope of being restored to a nearly normal life, freed of their medication requirements and the colonic cancer risk, can also be irresistible.

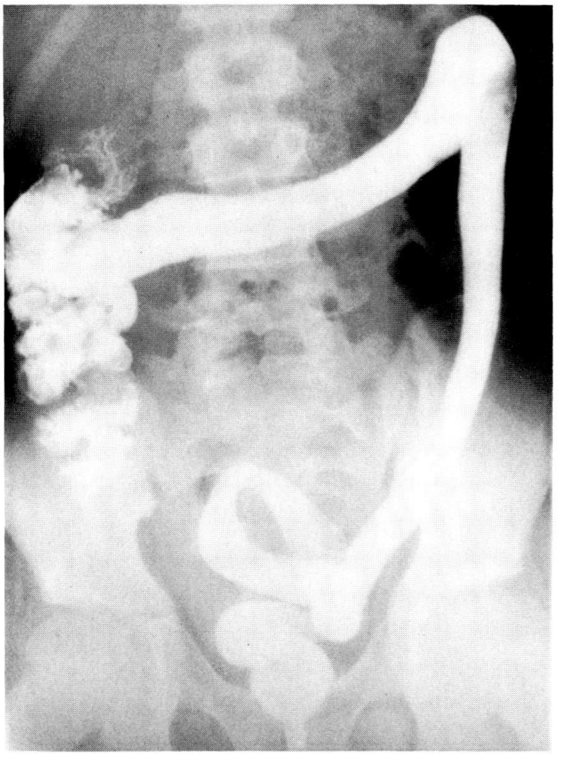

A

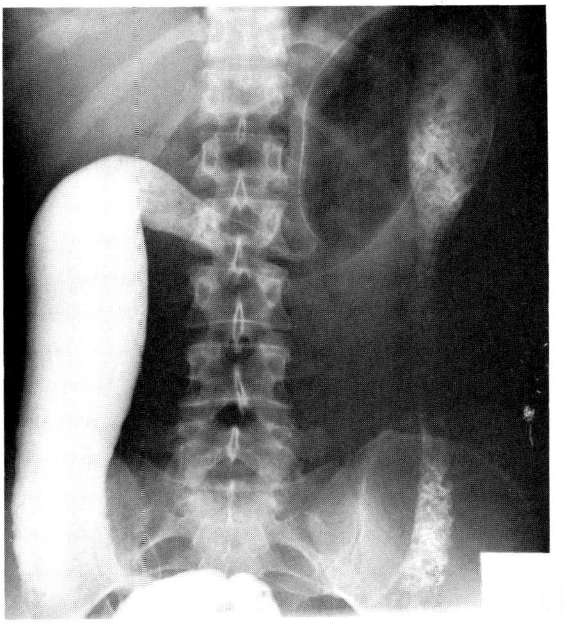

B

FIG. 5–3. A. Fixation of distal two thirds of colon; corresponding loss of reservoir capacity is inferable.
B. Smooth loss of haustrations noted through entire large intestine with stricture in the midtransverse colon.
C. Pseudopolyps are seen easily in air-contrast views of rectum and sigmoid. Haustrations are lost from most of the colon.

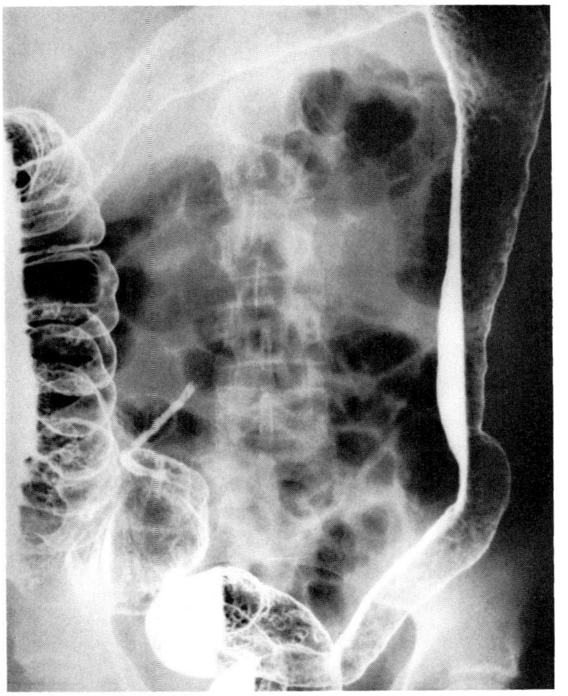

C

CHRONIC ULCERATIVE COLITIS AND CANCER

Ulcerative colitis is well established as a premalignant disease; colon carcinogenesis occurs most predictably in those affected by long duration of illness and large extent of colon involvement, also in patients whose illness developed prepubertally. Thus, the patient most likely to develop colon cancer has experienced more than 20 years of a colitis that commenced in childhood and involves the entire large intestine. Conversely, the most cancer-resistant colitis develops later in life, is of brief duration, and is limited to the rectum. The high mortality of colon cancer complicating colitis may relate to the biologic behavior of these tumors or to their penchant for simultaneous, multifocal development; or it may be due to the fact that the usual clinical signs of cancer, such as rectal bleeding or changed bowel habits, are mistaken both by physician and patient for exacerbations of the colitis, thus delaying appropriate investigations. Superficial and plaque-like when early, the tumors may be difficult to diagnose radiologically, particularly when occurring in mucosa already deformed by chronic disease. Varying tumor-like complications of inflammatory bowel disease may occur simultaneously, such as benign and malignant strictures, true and "pseudo" polyps, as mentioned, and multiple carcinomas.

In Figure 5–4, symmetric narrowing of the rectum commanded first clinical attention; this narrowing was benign on biopsy, and its smooth tapering supports that finding. However, careful further inspection of the film reveals an additional irregular mass lesion, a classic adenocarcinoma, in the proximal descending colon.

Colonoscopy would be of no value here, because the instrument could not pass the stenotic rectum. An understandable clinical quandary arises when the clinician is unable to satisfactorily resolve the real nature of a colon stricture. Benign lesions may be irregular, cancers may be "smooth," and colonoscopes and their biopsy forceps may be unable to pass into or through a high-grade narrowing.

However, regular colonoscopy has its proponents as a mode of early cancer diagnosis in chronic inflammatory bowel disease. Furthermore, the finding of dysplastic, microscopic changes in proctoscopic biopsies of nontumorous rectum is felt by some to raise both the suspicion of a silent proximal cancer and the tempting possibility of earlier, easier presymptomatic diagnosis. The predilection for distal-bowel cancers (rectum and sigmoid) in the general population does not seem to occur in colitis patients.

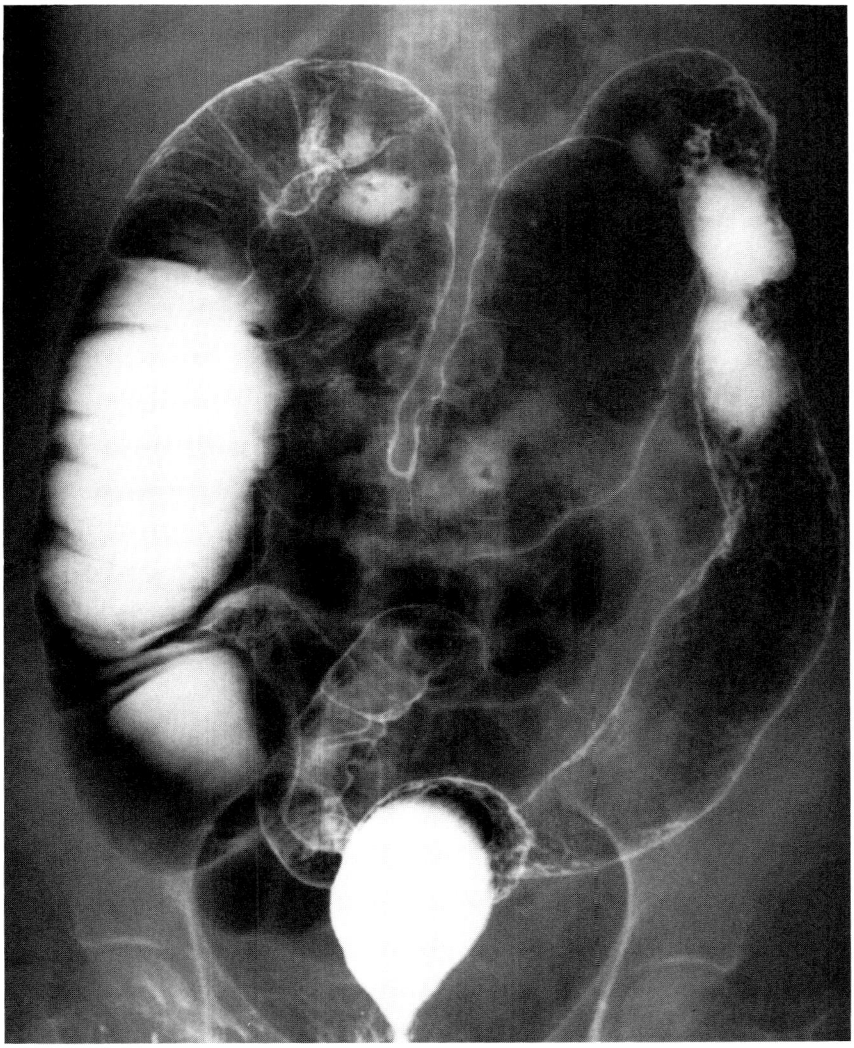

FIG. 5–4. Stenosis of the distal rectum and nodular lesion at the proximal descending colon in a patient with 20 years of disease. The rectal stricture prevents colonoscopy.

COLONIC PSEUDOPOLYPOSIS

Occasionally noted on the abdominal plain film when the colon is gas-filled, but best seen in the postevacuation barium enema, pseudopolyps may be multiple and tiny or single and enormous; they are made up of islands of preserved, hyperplastic mucosa and granulation tissue, and occur as a characteristic of long-standing inflammatory bowel disease. Both extremes are illustrated here (Fig. 5–5). Though any fixed polypoid filling defects, "pseudo" or real, summon up understandable concerns for cancer development in patients with long-standing disease, they are more an indication of the overall severity of the disease or of a distant previous attack, as they are sometimes found in asymptomatic patients. The clinician's job is to make certain the defects are just what they seem to be. Yet while pseudopolyps are not themselves a premalignant process, they develop in a disease with a potential for malignant degeneration, and they *can* obscure discovery of small cancers developing amidst a contorted, nodular, and creviced mucosa, concealing their development to both x ray and endoscopy. Because pseudopolyps can bleed independently of the activity of the colitis, they may warrant an attempt at electrocautery removal, particularly when they are large or when the bleeding is seen coming only from one or several pseudopolyps.

Pseudopolyps are frequently seen in the rectum at proctosigmoidoscopy, but are less easily demonstrated there on x ray because of the rectum's fixed walls below the peritoneal reflection. Unlike true adenomas, they lack the usual stalk or rounded apex and often show whitish patches of exudate at their tip. Brisk hemorrhage traced to a single pseudopolyp can be treated by colotomy or segmental resection, with the understandable attendant risk of surgical leak in bowel-to-bowel anastomosis in inflammatory bowel disease. Bowel obstruction from large or coalescent pseudopolyps has been reported.

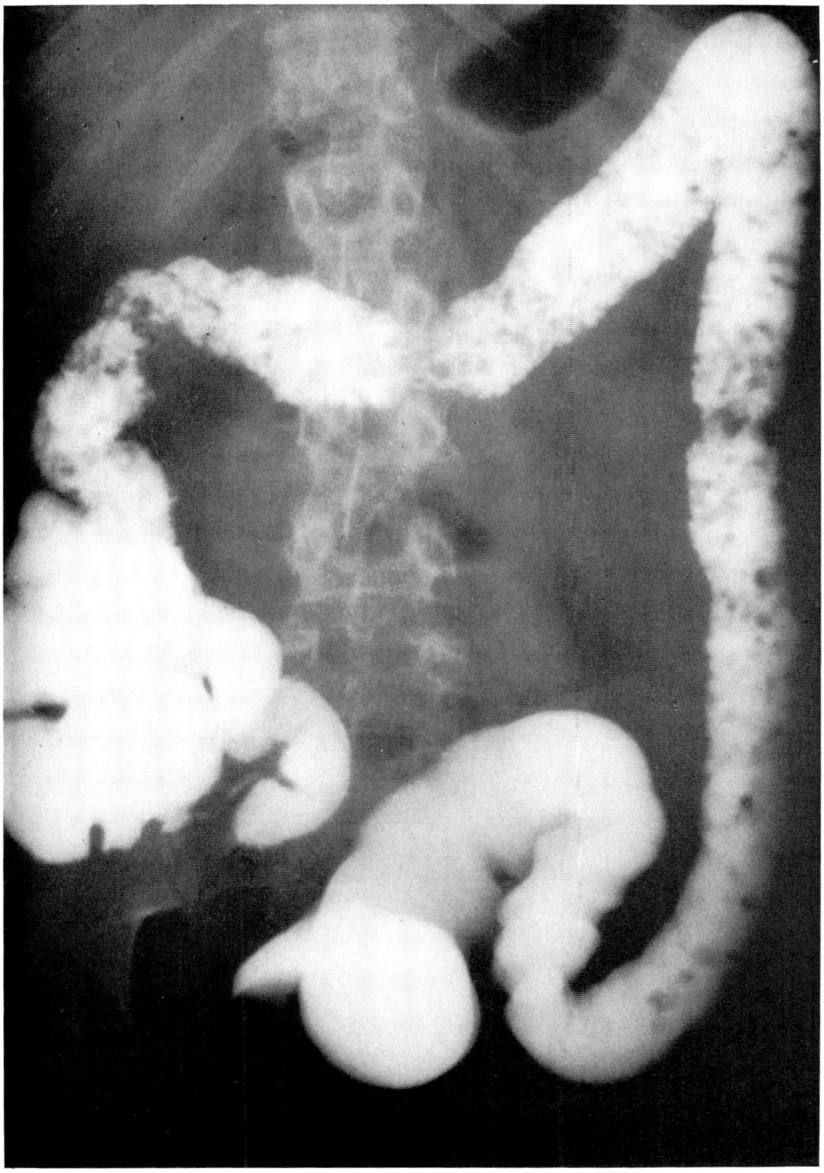

FIG. 5–5. Multiple rounded densities of varying size, virtually all nonpedunculated. Identification of a true neoplasm or malignancy in this chronically inflamed bowel is understandably difficult.

CHRONIC ULCERATIVE PROCTITIS

The concept has developed that ulcerative proctitis is a disease both qualitatively and quantitatively different from traditional ulcerative colitis. When the mucosal inflammatory process is confined to the rectum or, at most, the adjacent distal sigmoid, symptoms rarely exceed painless rectal bleeding, though in advanced or particularly virulent cases, urgency, tenesmus, pain, and fistula development do occur.

The typical barium enema x ray of an ulcerative proctitis patient is normal, but careful observations of the contour of the contrast-filled rectum may show some serrations in what is normally a smooth barium-mucosal interface. Chronicity results in the nondistensible circumferential contraction of the rectum seen here (Fig. 5–6), begetting a diminished reservoir capacity and perhaps a heightened sensitivity to its contents, with frequent urges to evacuate what prove to be only miniscule excretions. Lateral views show an increased, presumably fibrotic space between the anterior sacral surface and posterior wall of the rectum.

Satellite manifestations of chronic inflammatory bowel disease (spondylitis, arthritis, nephrolithiasis, pyoderma gangrenosum, gallstones, growth retardation, sclerosing cholangitis) are typically absent. However, by all other criteria, ulcerative proctitis is in fact simply a mild form of an ordinarily belligerent illness. Despite the generally benign nature of this limited inflammatory bowel process, it should be recalled that between 10 and 20% of patients whose colitis begins in and first seems limited to the rectum do eventually experience retrograde extension. As the amount of affected "real estate" increases, the other satellite manifestations of colitis become increasing evident, sometimes requiring total colectomy and ileostomy. One case of adenocarcinoma arising in the inflamed distal rectum of a patient with only proctitis is known personally. He had been intermittently ill for at least a dozen of his 24 years and mistakenly concluded that recurrent bleeding represented reactivation of his bowel disease.

An ulcerative proctitis diagnosis is easy by sigmoidoscopy. Intrarectal treatment with corticosteroids or the aminosalicylate analogs of salazopyrin is usually effective. Systemic steroids are occasionally required, and the intractable diarrhea or tenesmus may force performance of the rare proctectomy and colostomy or total proctocolectomy. Given their usually normal x-ray picture and mild symptoms, many patients with this illness are misdiagnosed as only having bleeding hemorrhoids.

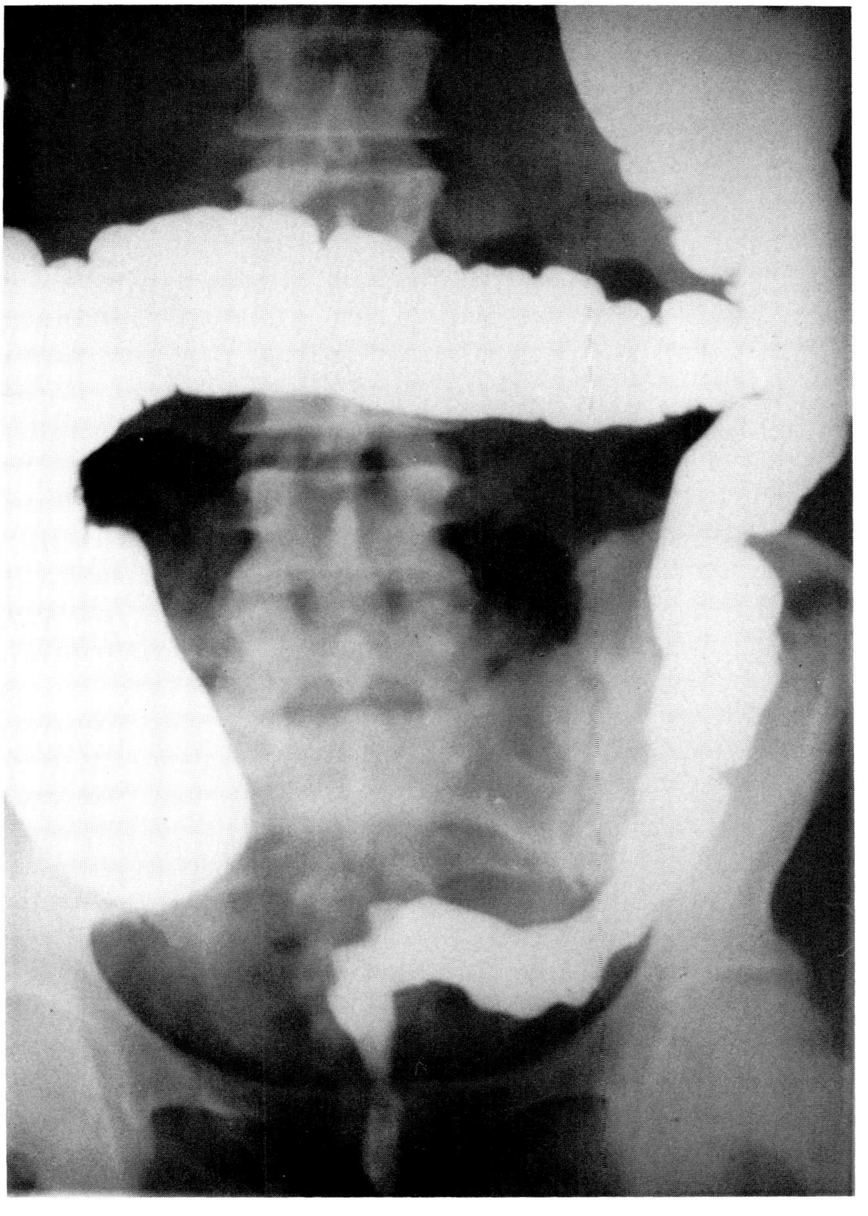

FIG. 5–6. Anterior view showing rectum circumferentially constricted up to and past the peritoneal reflection. Space between rectum and sacrococcygeal vertebra may be increased, while the remainder of the colon appears uninvolved.

CROHN'S DISEASE OF THE COLON

To most authorities, comparative clinical, anatomic, and radiologic studies successfully argue that the idiopathic colon-inflammatory diseases are separable into two somewhat overlapping forms; one is clearly "mucosal" (ulcerative colitis), and the other, Crohn's disease, more resembles the transmural, granulomatous ileitis first described in the 1930s. Viewed separately, the Crohn's colitis variant is agreed upon to more commonly involve proximal colon and adjacent small intestine, while typically sparing the rectum. Crohn's colitis regularly associates with internal and external fistulas, while narrowing the lumen with obstructive exuberant nodularity or strictures, often in a segmental discontinuous pattern. Its associated extraintestinal complications particularly involve the skin (cutaneous, particularly perineal ulcers), the skeleton (osteomyelitis, arthritis, spondylitis), and the genitourinary tract (calculi, ureteral blockage), while reportedly possessing a diminished penchant for carcinomatous degeneration, toxic megacolon, or vigorous bleeding.

Figure 5–7A through D illustrates some anatomic features of Crohn's colitis. In Figure 5–7A, the contour of the proximal two thirds of the bowel is normal, only to taper distally to a fixed, string-like, focal, mid-descending colon stricture. Barium's passage across it argues for its pliability, especially in a patient presenting with diarrhea rather than obstruction. Abdominal pain and lumbar kyphosis are both properly explained in Figure 5–7B. Barium enema (done just after an IVP) reveals thumbprint indentations along the course of the descending and transverse colon, which are consistent with a transmural inflammatory process. The fixed vertebrae assume the typical bamboo configuration of ankylosing spondylitis, which, when associated with inflammatory bowel disease, consistently exhibits the HLA B-27 chromosome marker. The bladder opacification is from IV dye, not barium sulfate. A "spot" film of the adjacent terminal ileum, ascending, and proximal transverse colon in Figure 5–7C shows the typical ovoid radiolucent nodules of Crohn's disease. The multiple streaks of barium entering the ascending colon from the ileum in Figure 5–7D are fistulas.

Medical management of both colitides is similar, employing systemic and topical corticosteroids and salazopyrin (and its derivatives) as anti-inflammatory agents, systemic antibiotics for infection, and metronidazole for both. Immunosuppressive therapy's value remains arguable, while the response to IV nutritional replenishment is often striking. Surgical therapy is another matter. In Crohn's colitis, segmental resection for focal stricture or ulceration seems to be more initially successful, despite a significant long-term recurrence risk at an ileocolic or colocolic anastomosis. Bowel diversion for fistula healing also seems to work better in Crohn's disease, particularly if the rectum appears normal.

The most compelling argument for distinguishing Crohn's disease and ulcerative colitis relates to decision-making when operating for "cure." In the patient with ulcerative colitis, proctocolectomy with ileostomy or ileoanostomy probably does the job, but the same operation in Crohn's disease is followed in one quarter to one half of patients by inflammatory recurrences in a previously healthy small bowel.

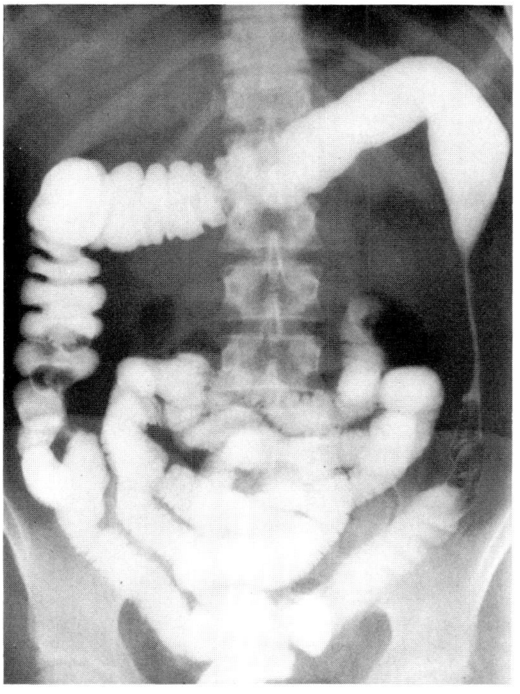

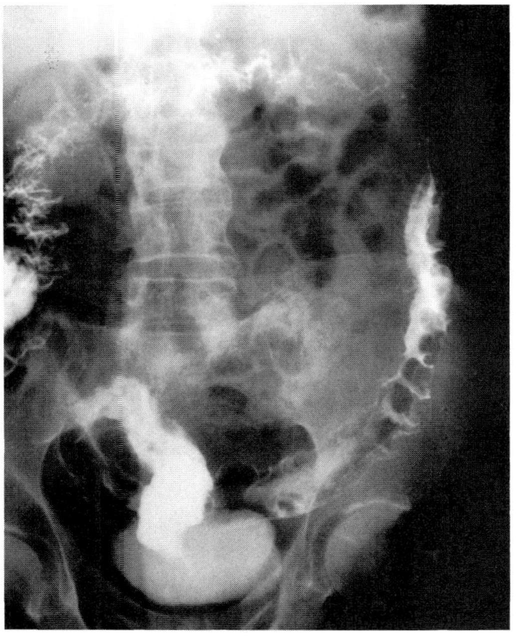

FIG. 5–7. A. High-grade stricture of mid-descending colon (a "skip" area) in a patient with alternating diarrhea and obstruction.

B. Barium enema (with IVP dye in bladder). Deep, edematous, thumbprint indentations seen throughout, maximal in mid-descending colon. Note "bamboo-configuration" of lumbar vertebrae, suggesting ankylosing spondylitis.

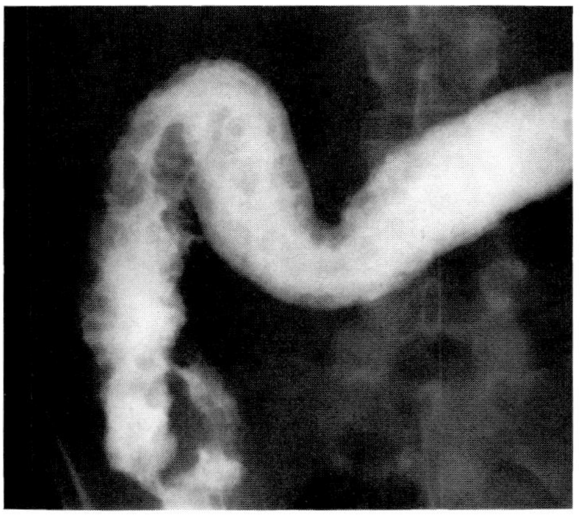

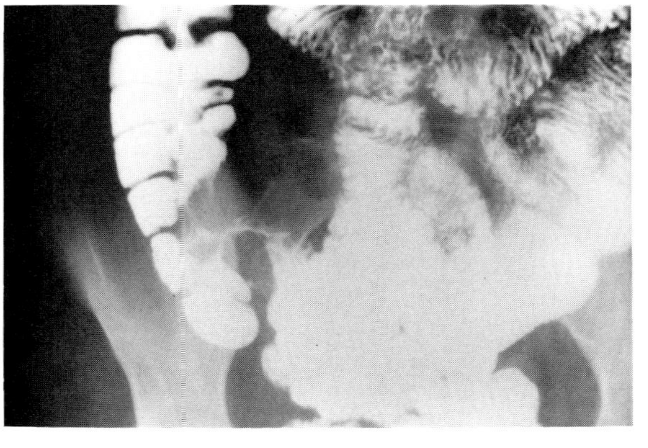

C. Edematous nodules of transmural involvement in proximal colon.

D. Multiple fistulous tracts from ileum into right colon.

RECTAL STRICTURE

Rectal strictures are relatively common and certainly easy to locate, yet each justifiably raises concern for cancer, especially when another cause is not clinically evident. Even if biopsies prove the strictures benign, cancer's possibility should remain suspect. Sampling error may accrue when too few specimens are retrieved or when the "bites" are too superficial. Even benign strictures, especially those developing in a chronically inflamed bowel, may become malignant. The usual etiologies of stricture include chronic inflammatory bowel disease (typically the Crohn's variant with primary or secondary rectal involvement), previous anorectal surgery, venereal infection, or prior pelvic irradiation for cancer.

Radiologically, most benign rectal strictures are smooth and regular, with preservation of mucosal detail over rounded proximal and distal margins (Fig. 5–8A). When they are high-grade or actively narrowing, constipation will develop, typically accompanied by changes in the character of stool, now extruded to a pencil or ribbon shape, without overt bleeding. Though common in advanced rectal cancers, tenesmus is usually a manifestation of either the pliable rectal edema or the narrowing secondary to infectious or idiopathic inflammatory bowel disease. Bleeding commonly occurs in patients with radiation enteritis, as the mucosal sites of bowel injury are rendered intensely vascular.

Most rectal strictures cannot be traversed by a rigid proctoscope, and even flexible instruments or dilators will find themselves blocked by the fixed, usually fibrotic stenosis. Well-lubricated, metal, olive-shaped instruments of gradually increasing diameter are required. Most inflammatory strictures can be managed by these manipulations, but unless the stricture is resected or deeply incised, repeat dilations will prove necessary. When there is a prominent inflammatory component, intrarectal corticosteroids in a liquid or foam vehicle can be dramatically effective as adjunctive therapy.

Benign strictures will rarely occlude to the point of colonic obstruction; at that point, surgical decision-making is difficult. There is an understandable temptation for circumferential excision and bowel-to-bowel anastomosis, but more conservative options include removing a wedge-shaped portion of the stricture, reanastomosis of mucosa, and, to the extent possible, preservation of the sphincter. In any surgery of this kind, there is always the risk of an anastomotic leak, resulting in a deep pelvic or buttock abscess. Likelihood of such a breakdown may be significantly lessened by a temporary bypassing proximal colostomy at the time of operation.

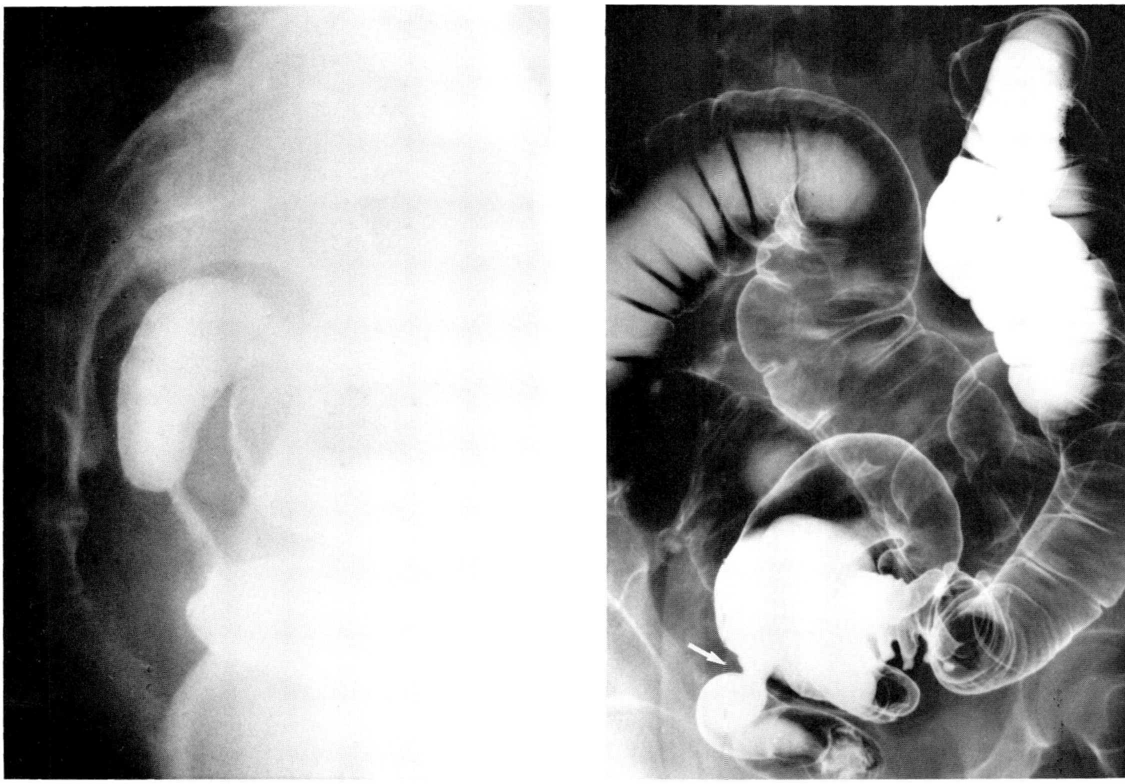

A B

FIG. 5–8. A. Lateral view of rectum, showing circumferential, smooth, high-grade stricture of the distal rectum in patient with chronic Crohn's disease.
B. Barium enema showing smooth stricture at the rectosigmoid junction ↑ in a patient irradiated for cervical carcinoma. Note the distensible rectum and absence of other evidence of inflammatory bowel disease.
C. Spot films of the stricture of the patient in Figure 5–8B. The film above demonstrates ease by which an overlapping loop of intestine obscures the stricture; the lower film with the patient slightly rotated reveals the lesion.

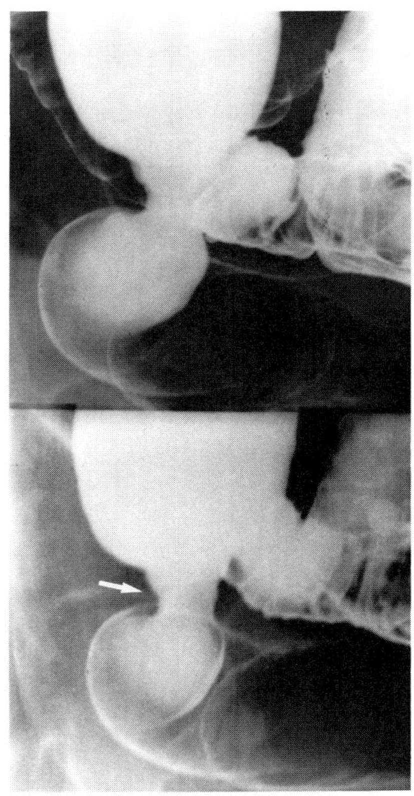

C

PERIRECTAL ABSCESS

A more satellite manifestation of an occasionally subtle distant bowel event, the perirectal abscesses evident in Figure 5–9A and B are often the first manifestation of inflammatory bowel disease, typically the Crohn's variant. Perirectal disease usually occurs in the absence of any radiologically demonstrable extravasation, but here (Fig. 5–9A) the barium sprays from and about the rectum like water from a lawn sprinkler. The clinical implications are obvious: a deep pelvic abscess communicating with a painful perineal bulge, fever, sepsis, and evident chronic disease. The track into the perirectal tissue is more often obscure, presumed to originate in an inflamed loop of ileum or large intestine whose proximal end is a transmural leak that opens and closes. The usual abscess is also radiologically inapparent but can sometimes be inferred from an increased, gas-containing presacral space (Fig. 5–9B). Abscesses of this magnitude often require transrectal or gluteal drainage with proximal colonic or small-bowel diversion, and sometimes complete rectal resection. Corticosteroids are probably of little value, and antibacterials, particularly metronidazole, occupy a minor but unquestionably secondary therapeutic function, particularly when the perineal skin is involved.

If a buttock abscess in a patient with inflammatory bowel disease is to be cured, the inflamed focus of origin must be identified and resected; hence, the entire bowel requires a radiologic survey. Perianal infections are far more common in patients with ileocolic or colonic disease than in those whose involvement is limited to the small intestine. As the illness responsible for the striking x rays is almost certainly an extensive and transmural enterocolitis, any attempt at isolated drainage without some bowel resection is almost certain to be unsuccessful and risks a recurrent deep pelvic abscess.

Many perirectal abscesses drain chronically as fistulas. Though a nuisance, most are bearable, and their referral for surgical cure should be ruminated carefully. Postoperative nonhealing is common, as is loss of sphincter tone, and the most "routine" excisions can eventuate in a colostomy or ileostomy. This form of pelvic inflammatory disease, though nongynecologic, can understandably impair fertility in women.

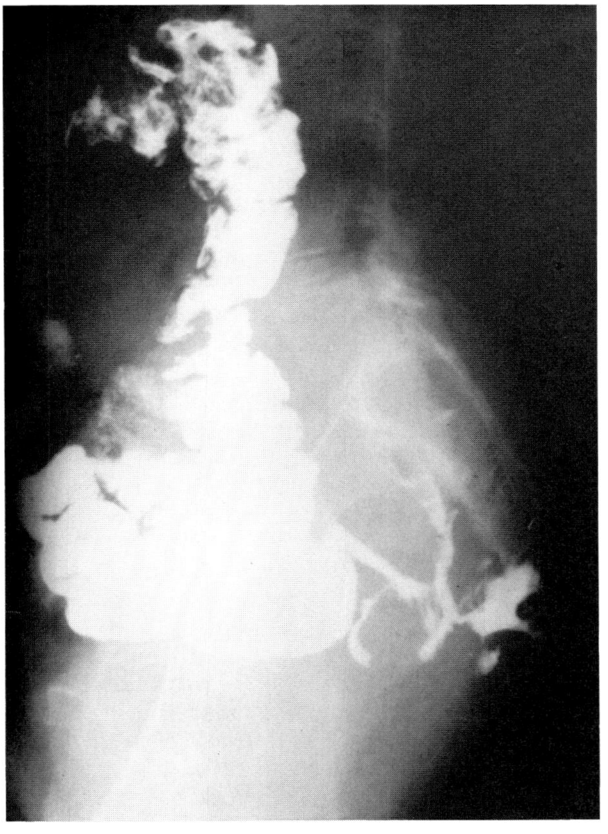

FIG. 5–9. A. Small-bowel series showing tracks of contrast spraying throughout the presacral area.

B. Extravasation of barium and a markedly increased air-filled retrorectal space, indicating a deep pelvic infection.

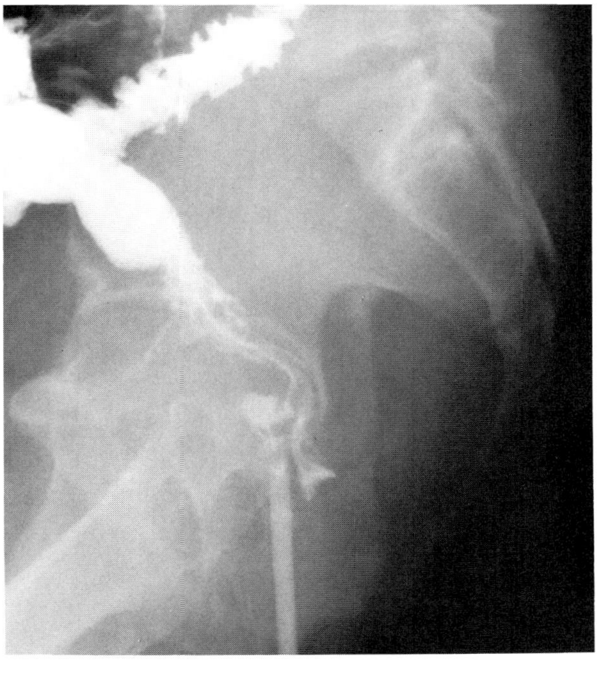

COLON CARCINOMA

It can be argued that the most important purpose of physician-patient interaction is the discovery of a lethal disease in curable or treatable form. Accordingly, the early identification of colon cancer may be the quintessential representation of ideal patient care. Between the subtlety of cecal cancer and clinical conspicuousness of rectal tumors rests the full literal, anatomic, and symptomatic spectrum of the remainder of large-bowel neoplasia. Acknowledging the occasional malignancy that appears with perforation or brisk hemorrhage, most colonic cancers announce themselves with anemia, by slow bleeding through surface necrosis, or by obstruction through progressive centripetal encroachment on the bowel lumen. Three typical examples are noted.

In Figure 5–10A, a large, presumably full-thickness, destructive lesion is clearly seen just proximal to the hepatic flexure. The normal caliber of the proximal and distal lumen argues that despite its considerable size, the tumor produces no alteration in bowel function, probably because of the relatively liquid nature of feces in the ascending colon. In this patient, a deteriorating tennis game led to his physical examination, which revealed pallor and iron-deficiency anemia. Barium enema followed. In tumors of this size, serosal involvement is expected, usually with associated blood-vessel or lymphatic invasion.

The patient of Figure 5–10B presented with progressive constipation alternating with episodic diarrhea and occasional passages of visible blood. Conventional sigmoidoscopy was negative. Barium-enema fluoroscopy was halted when the dilated column was found blocked at the mid-descending colon, illustrating the valve-like nature of some bowel tumors. The patient's constipation was caused by incomplete antegrade obstruction; retrograde flow of barium was completely obstructed. The absence of adjacent diverticula make the diagnosis a near certainty.

There is nothing unique about malignant tumors in the transverse colon except that they occur less frequently there than in either ascending or descending colon. These tumors may appear with bleeding or obstruction, and unless the center of the transverse colon dips into the pelvis, they are easily visualized on either barium-filled or air-contrast views. This x ray (Fig. 5–10C) is noteworthy because the tumor demonstrates features of both a benign and a malignant lesion: its clearly exophytic, lobulated, and non-ulcerated shape argues for adenoma. However, a mural attachment as broad as it is high suggests cancer and warns that attempted electrocautery removal conveys as much current to the bowel wall as to the lesion's attachment, risking perforation. Removal of a lesion of this contour requires colotomy or segmental colectomy. The only role for colonoscopy may be to search for additional benign or malignant lesions or to ablate tumor mass in a patient too ill for laparotomy.

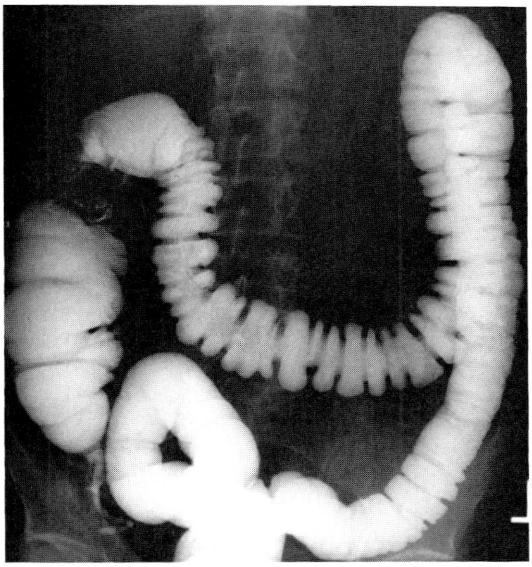

A

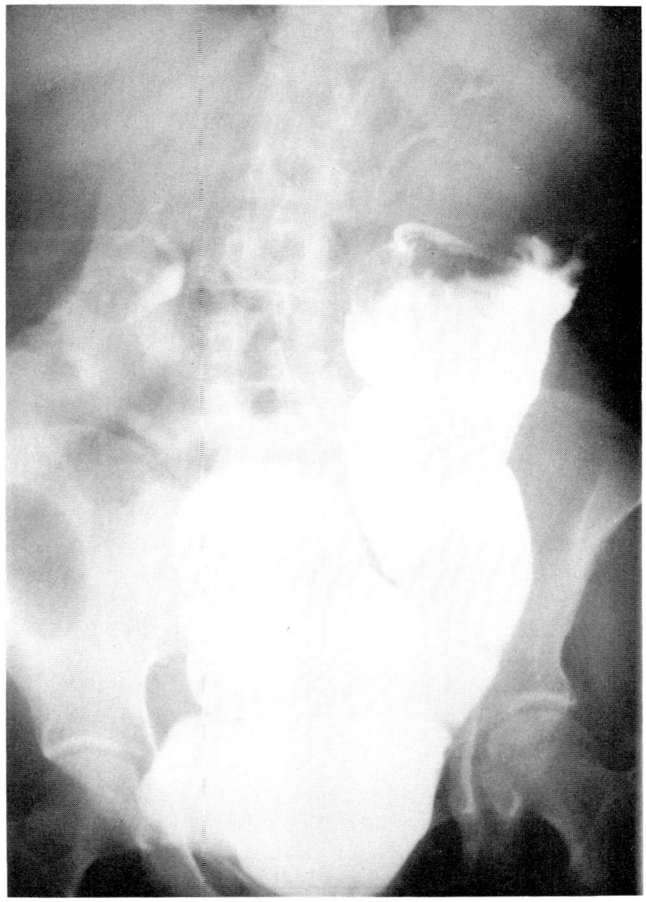

B

FIG. 5–10. A. Easy depiction of a large, circumferential non-obstructing, bleeding malignant tumor of the distal ascending colon.
B. Large tumor of descending colon, producing complete retrograde obstruction to barium but no evident antegrade blockage. IVP dye is seen filling the left renal collecting system.
C. Lobulated, sessile polypoid carcinoma on antimesenteric border of the distal transverse colon.

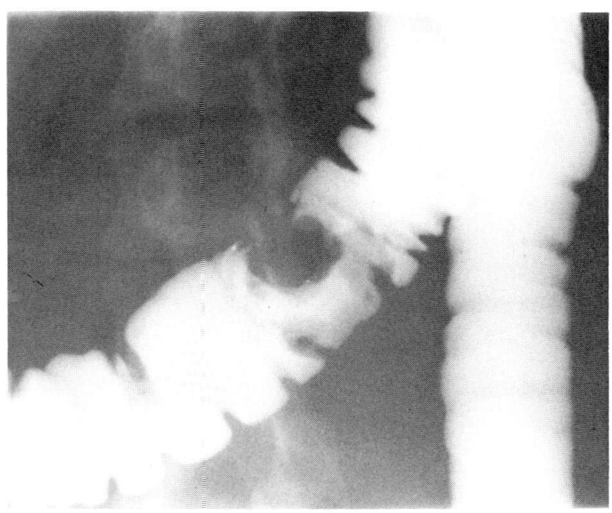

C

RECTAL CANCER

The charming aphorism, "he who doesn't put his finger in it, puts his foot in it" may lead to the mistaken belief that a diagnosis of rectal cancer can or always should be made on digital examination or proctosigmoidoscopy, and rarely if ever on barium enema. Even patients with biopsy-proven rectal cancer require colon x rays to search for synchronous lesions or fistulae, measure a lesion's size, or estimate the length of rectum beneath the tumor's lower edge, helping the surgeon decide between an abdominoperineal and low-anterior resection.

These PA and lateral views (Fig. 5–11A and B) define a classic, irregular, "applecore" circumferential lesion. The x rays further allow the physician to infer something about a patient's fears. A tumor of this magnitude and low location has certainly produced months of visible rectal bleeding, changing stool caliber, and constipation, the inescapable potential significance of which could only be repressed or denied with enormous neurotic energy. Circumferential rectal lesions are almost always primary carcinomas, but, occasionally, prostatic or ovarian cancer will surround the outside of the rectum. The compromised lumen is then usually smooth and nonulcerated (Fig. 5–11C). Obviously, any such film should be further examined for hepatomegaly or ascites, bony involvement, and, in a corresponding chest x ray, pulmonary metastases.

Since it is so easily diagnosable and eradicable by appropriate surgery, rectal cancer should be lethal in only a small minority of patients who have access to and use their healthcare opportunities. Because the most defensible raison d'etre of regular physical examinations is the early detection of a treatable, serious disease, the first x rays indicate that the patient has failed the system, or vice-versa. A lesion of this extent, years in the making, indicates that no rectal examinations have been performed on a patient who deserved them. Certainly, a diagnosis of new onset "bleeding hemorrhoids" mandates colon x rays, even if visual, instrument, or digital examinations are considered confirmatory.

The value of preoperative perineal irradiation in all rectal cancer patients remains unanswered, as most of the data suggesting improved survival in pretreated patients are found from surgical specimens whose particular stages of intermediate invasiveness were impossible to predict preoperatively. Moreover, the complications of x-ray injury to bowel, bladder, skin, and pelvis are significant, chronic, and difficult to treat.

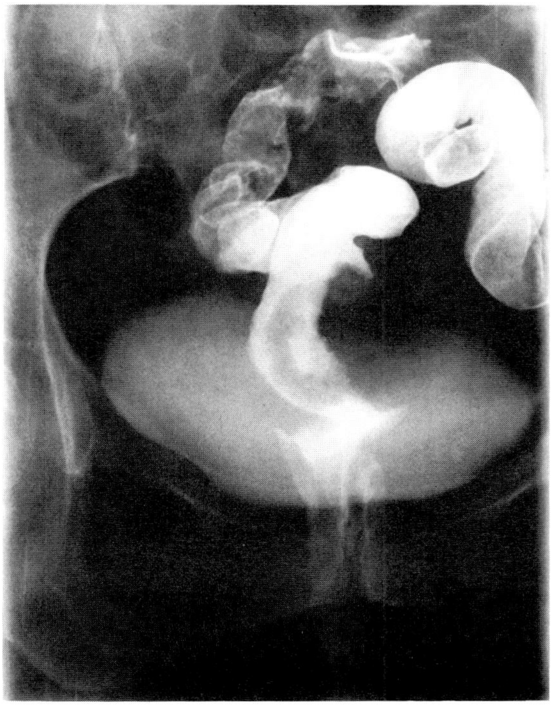
A

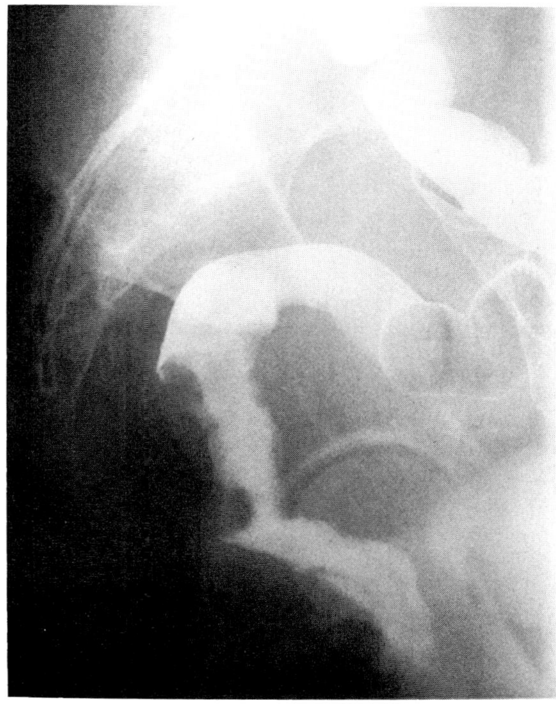
B

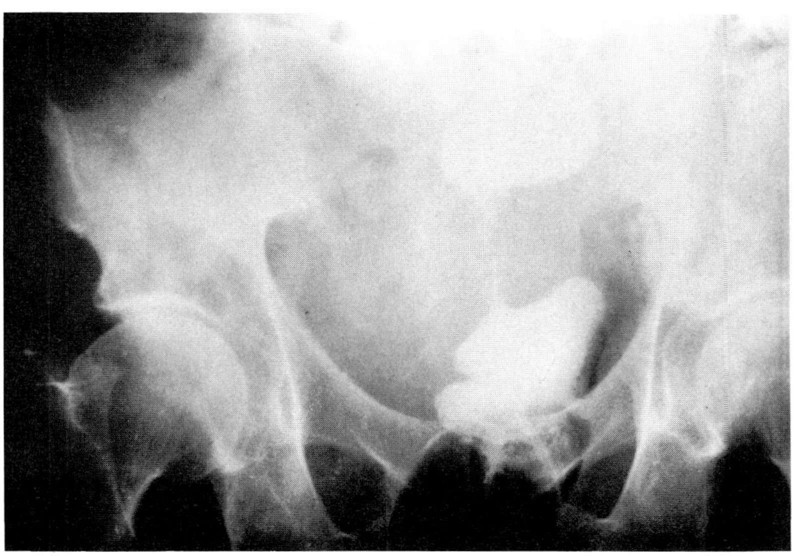
C

FIG. 5–11. A and B. PA and lateral views of extensive circumferential "applecore" lesion of the rectum, extending too far below the peritoneal reflection for safe low anterior anastomosis. Only 2 to 3 in. of normal rectum are seen below the inferior margin of the cancer. Bladder opacification is from IVP dye, not a fistula.
C. Prostate carcinoma involving rectum. Extrinsic encirclement with smooth stenosis of rectum, producing near-total retrograde obstruction.

CECAL CARCINOMA

Oddly one of the commonest, most elusive, yet potentially curable causes of cancer death, cecal carcinoma earns its reputation because of the inherent difficulties involved in its nonsurgical diagnosis. The first portion of colon soiled by ileal output, least accessible to enema cleansing, and arduous to reach by colonscopy, the cecal mucosa is the hardest area of the large bowel to visualize clearly or with confidence. Furthermore, depending on its contour and the right mesocolon's length and mobility, the cecum itself may avoid identification. Pear-, acorn-, or funnel-shaped, it can be in either upper or lower abdominal quadrants. An empty, bulbous portion of midascending colon resting in the right lower quadrant may mimic a normal cecum, while a proximal cecal carcinoma is rotated counterclockwise behind a screen of barium-filled ileal loops. Finally, since the cecum is expansile, mostly dependent from a lumen containing a liquid fecal stream, a cancer contained there can grow large without causing changes in bowel function or hematochezia. Exertional dyspnea, abdominal pain, fullness, mass, pallor, or even iron-desaturation-absent anemia may be among the first hints at this slow leak of life.

The operation (right colectomy) is relatively simple. Lives are saved only when it is performed before the disease is obvious. Thus, the smart (i.e., skeptical) clinician considers cecal cancer when pondering "positive" stools or iron-deficiency anemia in adult males and postmenopausal women with so-called "negative" x rays, and even in patients receiving nonsteroidal inflammatory agents in whom gastritis seems the logical explanation. Aspirin can make cancers bleed, and there is no rule that mandates that a patient can have only one disease at a single time.

In this first film (Fig. 5–12A), a normal but mobile ileum obscures the cecum, allowing the inexperienced, hurried, or nonchalant radiologist to mistake it for the portion of normal mid-ascending colon seen immediately above the ileum. Irregularity of barium can be seen *behind* the ileum, but only when its loops are manipulated medially or the patient is rotated, as in Figure 5–12B, does the classic applecore lesion reveal itself. Such film needs no colonoscopic confirmation, for even if the cecum is reached, biopsies may fail to deliver up malignant tissue. Provided the patient is not already dying of metastases or some other illness, this x ray makes absurd any therapeutic position short of laparotomy. This is not Crohn's disease, appendicitis, trichuriasis, or an ameboma; this is cancer. The smooth oval lucency of Figure 5–12C is a typical benign ileocecal valve.

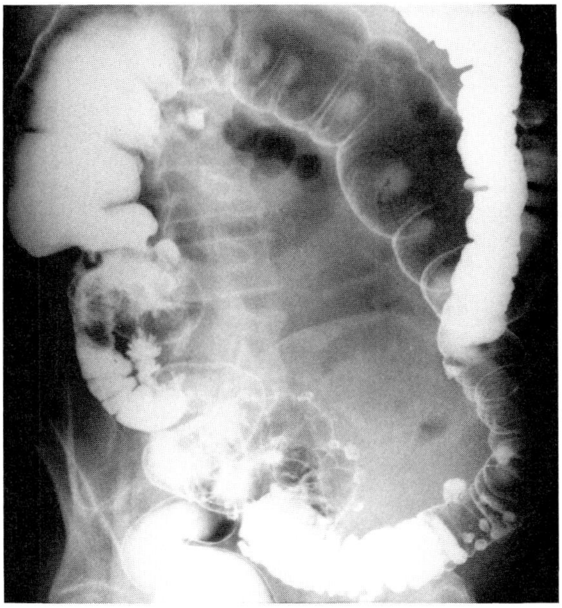
A

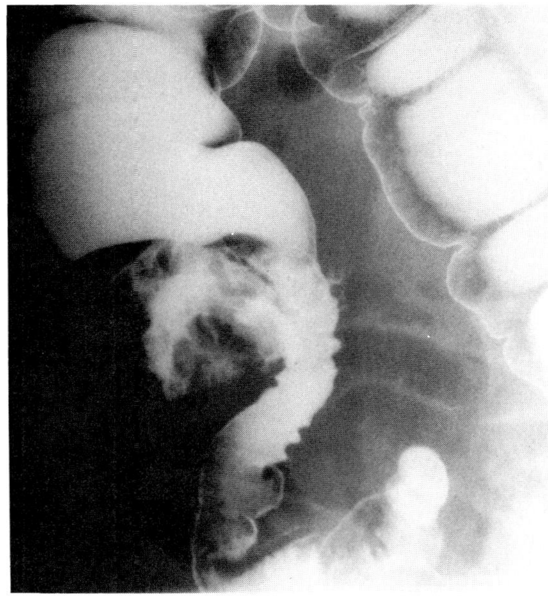
B

FIG. 5–12. A. Incompletely filled-out cecum partially obscured by loops of ileum. B. With ileal loops deflected medially, a typical fungating mass with a central core is identified. Note the absence of obstruction to the upward migration of barium. C. A smoothly rounded, almond-shaped radiolucency on medial border of cecum is an enlarged, probably lipomatous ileocecal valve, not to be mistaken for a cancer.

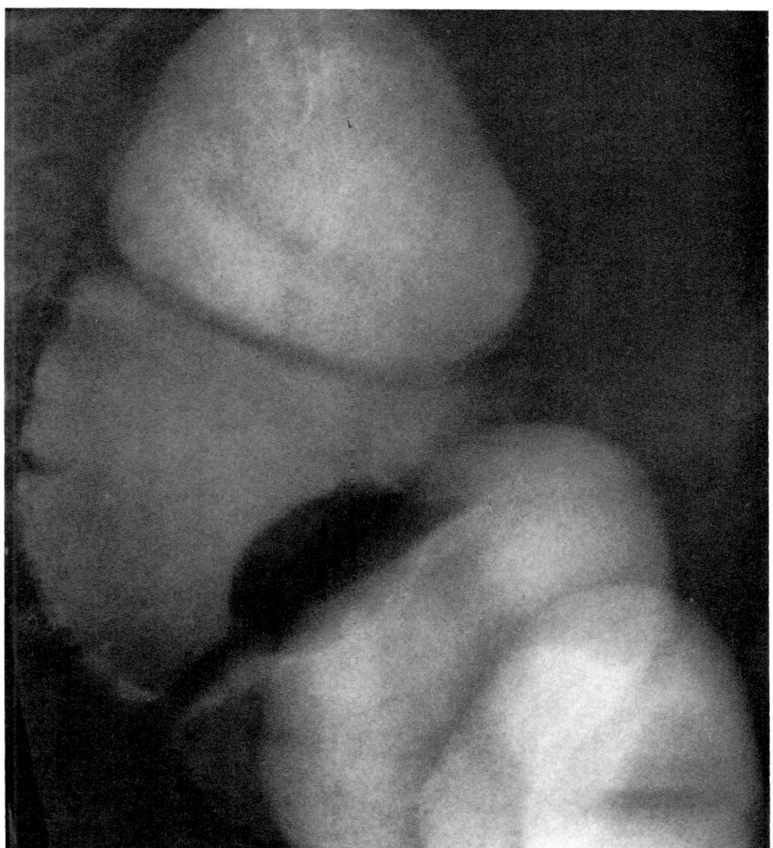
C

THE POORLY PREPARED (OR EXAMINED) GUT

Careful medical practice necessarily includes a physician's ongoing, admitted uncertainty, clearly a somewhat neurotic trait but one directed selflessly at securing the benefit of thoroughness for one's patient. In diagnostic medicine, most of the worries relate to cancer and must begin with any middle-aged patient's medical evaluation, perhaps even particularly for those who indicate their desire for a "routine" physical. Initial, seemingly remote clues might include a hematocrit of 40% in a man whose usual packed-cell volume exceeds 45%. The finding of microcytosis or hypochromia on a blood smear, new onset fatigue, or even unexplained hypoferremia all argue that the patient may be bleeding from an intestinal cancer. Until that is disproved, scrupulous digestive-tract examinations and continued diligence (if nothing is found at first) are necessary. Moreover, it cannot be overemphasized that finding one nontumorous explanation for bleeding doesn't mean the patient cannot have another cause elsewhere. Hemorrhoids and hemorrhoidal bleeding are common enough, but neither diagnosis excludes rectal cancer. The increasing use of aspirin for stroke or myocardial infarction prophylaxis will enlarge the harvest of erosive gastritis, but finding or assuming that diagnosis in an anemic aspirin-taker does not, for example, eliminate the need to consider a cecal neoplasm. Plainly, patients can have "fleas *and* lice at the same time."

Among the undertaker's and plaintiff's lawyer's allies are the poorly prepared large intestine, the inadequately unfolded bowel loop, and the barium-filled stomach. Some patients do not take laxative preparations, others vomit them, and they don't work adequately in everyone. Figure 5–13A shows an exceptional example. But whether the amount of residual stool in the colon is small or large, solid or liquid, if the mucosa cannot be cleared adequately and visualized "on edge," the preparation has been inadequate and the test must be repeated. Today, most radiologists affix a poor-preparation caveat on their barium-enema reports, describing an "inability to rule out small polypoid lesions." Either for himself or his patient, the clinician cannot choose to ignore this, even at the risk of the patient's displeasure. The doctor must be equally skeptical of a study in which exposures are made where overlapping loops of bowel are not adequately separated. Figure 5–13B faintly hints at a retrorectal portion of sigmoid whose left-hand edge shows the encroaching shoulder of a malignant tumor. With that portion of bowel remaining obscured, the examination had been interpreted as normal.

The barium-filled stomach will show only large lesions. A mound of mostly smooth tumor (Fig. 5–13C), easily seen after air is swallowed, could have been mistakenly interpreted as a peristaltic wave if contrast had not been partially cleared.

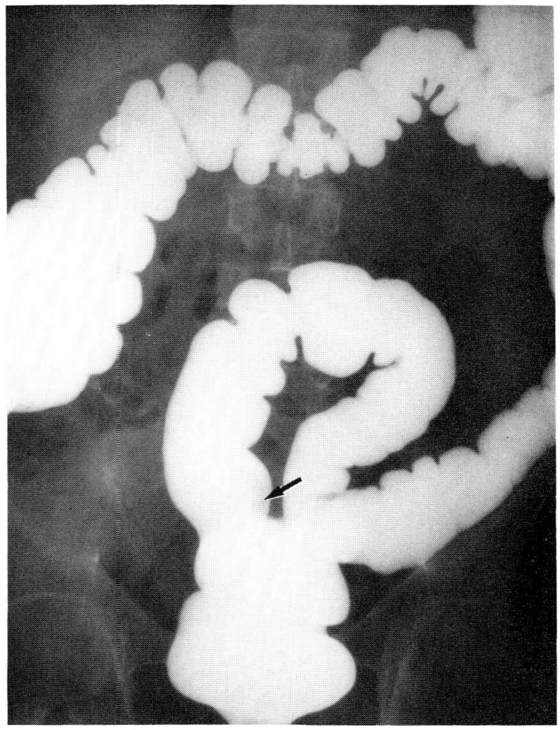

B

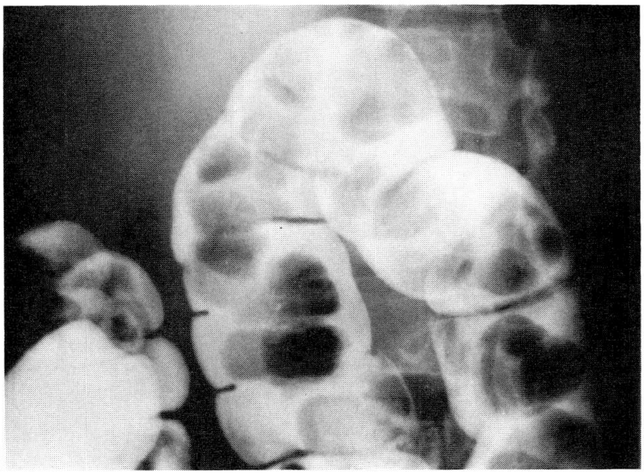

A

FIG. 5–13. A. Poorly prepared colon—no laughing matter, this spot film of the splenic flexure contains spheres of unevacuated feces, any of which could be a polypoid tumor. Any variation on this abnormality, however trivial, argues for repeating the x ray or performing colonoscopy.
B. The retrorectal location of this sigmoid tumor, of which only an edge is visible, is a favorite location of a colon carcinoma in the patient with a "negative" film.
C. Rounded fullness on greater curvature of gastric antrum. Air-contrast visualization of mucosal irregularity suggests cancer.

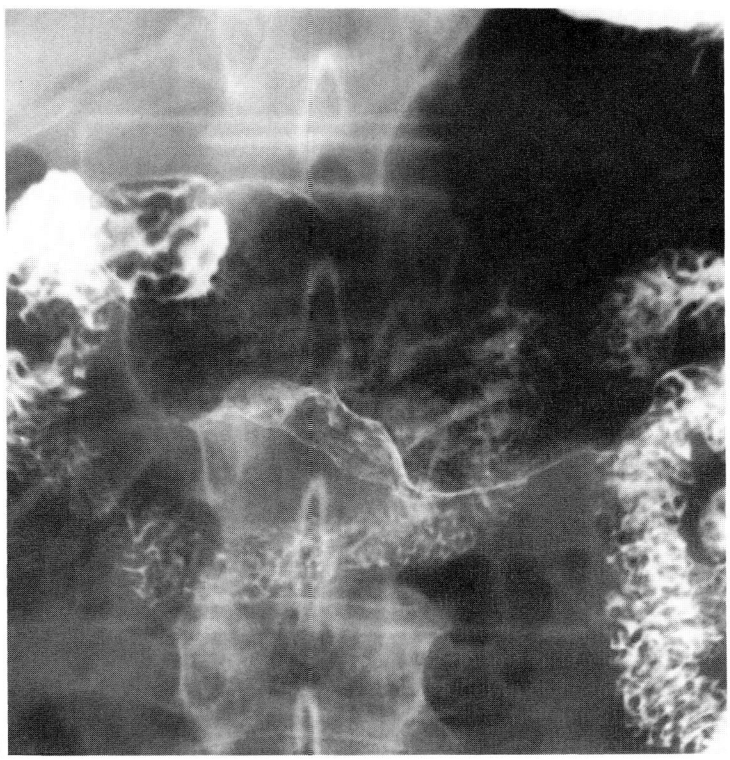

C

THE COLONIC POLYP

In an earlier era, the biologic and clinical implications of the discovered colon polyp were argued endlessly and resolved only at pain or risk to their owner. Were filling defects that looked like polyps cancerous or premalignant? Did a visible stalk diminish, or large size increase, the risk of malignancy? Were one or more polyps revealed at x ray or sigmoidoscopy harbingers of other, less visible synchronous polyps or cancer? Most of the light shed on those questions was conveyed by flexible glass bundles, and as large-bowel neoplasia can be biopsied or removed endoscopically, several issues seem partially resolved.

For instance, we known now that many polyps and some cancers occur in multiples. They can precede, coexist with, or follow one another. The patient with benign, particularly multiple polyps is at increased risk for colon cancer, and seems to need ongoing x-ray or endoscopic surveillance. While most polypoid cancers were never adenomas, many larger (greater than 1.5 cm) adenomatous polyps have an apical focus of noninvasive carcinoma. Finally, occasional stalked, carcinomatous polyps, when transected, indeed reveal malignant cells gliding down their mural attachment.

The typical descending-colon location, the often friable, spherical head, and the long stalk of the classic lesion illustrated here (Fig. 5–14) argue that it is an adenomatous polyp (or tubular adenoma). As such a polyp enlarges, it is mistaken by the colon for excreta and tugged distally, causing its stalk to lengthen. Best seen when barium is thin or partially evaluated in double-contrast technique, yet having little mass and extraordinary radiolucency, polyps rarely deform or stiffen the colon wall or obstruct its contents. Thus, polyps are missed easily, and their evasiveness extends to colonoscopy. Small polyps or cancers can nest behind a valve or haustration, lie submerged in a lacuna of opaque, liquid stool, or refuse to oblige the examiner by bleeding during endocopy.

The size of a polyp seen on x ray is only modestly helpful to the clinician. While polypoid lesions under 1.5 cm are rarely malignant, logic argues that nearly all colon cancers must exist sometime in their natural history in small, curable form. As tumor growth into the lumen partly parallels its centrifugal invasion, colonoscopy seems an unavoidable adjunct to the barium examination.

Yet, while settling old arguments, progress creates new ones. The enthusiastic colonoscopist assures us that a direct color image or a biopsy of mucosa is superior to black-and-white transparencies, and that only the resected polyp can be certain to bode no ill for its former host. The radiologist counters that as he has more ounces of barium than there are centimeters of colonoscope, no portion of a lengthy, tortuous large intestine can elude him. Furthermore, his radiopaque liquid flows easily through strictured or fixed loops of bowel that might block or be perforated by a heavy endoscopic instrument.

No discussion of colonic polyposis is clinically useful without some mention of this condition's burgeoning medicolegal impact. Sadly, it now generates at least as much lawyerly as medical debate, assuring decades of profit for malpractice lawyers and professional testifiers, and quizzical inspection of ancient barium enemas by innumerable future juries. Such lawsuits emerge primarily on the issue of preventable death through negligent failure to diagnose or predict colon cancer in the patient who has or once had colonic polyposis. Unfortunately, diligence can prove as expensive as nonchalance, as colonoscopy with or without polypectomy is attended by a low but ineradicable danger to the patient. Hemorrhage complicates polypectomy when transection is preceded by insufficient stalk coagulation, and perforation may occur if excessive current passes onto the bowel wall or if the instrument is inserted too forcibly into a weakened or stenotic lumen or lured, siren-like, into a wide-mouthed diverticulum.

For both the colonoscopist and the clinician facing the viewbox (and a potentially worrisome future), the continuing question is whether this x ray or that endoscopy was adequate to exclude neoplasia. In either case, the answer mandates thorough pre-examinational bowel cleaning, deliberate and careful inspection, and distrust of, or willingness to repeat, the "negative" study.

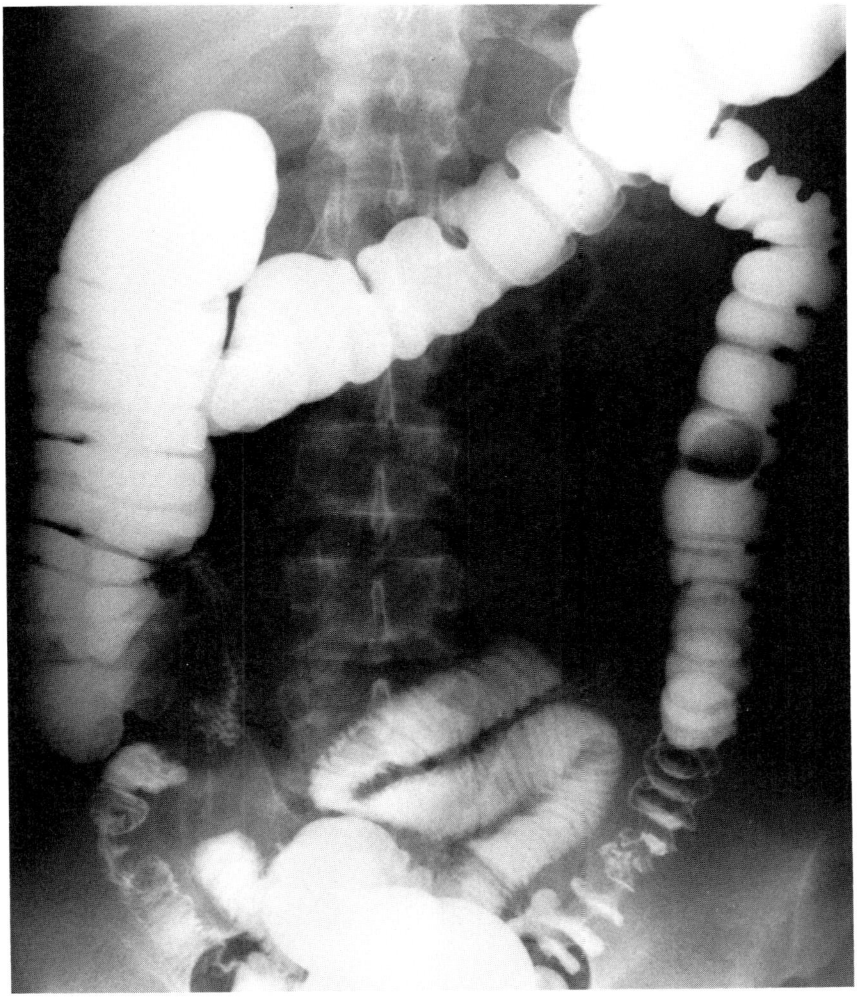

FIG. 5–14. Spherical, smooth, lucent lesion of mid-descending colon, with radiolucent stalk seen inferiorly.

FAMILIAL MULTIPLE POLYPOSIS

This disease is well described; in fact, nearly everything factual needed by the clinician is known about this illness, apart from specific therapy for the individual patient. Transmitted as an autosomal-dominant disease, it consists of multiple adenomatous colon polyps (often numbering in the hundreds) emerging exuberantly from the mucosa and extending from the cecum to the distal rectum. The polyps themselves are typical, varying in shape, age, and size. Most are asymptomatic; some are large enough to obstruct the bowel, while others produce only low-grade bleeding. Only their eventual, certain, individual or multifocal degeneration into carcinomas make the condition unique. Accordingly, management is always surgical. While some enthusiasm might be aroused by the colonoscopist's assurance that he can remove any and all lesions by colonsocope, the ultimate cost of multiple examinations with polypectomy and the high likelihood of missing one or several malignancies argue strongly for colectomy.

However, the best type of surgery required is debated; there are several options. The first and in some ways simplest option is total proctocolectomy with continent or conventional ileostomy; second choice is an ileoanostomy with a perineal-ileal reservoir; finally, there is ileoproctostomy with preservation of the rectum. This last option would seem permissible only in the atypical patient whose rectum contains few or no polyps; it also, of course, mandates regular proctoscopic surveillance for the patient's lifetime, with the nervous understanding that an eventual rectal cancer will certainly require abdomino-peritoneal resection, and might well be discovered too late.

Barium enema in these patients (Fig. 5–15A and B) shows multiple, rounded, radiolucent defects throughout the colon. The lesions are often sessile or, less commonly, pedunculated. The x ray is usually appended with a history of either a first-order relative dying from colon cancer, perhaps with a similar polyp antecedent, or, in the setting of a radiologic survey, of a family member of a patient with known colonic polyposis. Absent a known genetic predisposition, the lesions are identified in the evaluation of rectal bleeding, whether latent or obvious.

FIG. 5–15. A. Air-contrast barium enema showing innumerable polyps. B. Polyps better seen on lateral view of an air-filled rectum with barium coating dozens of visible, spherical mucosal excrescences.

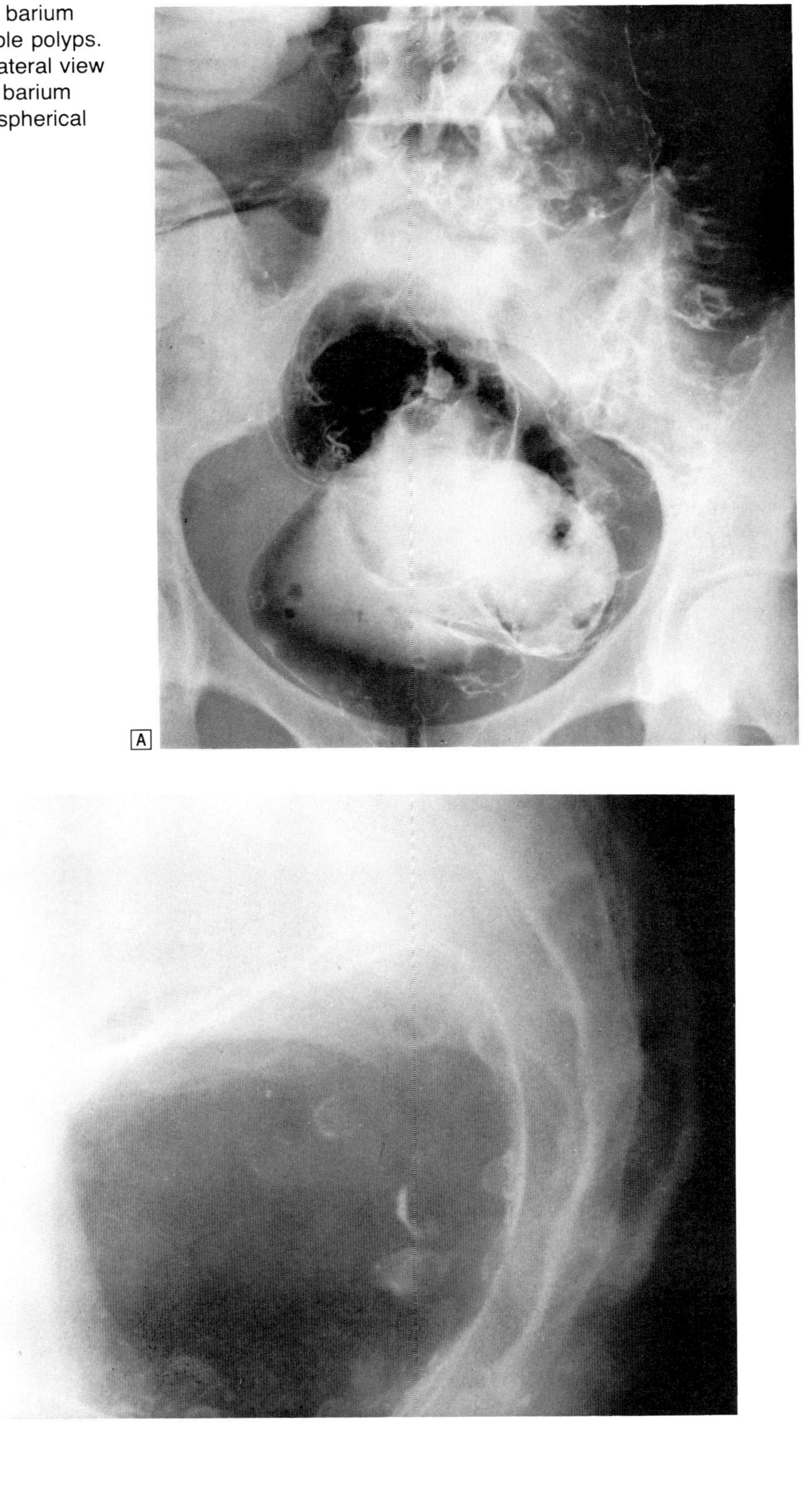

VILLOUS ADENOMA

These lesions are most commonly recalled as a cause of a severe, secretory, watery diarrhea with iron-deficiency anemia, seen typically in elderly patients and often associated with significant potassium deficiency with all its metabolic and muscular complications. Their villous character gives them a tremendous surface area and blood supply; hence, they function as a friable form of intestinal glomerulus, secreting an electrolyte- and blood-rich stool. Anatomically, the lesions are lacy and broad in appearance. Even when sessile or malignant, their typically soft, fleshy texture rarely deforms a barium column. Their malignant potential increases with their size; sessile large adenomas are almost always entirely or focally malignant. The treatment is surgical removal. If the lesion is pedunculated, it may be accomplished via colonoscope.

Despite the clinical picture commonly attributed to them, most villous adenomas are asymptomatic and not associated with diarrhea or hypokalemia, but often with blood loss. They may be multiple or exist in association with a separate synchronous cancer. Suspicion of their presence, even when the barium enema is negative, mandates careful colonosopic examination where they are seen to bleed easily. The frequent focal development of cancer within a large villous adenoma and their often sessile position on the bowel wall argue for operative colotomy or segmental resection. Colonscopy in these lesions is more a diagnostic than therapeutic tool.

Greater than half of all colonic villous adenomas are located in the rectum or sigmoid, making the diagnosis somewhat easier and diarrhea more metabolically significant. Since these adenomas are closest to the point of fecal exit, the small amount of colon distal to them will resorb their secretions only slightly. Hence, when they are functional, their metabolic significance is often enormous. There have been reports of hypokalemia-induced quadriparesis or shock, particularly in the elderly.

Because colonic villous adenomas are, in truth, merely a form of adenomatous polyp, the same carcinoma caveats that pertain to their more prosaic relatives apply. There may be other polypoid lesions present, and a small number of them can very well be cancerous.

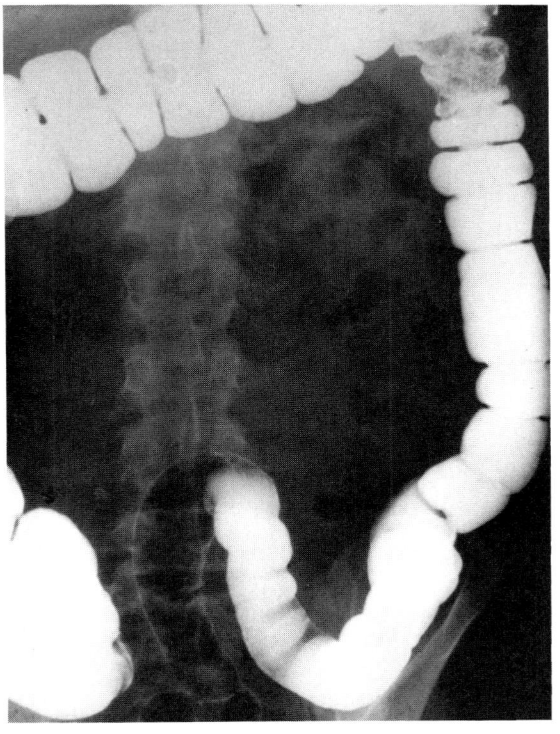

FIG. 5–16. A. Lacy mottling of barium noted over a rounced, focal defect of upper descending colon. Despite large size of lesion, the colon wall is not altered, nor is barium blocked.

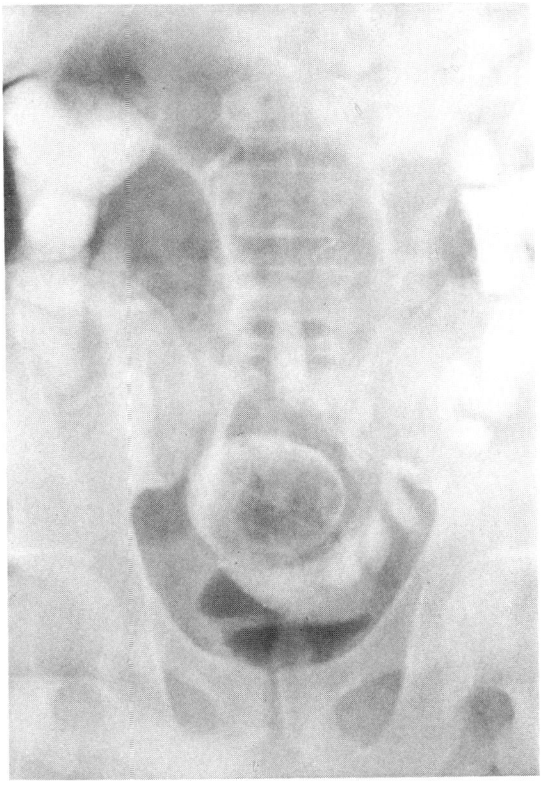

B. Enormous spherical "lucent" lesion of rectosigmoid. The distal location increases its metabolic implications (hypokalemia or diarrheal dehydration).

DIVERTICULOSIS—GENERAL REMARKS

Diverticulosis results from an aging and weakened colon's seemingly paradoxic, exaggerated capacity for both storage and contraction. Portions of bowel wall uncovered by smooth muscle passively herniate, forming these separate, often multiple saccular extrusions. Because its smooth-muscle development and intraluminal pressures are the highest, the sigmoid understandably has the greatest number and density of diverticula. However, they can occur anywhere, from cecum to the peritoneal reflection above the rectum. When diffuse, they are typically asymptomatic. Figure 5–17A and B shows the unusual capacity of diverticula for development, implying that the diverticula themselves sometimes account for a substantial portion of the bowel's reservoir function.

Several important issues deserve mention. Because diverticulosis can obscure mucosal visualization by barium, the question of a simultaneous carcinoma is commonly raised and is sometimes difficult to resolve. A classic example emerges when investigations of occult GI bleeding or abdominal pain disclose only diverticulosis. Though aware that diverticula sometimes bleed slowly, the careful doctor knows further that his patient may have "fleas and lice at the same time" and fights the temptation to think that he has done enough searching. Yet along with its rewards, clinical competence may have a price; a fragile bowel wall may be perforated from the pressure of an extra or incorrectly timed barium column or a colonscope. Thus, other studies, or more than one x-ray examination, perhaps done more carefully and separated by several weeks, may be required.

Another issue is the complication of diverticulosis by inflammatory bowel disease. Since the diverticulum, by definition, lacks a muscular layer, it is more predisposed to perforation when leukocytic infiltration and mucosal necrosis occur from any type of colitis.

Clearly a disease of Western man living in an industrialized society, diverticulosis is rare in populations subsisting on vegetarian or high-roughage diets. Hence, the high-fiber admonitions of contemporary physicians to patients with diverticulosis seem physiogically supportable.

Finally, a remark on noninflammatory abdominal pain and diverticulosis: When limited to or clustered about the sigmoid colon, diverticula seem to associate with hypertrophy of bowel smooth muscle there and may induce the bowel spasm and constipation suggested as causes of the irritable-colon syndrome.

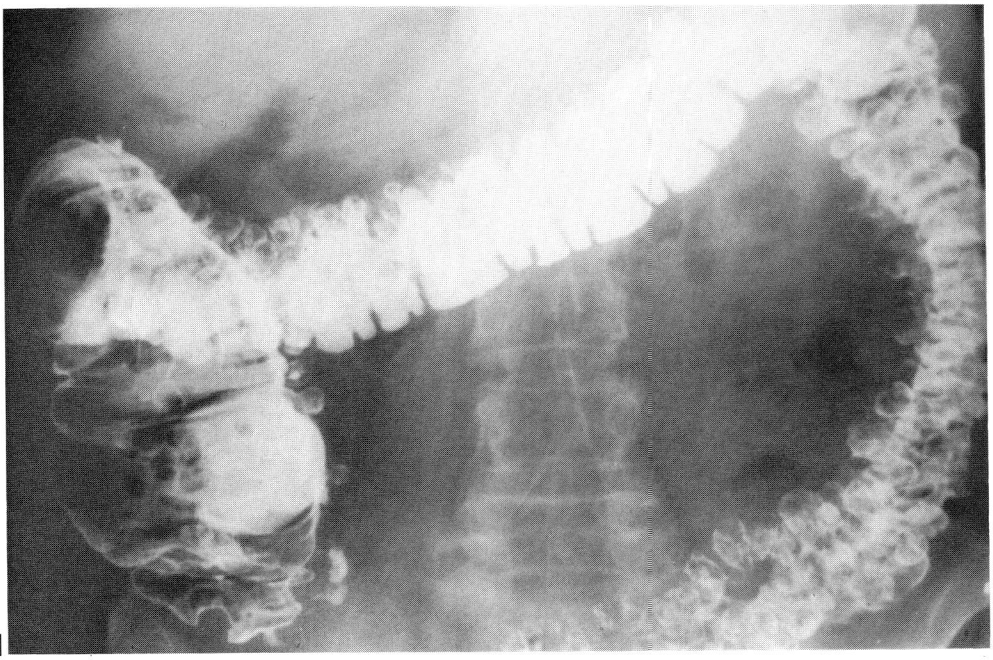

A

FIG. 5–17. A. Filled barium x ray of patient with pan-colonic diverticulosis. B. Plain film, one week later (same patient), showing failure of diverticula to empty.

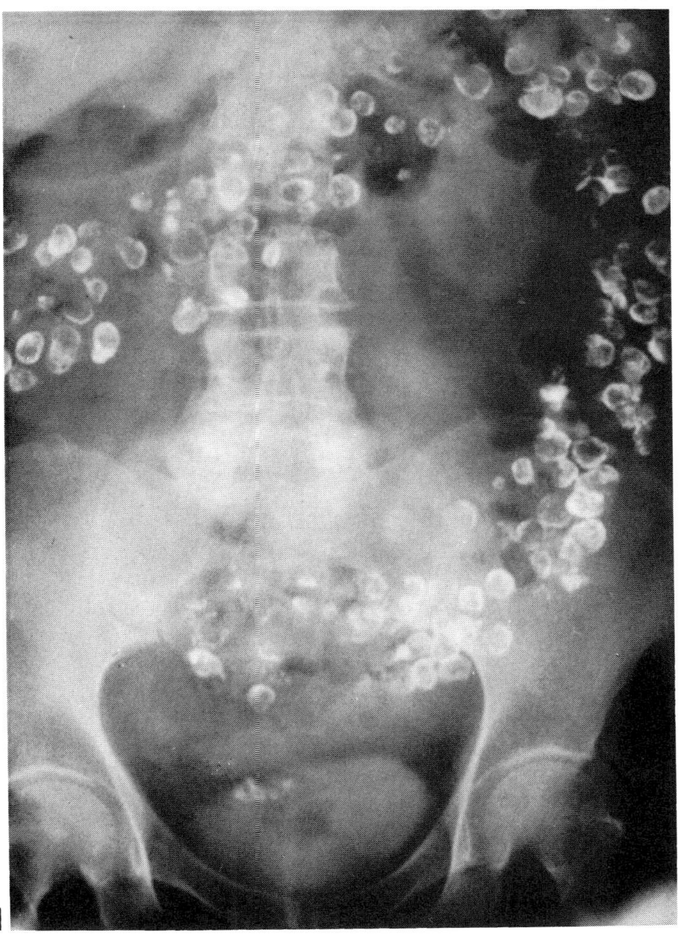

B

DIVERTICULOSIS AND BLEEDING

Probably emerging from a vascular break in the neck of a single, expanding colon diverticulum, and likewise a curse of the elderly, the bleeding of colonic diverticulosis is typically massive and sudden. It usually begins with some cramping but is followed by otherwise painless yet continuous evacuation of voluminous bloody, purplish stools with clot. The hypotension that commonly follows diminishes colon blood flow and probably helps terminate the emergency, which often ceases spontaneously and just as abruptly.

When hemorrhage recurs, continues, or accelerates with a significant transfusion requirement, only the correct diagnosis and surgery are life-saving. Despite the dream of visualizing the single bleeding diverticulum, which would allow specific segmental resection, cleansing enemas usually fail to prepare the bowel adequately for any useful endoscopic examination, except when a view of unobscured rectal mucosa discloses the rare ulcerative proctocolitis that appears with gross hemorrhage. The color or character of bloody feces cannot be relied upon to localize the bleeding source. Unless it discloses the rare clear-cut, focal extravasation (as in Figure 5–18) or a conspicuous AV malformation, angiography may consume time, blood, and opportunity without being of help. This also seems true of radionuclide bleeding scans. Moreover, the repetitive infusion of intravascular dye may injure old kidneys already affected by arteriosclerosis or a mercurial blood pressure.

The question of how much colon is to be removed is answered with knowledge of both of the presence and location of colonic diverticula. If barium enema reveals a cluster in only one area, segmental resection seems justified. Conventional x rays of bleeding and nonbleeding diverticulosis, however, are identical. If diverticula occur in both the right and left halves of the large bowel, how much colon is to be resected to guarantee surgical hemostasis? Paradoxically, the largest operation, subtotal colectomy and ileoproctostomy, seems also the most conservative.

The disproportionally high frequency of bleeding from the less common ascending colon diverticula deserves attention. While the blood vessels of the proximal colon could be more fragile, some right-sided bleeding in generalized diverticulosis may actually arise from adjacent, concomitant arteriovenous malformations, which typically favor the ascending or proximal transverse colon and are, of course, invisible to conventional x rays. More importantly, resecting the wrong half or third of the colon, simply because it contains *most* of the diverticula or a nonbleeding angioma, risks a second operation whose added mortality far exceeds that of a single, definitive procedure. Happily, ileoproctostomies are rarely associated with disabling diarrhea.

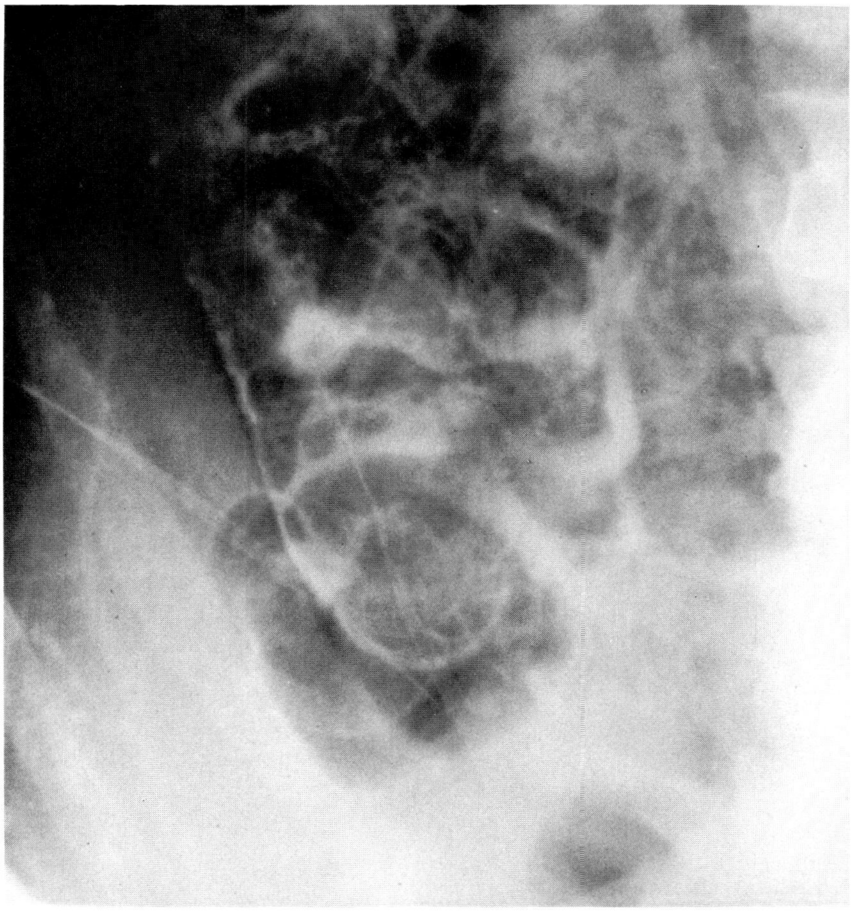

FIG. 5–18. Extravasation of intra-aterial dye into the cecum and ascending colon, identifying site of hemorrhage in a patient with universal diverticulosis. Right colectomy was curative.

If impacted with stool, or thinned, a diverticulum can perforate, usually at its base, thus producing a localized peritonitis. Figure 5–19A shows segmental, spastic, or fixed narrowing of diverticula-bearing bowel, almost always over the sigmoid, occasionally with actual obstruction to the retrograde flow of barium. On careful inspection, indentation of the diverticula's normally flask-like base is noted. An associated, smooth, extrinsic deformity on the bowel suggests a pericolic or mesenteric abscess. Occasionally, "blind" fistula, seen as streaks of barium, extend out from or connect into adjacent diverticula. Under rare and understandably frantic circumstances, contrast may be seen leaking (Fig. 5–19B) into an adjacent hollow organ or the free peritoneum, the latter identifying a surgical emergency.

Left lower abdominal pain, fever, leukocytosis, and a tender mass in a middle-aged or elderly person almost always indicate diverticulitis. But a perforative carcinoma, focal inflammatory bowel disease, or an ischemic event must be considered. The diagnostic gold standard is still the careful barium enema, attended by a forewarned, meticulous fluoroscopist, so that in the event of perforation, either induced or documented, contrast infusion can be halted and the responsible physician and surgeon alerted immediately.

The usual initial treatment of uncomplicated diverticulitis is carefully medical, with the replacement of a solid diet with fluids, the parenteral administration of broad-spectrum (or multiple) antibiotics, and, for the cautious, a surgical consultation. Though most attacks resolve medically, diverticulitis must be treated with the greatest respect by the internist or generalist, who must be conscious that it is a form of peritonitis and a potential source of sepsis, fistulas, or intra-abominal abscess.

These complications, as well as recurrent attacks, argue for surgery, which, if done electively in a stable patient whose operation has been preceded by a period of bowel "sterilization," can be completed by single-stage resection of the inflammatory mass and primary anastomosis. But if diverticulitis is complicated by abscess, communicating fistula, or perforation, immediate anastomosis risks early breakdown by infected sutures, and temporary colostomy is considered safest by most surgeons. Some patients thought to need an operation will spontaneously drain necrotic or infected abscess contents back into the colon lumen for rectal expulsion. Because hemorrhage typically occurs from uninfected diverticula, diverticulitis and significant rectal bleeding rarely occur together.

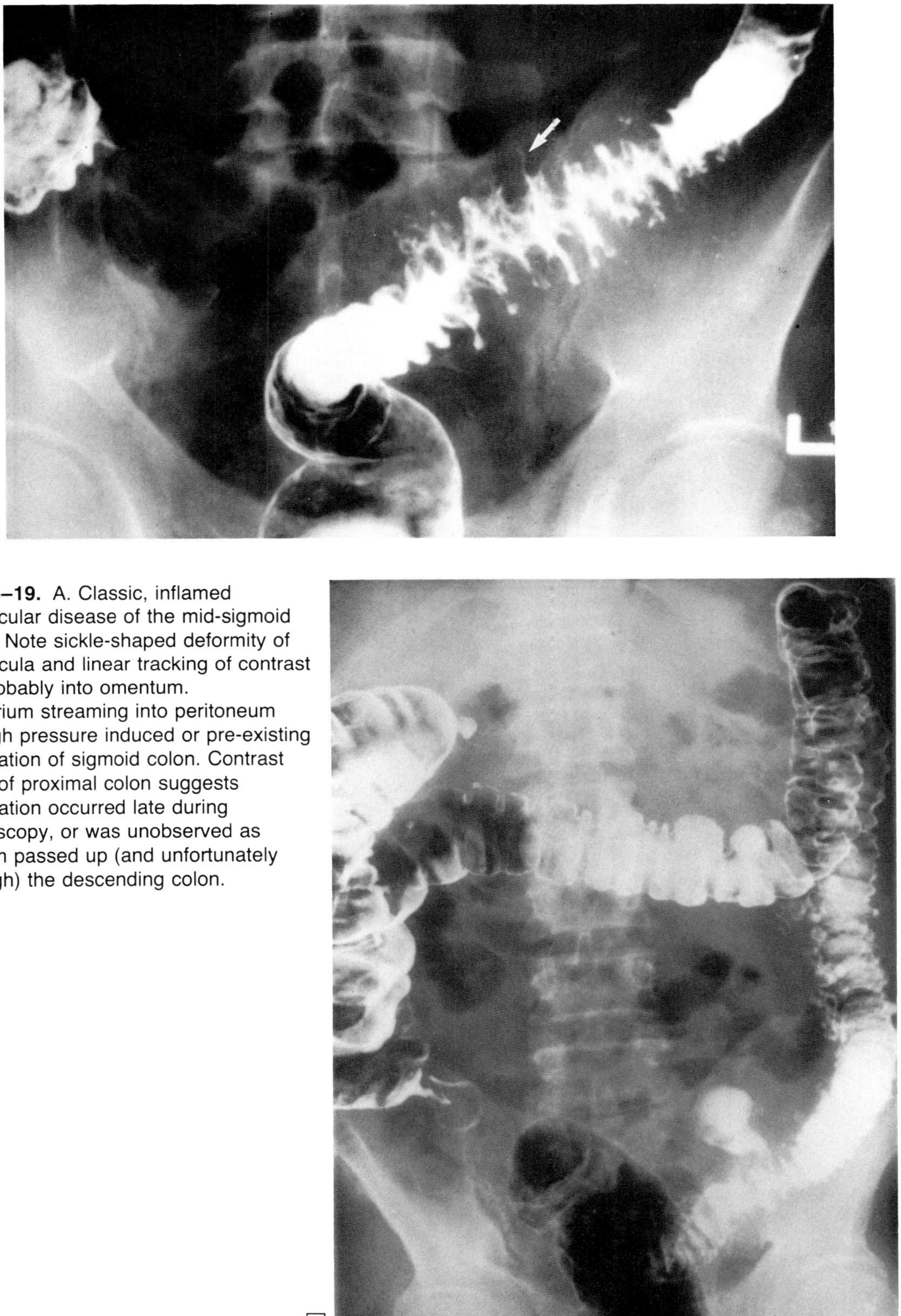

A

B

FIG. 5–19. A. Classic, inflamed diverticular disease of the mid-sigmoid colon. Note sickle-shaped deformity of diverticula and linear tracking of contrast ↑, probably into omentum.
B. Barium streaming into peritoneum through pressure induced or pre-existing perforation of sigmoid colon. Contrast filling of proximal colon suggests perforation occurred late during fluoroscopy, or was unobserved as barium passed up (and unfortunately through) the descending colon.

ACQUIRED MEGACOLON—LAXATIVE ABUSE

Like any overused muscle's tendency to hypertrophy, the large intestine regularly thrashed by oral laxatives will eventually dilate and lengthen, further increasing its capaciousness. This barium enema (Fig. 5–20) displays the typical, probably irreversible result of decades of hypercatharsis, administered in the obsessive notion that daily or voluminous evacuations were necessary for health, hygiene, or beauty. Given the recent surge in (or awareness of) bulemic disease, x rays like this will undoubtedly increase in frequency.

This typical film shows an elongated, dilated, much-folded colon whose loss of haustral markings is conspicuous and reminiscent of the contracted version seen in chronic ulcerative colitis. Large volumes of residual colonic fluid are often noted diluting barium within the lumen. Offending agents include casanthranol, phenolphthaline, castor derivatives, and, less commonly employed, magnesia or bile salts. Since laxative takers tend to be closed-mouthed about discussing (but not taking) their drugs, pills found within a widened barium column should also come as no surprise to the clinician or radiologist. Chronic use of phenolphthaline laxatives is often associated with brownish pigmentation of the rectal mucosa, as seen on proctoscopy (melanosis coli); this association may be a way of confirming the diagnosis in a patient who denies laxative use.

As it does in the chronically constipated patient, protracted diarrhea, including that of the malabsorption syndromes, may lead to colon enlargement and redundancy. This megacolon favors volvulus developing either in ascending or sigmoid colon. Serious mineral depletion, malnutrition, and dehydration may develop in laxative takers.

Differential diagnostic considerations include the adult form of Hirschsprung's disease, hypothyroidism, chronic habit constipation, idiopathic pseudo-obstruction, or any organic distal colonic stenosis. But the major disability is usually both psychic and physiologic, with an understandable dependence on increasing use of laxatives and enemas. Regardless of whether the laxatives are the cause or the result of an anatomic or autonomic abnormality, subtotal colectomy is often required, just as it is in cases of idiopathic megacolon or recurrent pseudo-obstruction. Taking refuge in the "cookbook" approach by reserving major operations for so-called "real disease" will leave many of these patients perpetually disabled.

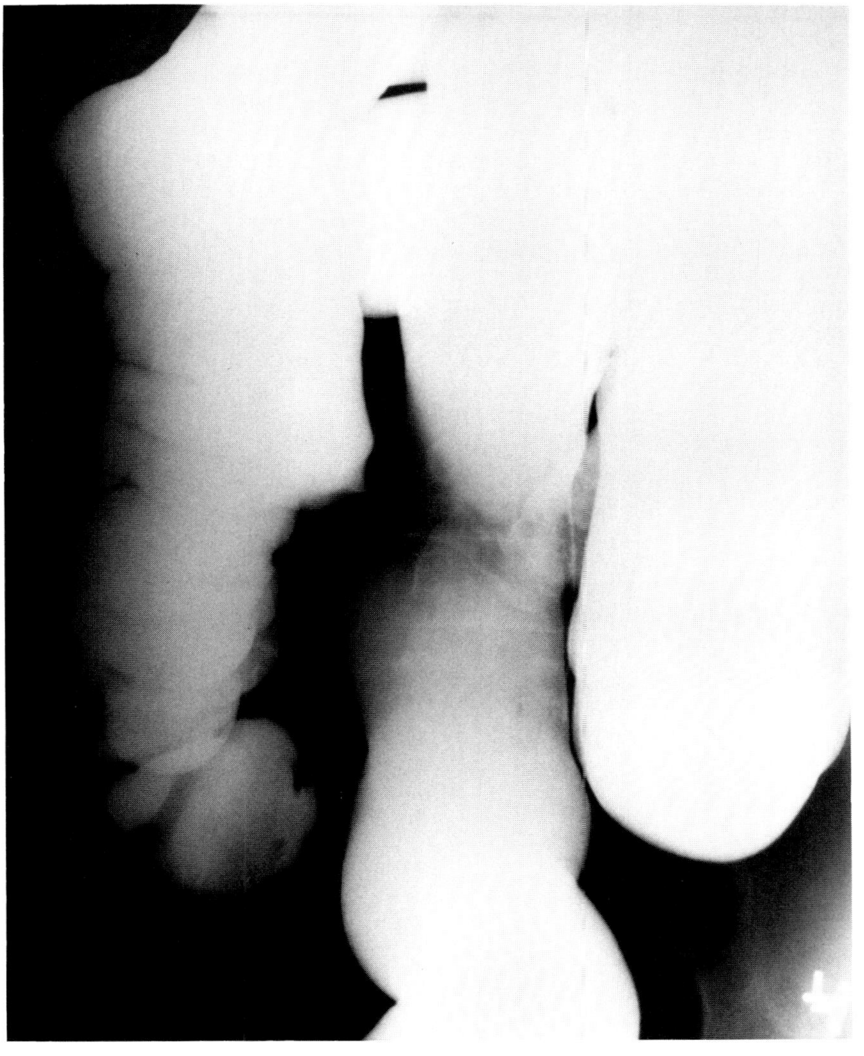

FIG. 5–20. An enormous, barium-filled colon virtually filling the peritoneal cavity. An elongated sigmoid extends almost to the diaphragm, returns to the pelvis, then swinging into the left upper quadrant.

HIRSCHSPRUNG'S DISEASE

This congenital, aganglionic megacolon usually becomes apparent in the neonatal period by the simultaneous appearance of abdominal distention and failure to pass meconium or feces. However, a few patients, particularly those with a small denervated segment, present in adulthood. The linkage of anatomy and physiology in Hirschsprung's disease is essentially absolute. The intramyenteric ganglia are always absent from the area of the internal anal sphincter and proximally to a variable degree; the extent is demonstrable by microscopic examination of deep, occasionally near-full-thickness biopsies taken per rectum.

When the normal rectum distends with feces or gas, the internal anal sphincter relaxes and the external anal sphincter contracts. The contrary Hirschsprung pathophysiology is confirmed by failure of the internal anal sphincter to relax with rectal distention and is easily determined by laboratory balloon manometry. The dysmotility is reminiscent of the failure of the distal esophageal sphincter to relax in esophageal achalasia, a disease also associated with intramural neural loss.

Hirschsprung's disease can be managed by operative resection of the aganglionic segment and "pull-through" of normal rectum to the external sphincter. Some degree of late postoperative fecal incontinence often remains, but colostomy is usually unnecessary. Though rarely first evident in adulthood, Hirschsprung's disease should be considered in the differential diagnosis of any severely obstipated patient when contemplating the megacolon of recurrent "pseudo-obstruction" or in patients with chronic laxative abuse.

The barium enema (Fig. 5–21A) clearly reveals a pliable narrowing of the most distal anorectum, immediately below a massively dilated, feces-filled large intestine. The plain film of the abdomen (Fig. 5–21B) often displays the distended mottling of a diffuse fecal impaction. Almost certainly involving a herculean effort, bowel movements may occur as infrequently as once every 3 to 4 weeks, followed by a predictable 10 to 20 lbs. of weight loss.

In preparation of such a patient for barium enema, or in attempts at symptom relief, the cleansing-enema requirements should be monitored carefully as they may be substantial, risking both excessive colonic fluid absorption and total body-water overload.

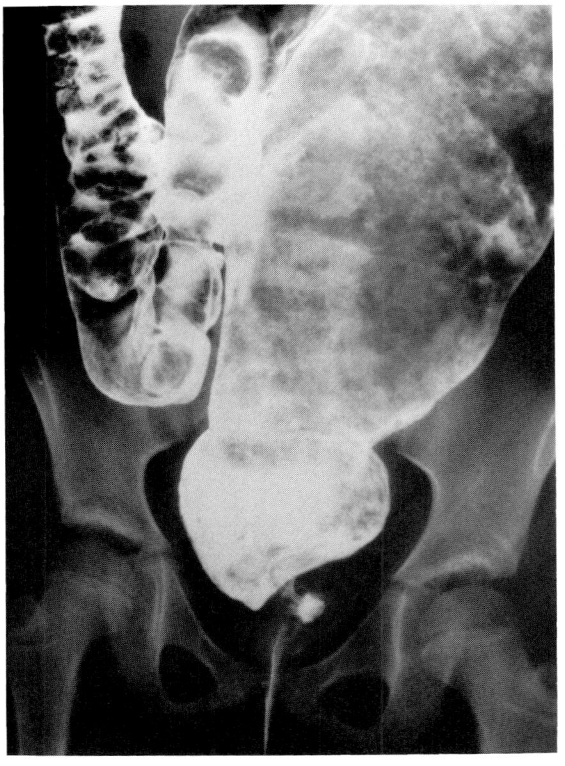

FIG. 5–21. A. Barium enema with constricted rectal segment below a wide, smoothly dilated and lengthened sigmoid.

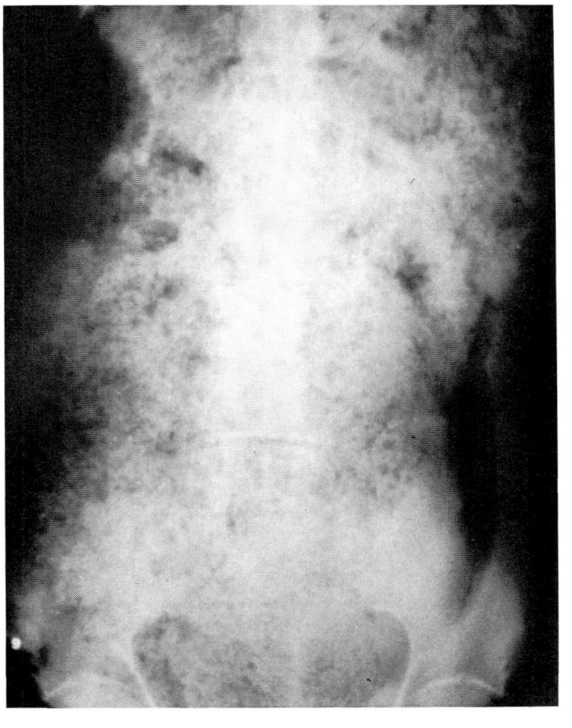

B. Plain film of abdomen showing intraluminal feces filling virtually the entire peritoneal cavity.

SIGMOID VOLVULUS

This form of large-intestinal blockage is manifested radiologically by clockwise or counter-clockwise torsion of a redundant sigmoid, probably occurring on a correspondingly lengthy mesentery. Resulting bowel obstruction may be acute and complete or partial and spontaneously remitting. It is often preceded by the megacolon of chronically constipated patients. Accordingly, it is seen frequently in the elderly, debilitated, and bedridden. Paradoxically, it is also the commonest cause of bowel obstruction in nonindustrialized nations. Thus, it may also be a distant manifestation of a vegetarian diet or chronic diarrheal disease. Whether the cause is dietary, an intestinal parasite, chronic laxative abuse, a bile-salt-wasting syndrome, or an inflammatory or atrophic intestinal disease, long-standing diarrhea frequently results in the colonic elongation that renders it more disposed to this form of rotation.

The most reliable radiologic sign is that of an obstructed sigmoid with two distended, often parallel air-filled limbs extending obliquely out of the pelvis in a more or less "coffee-bean" pattern (Fig. 5–22A). Once the diagnosis is suspected, immediate management is digital emptying of the rectum, should an impaction be present. Decompressing the volvulus by derotating its distal kink may be accomplished by careful introduction of a rigid sigmoidoscope or with a barium column infused under gentle pressure with scrupulous fluoroscopy. If these initial maneuvers are unsuccessful, exploration and manual derotation of the distal colon are mandatory. Even if not yet gangrenous or perforative, an exceedingly redundant sigmoid (Fig. 5–22B) should be resected if future, similar emergencies are to be avoided.

Volvulus of the sigmoid is rarely caused by malignancy, but in any illness in which large bowel obstruction is preceded by either chronic constipation or diarrhea, that possibility needs consideration.

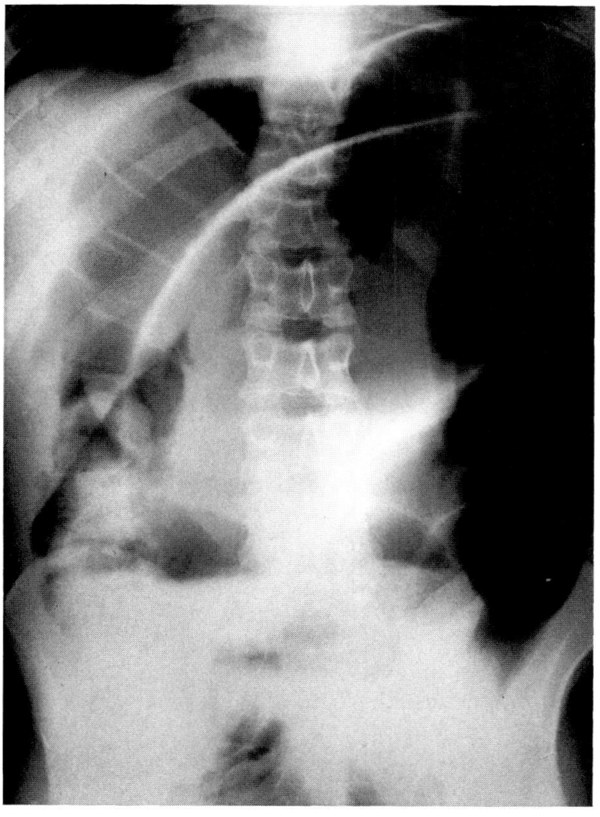

FIG. 5–22. A. Upright plain film revealing typical "coffee bean" configuration of an acutely obstructed, redundant sigmoid colon.

B. Air contrast barium study after non-surgical relief of volvulus. The deflated "coffee-bean" contour of the markedly redundant sigmoid remains, warning of likely recurrence.

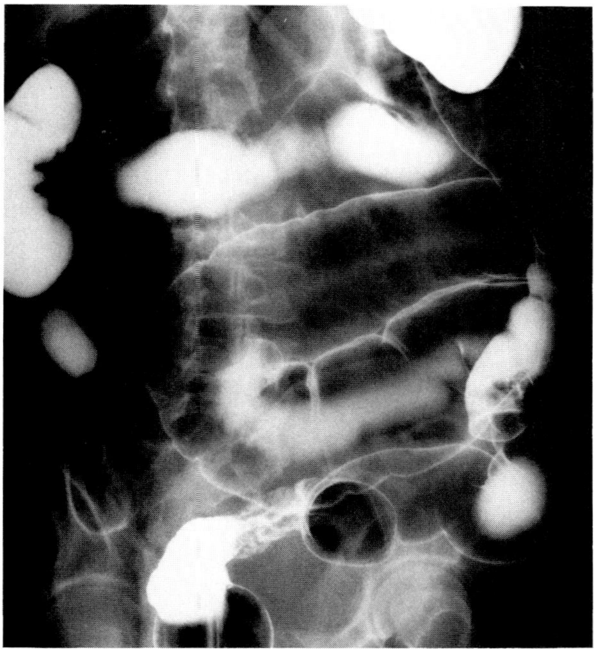

CECAL VOLVULUS

The occasional misplacement of an inflamed appendix's tenderness is not the only clinical consequence of the right colon's frequent exaggerated mobility. Because of a redundant mesentery or malrotation, the proximal colon and cecum may travel to any portion of the abdomen, occasionally twisting on its anchor to cause an occlusive obstruction. Cecal volvulus, for the most part, is a misnomer given the cecal distention associated with right-colon volvulus. The x rays (Fig. 5–23A and B) that give the syndrome its name reveal here a large, spherical, or ovoid abdominal shadow, with a horizontal air-fluid level, connecting the walls of obvious thinly stretched bowel. Tender distention and tympany in the right lower quadrant are usually evident. If there are no or few air-fluid levels in the distal small bowel, the ileocecal valve is assumed to be competent, which unfortunately prevents regurgitative decompression into the ileum. A true closed-loop obstruction is thus created, increasing the likelihood of cecal rupture.

The colonic dilatation occurring in chronic laxative abuse, constipation, or diarrheal disease does not seem to be a precursor of volvulus of the right colon, as it clearly is in the sigmoid. Likewise, there is no likely derotative remedy by cathartic enemas, a retrograde barium column, or a sigmoidoscope. Moreover, the air instillation required in the passage of a colonoscope would further distend the cecum.

If the patient gives a history of recurrent, similar previous attacks with spontaneous decompression, the treatment is clearly operative. Depending on the surgeon's perceptions at laparotomy, an attempt could be made to either derotate the right colon first or to precede that by aspiration and decompression of the cecum. If there are no signs of peritoneal irritation, and if ischemic changes have not yet occurred, then simply suturing the cecum back into its rightful place in the right lower quadrant will prevent recurrences. Nasogastric tube decompression should probably be employed, but it must be recognized as only a token act. The bowel obstruction is too distal for aspiration of gastric contents to be helpful.

Occasionally, a carcinoma of the proximal ascending colon will complete its slow centripetal growth by producing an air-distended, obstructed cecum, but this issue is likewise resolved at surgery. In those patients with an exceedingly long right colon, the cecum may not seem to fit into the right lower quadrant, and occasionally flops upward and posteriorly onto the ascending colon. Involving only cecal mobility, this abnormality rarely creates or resembles bowel obstruction.

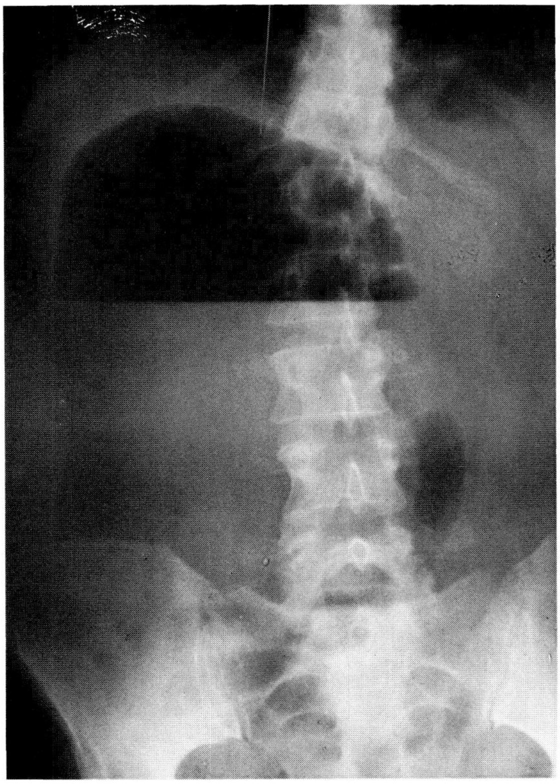

FIG. 5–23. A. Upturned, obstructed, and widely distended cecum with a right upper quadrant air-fluid level.

B. In the recumbent position, the obstruction is equally evident, particularly the twisting of the upper ascending colon.

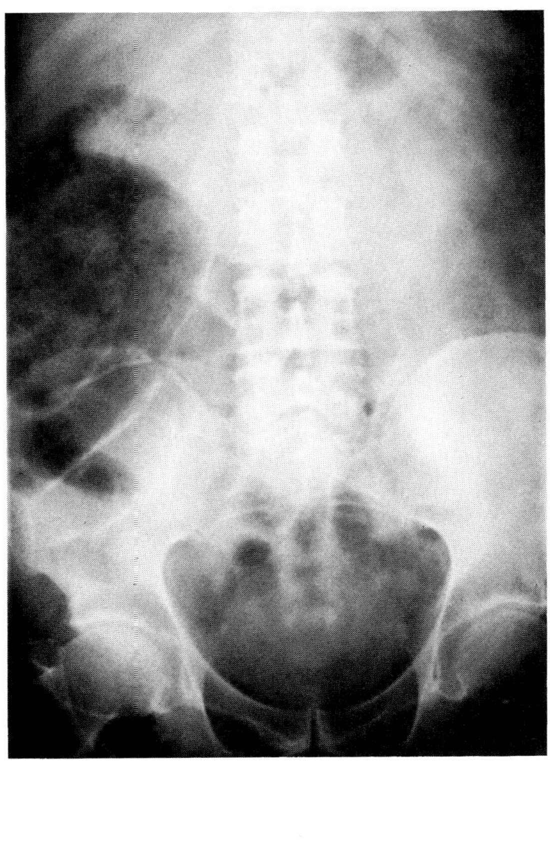

Radiologically, the cecum and rectum are the favored residences of an ameboma, the term employed to describe a heaped-up, focal, intramural proliferative hive of Entamoeba histolytica. While the x-ray changes are not specific, deformed mucosa in those areas should raise the possibility of amebiasis, particularly in patients with a clinical or travel history consistent with parasite infestation. The cecum's normally smooth acorn shape tends to become ragged and conical (Fig. 5–24A and B) in amebiasis, with its edges tapering inferiorly. Pre-existing inflammatory bowel disease does not exclude intercurrent development of amebiasis. Accordingly, microscopic stool examinations are reasonable, even for patients with established idiopathic enterocolitis in exacerbation, using the logic employed in a search for Clostridium difficile toxin in a similar setting.

Hepatomegaly suggests associated amebic hepatitis or amebic liver abscess (usually in the right lobe). Elevation or tenting of the right hemidiaphragm seen on chest x ray warns of an expanding liver abscess, threatening erosion into the thorax. Any attempt at surgical drainage should be preceded by vigorous antiprotozoal therapy, as inadvertent dissemination of viable trophozoites into a body cavity can be fatal.

Despite the large number of stool parasite examinations performed, the disease is probably underdiagnosed. Because their symptoms are often similar, and amebiasis is so easily managed with generally non-toxic, inexpensive agents, empiric amebicidal therapy in selected patients with recurrent inflammatory bowel disease seems inarguable. To some, a protozoan superinfection is inferred by the response of occasional patients with Crohn's disease to metronidazole.

While x ray is useful in a diagnosis of amebiasis, fecal contamination by instilled particulate barium will delay visual identification of both trophozoites and cysts. Physicans should not forgo an opportunity for diagnosis in patients who need their stools inspected, yet may have "just gone to the bathroom." Such patients can be provided with preservative containers to be inoculated during laxative preparation for x ray. Diagnosis can also be accelerated by prompt microscopic examination of liquid stool or mucus aspirated at proctoscopy. Positive rectal biopsies suggest heavy infestation and are usually found in patients in whom the diagnosis is already strongly suspected. Indirect hemagglutination testing is particularly valuable where there is hepatic involvement.

While amebiasis occurs mostly in immunocompetent heterosexuals, it can be transmitted venereally along with innumerable other protozoa, fungi, and bacteria included in the "gay-bowel" syndrome and AIDS (e.g., Endolimax nana, Giardia lamblia, Isospora belli, Cryptosporidium, Salmonella, and Shigella). The rapidly absorbed metronidazole has replaced emetine in therapy of tissue-invasive amebiasis; the poorly absorbed drugs (paramomycin or di-iodohydroxyquin) may be more effective when infestation is restricted to the bowel.

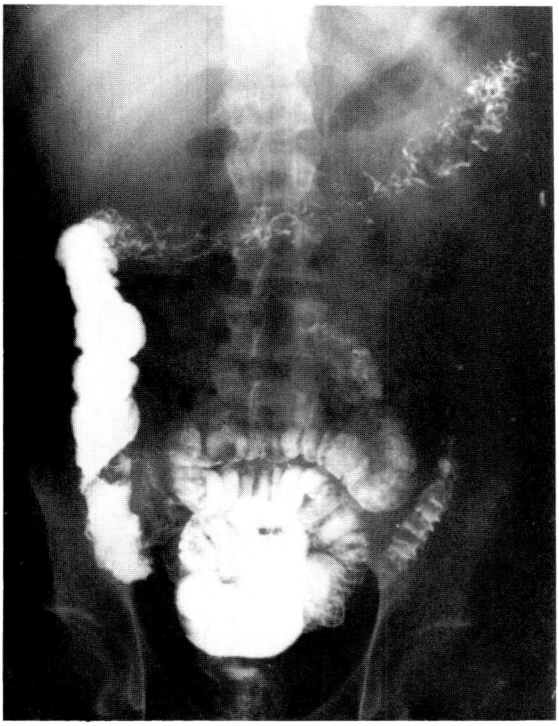

FIG. 5–24. A. Shaggy distortion of cecal mucosa is noted in the right lower quadrant. The cecum appears more cylindrical or conical than acorn- or pear-shaped.

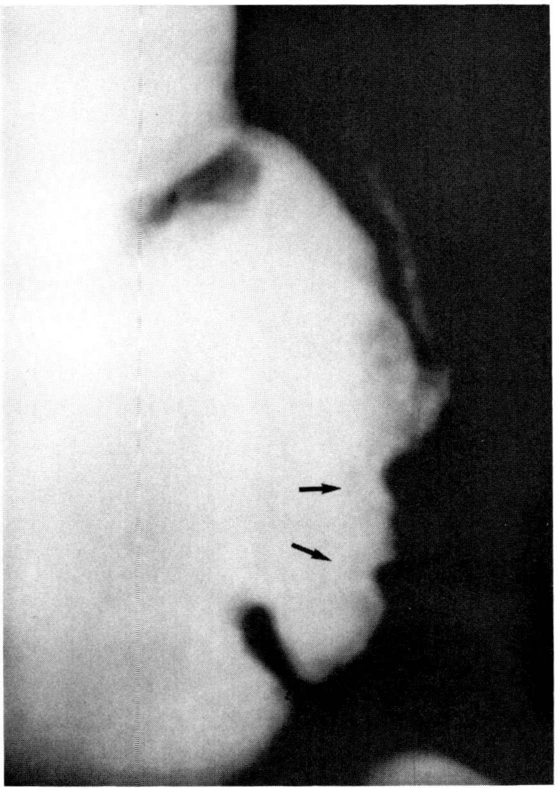

B. An intramural mass lesion (ameboma) is apparent on closeup view of the cecum.

ISCHEMIC COLITIS

While acute infarctions of the large intestine are not terribly common or even frequently identified, their bedside presentation, clinical setting, and radiologic findings seem notably uniform. Understandably, the background will usually include a patient of advanced age with narrowed intestinal or aortic vessels, or perhaps with an augmented potential for cardiac embolization or hypercoagulable blood. An antecedent paraproteinemia, thrombocytosis, atrial fibrillation, ventricular aneurysm, or severe abdominal aortic arteriosclerosis are examples. Though neither sick nor elderly, young women taking oral contraceptives develop colon infarctions with a frequency sufficient to warrant their inclusion among those at risk.

Unlike patients with typical superior mesenteric vascular insuffiency, there is rarely a prodrome of abdominal angina. Rather, ischemic colitis usually begins abruptly, with severe, cramping abdominal pain, often associated with watery, blood-tinged stools resulting from mucosal necrosis. The infarctions are generally focal and single. Probably because of the plethora of collateral colonic arteries or simultaneous venous infarction, the ischemic areas appear radiologically hyperplastic rather than thinned. Though bloody diarrhea is characteristic of infarcted colon, serial hematocrits generally show a paradoxic transitory increase, as if the patient were becoming dehydrated, as the diseased bowel sequesters lost intraluminal tissue fluid in excess of blood cells.

At the bedside, more common alternative considerations include acute inflammatory bowel disease and diverticulitis. When the rectum or rectosigmoid is infarcted, sigmoidoscopically visualized hemorrhage or ulceration may suggest inflammatory polyposis, while intramural bleeding is likely to obscure underlying cyanosis. The biopsies are similar, except when small vascular thromboses are present, favoring the ischemic process. In diverticulitis, it's helpful to recall that the rectum is endoscopically normal and that luminal bleeding is rare. When the ruminated diagnoses include inflammatory or perforative diseases, the employment of antibiotics lethal to aerobic and anaerobic colon bacteria seems imperative, and the patient's abdomen must be considered potentially operable until there is clinical stabilization.

X rays, such as those seen in Figure 5–25, show a solitary, cobblestone, or "thumbprinting" stenosis, often visibily silhouetted against bowel gas on an abdominal plain film, further confirmed by barium enema. Ileus is a common accompaniment. Unlike the gangrenous progression of midgut infarctions, the clinical and x-ray events in ischemic colitis typically resolve, though some permanent bowel narrowing may remain.

While in the strictest sense a definitive diagnosis seems to demand arteriography, the finding of even severe aortic or mesenteric stenosis does not establish a diagnosis of ischemic colitis. Moreover, manipulating a catheter into the narrowed tributary of an already caked, sclerotic aorta risks causing or worsening the very event one is considering.

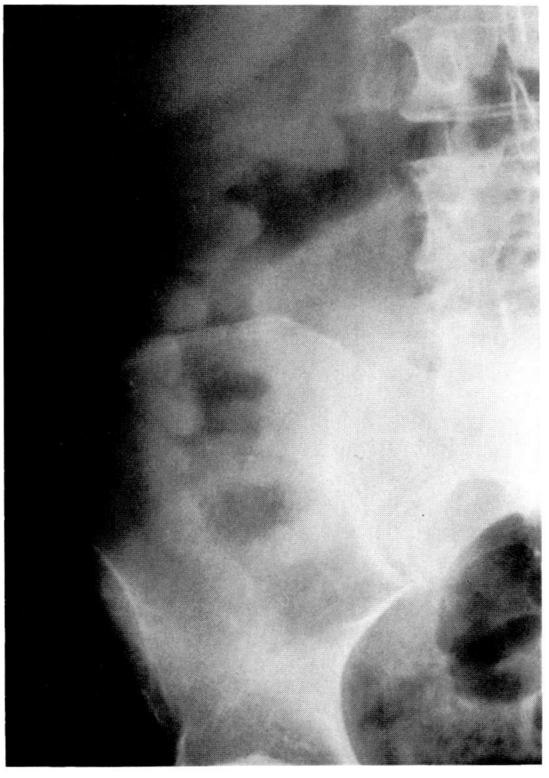

FIG. 5–25. A. Thumbprint indentations on antimesenteric border of ascending and proximal transverse colon, visualized against the air shadow of a focal ileus. Infarction of a branch of the superior mesenteric artery occurred in a previously healthy female on oral contraceptives.

B. Focal circumferential thumbprinting of mid-transverse colon on barium x ray. This broad scalloping occurs also in infiltrative malignancy and focal Crohn's disease.

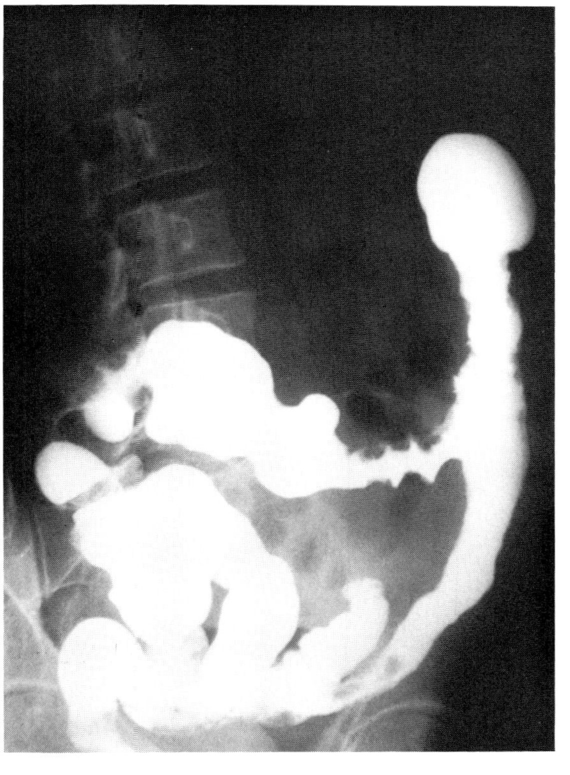

PSEUDOMEMBRANOUS COLITIS

This is a disease of medical progress, with clinical features of medical antiquity: a cholera-like secretory diarrhea with an almost diphtheritic membrane lining the colon. Because pseudomembranous colitis is usually acute, often suspected by history and partially confirmed at proctoscopy, and because barium enemas are best avoided in patients with fulminant diarrhea, this disorder typically isn't (and sometimes shouldn't be) seen on contrast study. Intractable and innumerable dehydrating, nonbloody, purulent stools characteristically follow the oral administration of antibiotics, particularly those effective against gram-positive organisms (e.g., clindamycin, erythromycin, ampicillin, cephalosporins). However, this disease, as well as simple diarrhea, can develop after any antibiotic given by any route, or with no antibiotic antecedent.

Most inflammatory changes are on the mucosal surface (*intra*luminal). The typical barium enema discloses multiple, elevated plaques of coagulated granulocytes lining the mucosa, always best seen on air-contrast views in the sigmoid colon (Fig. 5–26A). The right colon is rarely involved. To the sharp-eyed observer, barium is sometimes seen dissecting, under a coalescent "pseudomembrane" of coagulated leukocytes and fibrin, parallel to the rectal lumen. (Fig. 5–26B). Toxic megacolon has been described; in debilitated patients, pseudomembranous colitis can be fatal. Repeatedly (but not invariably) implicated, the causative agent seems to be the toxin of Clostridium difficile found in the feces. In addition to vigorous rehydration and mineral replacement, treatments include oral vancomycin, trimethoprim-sulfamethoxazole, and, rarely, corticosteroids.

The most important alternative consideration is acute ulcerative colitis, in which the colonic mucosa may be undermined sufficiently on x ray to suggest a pseudomembrane, but the "plaques" are not seen, and gross bleeding characteristically occurs. To confuse matters somewhat, flare-ups of ulcerative colitis have been associated with the appearance of Clostridium difficile toxin in the stool; this relationship, if any, is not understood.

Another form of pseudomembranous colitis is caused by bowel ischemia complicated by intestinal staphylococcal overgrowth. This variant of pseudomembranous colitis may also be preceded by antibiotic therapy, but usually in the volume-depleted, wasted, often diabetic patient, with an antecedent bowel obstruction or ileus. There, the stool gram-stain reveals sheets of staphylococci in addition to leukocytes and tissue macrophages, and the x ray may disclose the ominous intraumural gas of bowel-wall necrosis. While the cause and treatment of both diseases include specific bacteria and antibiotics, the outlook in "staphylococcal colitis" is understandably far worse.

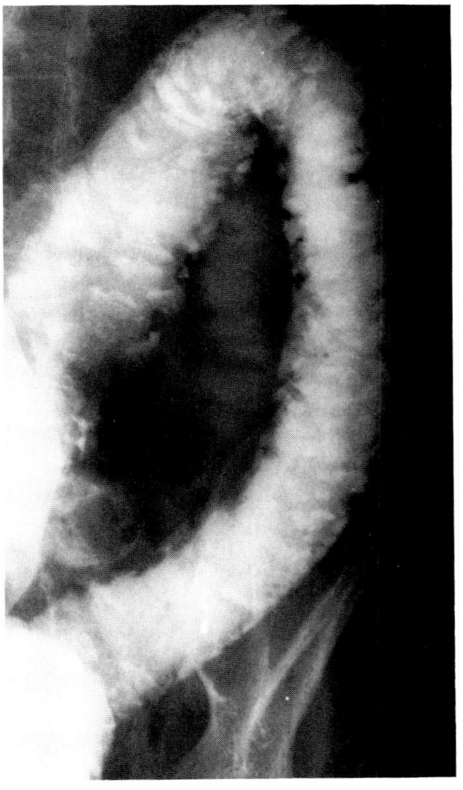

FIG. 5–26. A. Multiple lucent, ovoid islands of fibrin deposited on mucosa. Generalized shaggy appearance of colonic mucosa in the rectum, with barium tracking underneath a coalescent membrane. (Courtesy of Dr. Robert K. Zeman.)

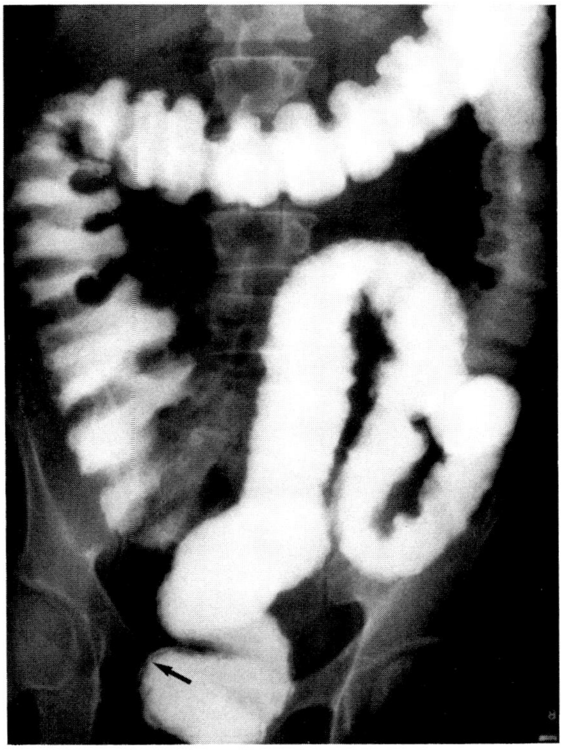

B. Lucent membrane seen in rectum *between* mucosa and lumen.

PERIAPPENDICEAL ABSCESS

Belying the principle that the diagnosis of appendicitis must be "all-or–nothing," a periappendiceal abscess confirms the existence of "chronic appendicitis," a euphemism for an inflamed yet incompletely perforated appendix with an adjacent loculated abscess. Without dispersion of intestinal contents into the peritoneal cavity, the relatively indolent symptoms of periappendiceal abscess include intercurrent fever, right lower quadrant pain and tenderness, with an occasional mass, and leukocytosis. On reflection, its radiologic manifestations (Fig. 5–27) seem perfectly logical: the abscess itself constitutes a space-occupying lesion, which deflects the ileum as it enters the ascending colon, while the cecum itself is squeezed from without, giving it an rightward-indented, occasionally conical appearance. Because the abscess is typically behind and below it, the ileum is usually pushed superiorly and anteriorly. The appendix, naturally enough, will not fill with barium; a fecalith on the plain film of a patient with a chronic periappendiceal abscess must be quite rare.

The sonogram and CT scan of the right lower quadrant are often of great help, disclosing not only a mass but a localized air-fluid level or extraluminal bubbles. Other diagnostic considerations include perforated cecal diverticulosis, amebiasis of the cecum, Crohn's disease, and, of course, a cecal or appendiceal cancer with or without perforation. The major obstruction to accurate diagnosis is the clinician's understandable refusal to recognize that appendicitis is not necessarily an acute disease. The usual compendium of peritoneal signs may be incomplete, and previous empiric management with an antibiotic may stabilize or sterilize the abscess itself. The mobility of the cecum may delay diagnosis further; the appendix and cecum can travel from right lower to right upper quadrant, and occasionally to the left upper quadrant.

Once the diagnosis of appendicitis, whether acute or chronic, is raised seriously, surgical appendectomy, with drainage of an abscess if present, seems the most conservative approach. The occasional removal of a normal appendix does not indict the physician as aggressive, as the implications of an untreated abscess potentially dissecting into the pelvis, blocking the right ureter, or inducing a portal bacteremia are ample justifications to operate. Since the removal of the appendix is so easy, a postoperative periappendiceal abscess usually implies that a purulent collection was missed at surgery or was a complication of the operation itself.

FIG. 5–27. A. I. Identation deformity on cecum, II. Separation of terminal portion of ileum from the large intestine, III. Swinging of the ileum around a radiolucency into the ascending colon, and IV. Nonfilling of appendix.
B. Fecalith visible in right lower quadrant, proximal to the barium-filled cecum.

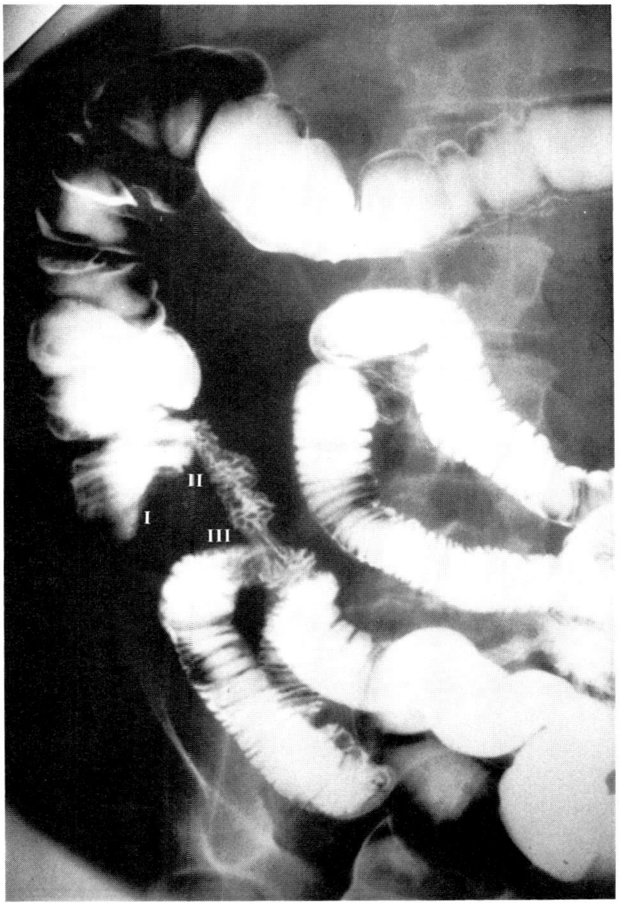

A

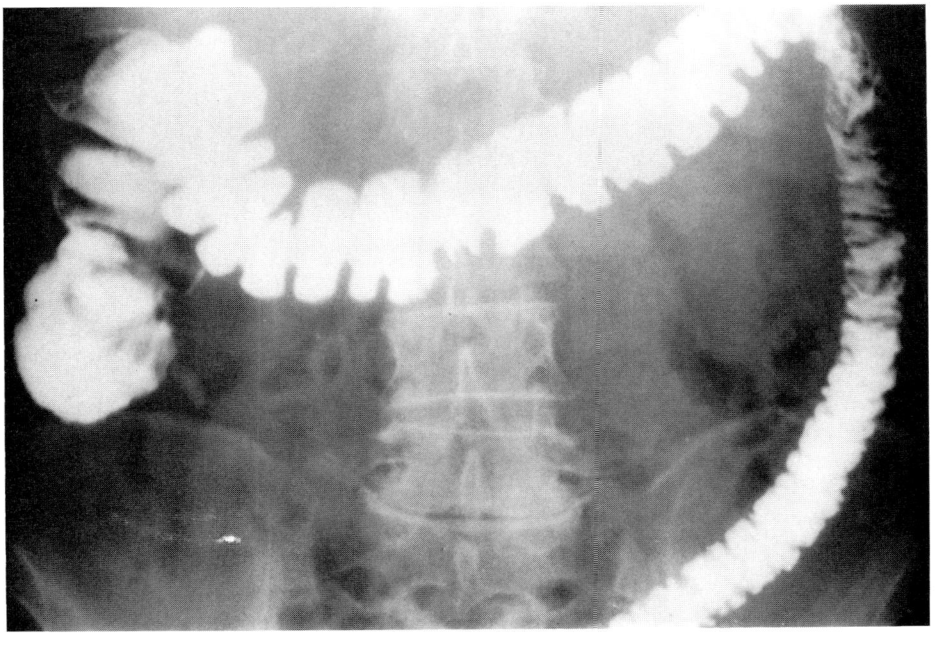

B

PNEUMATOSIS CYSTOIDES INTESTINALIS

This rare, clinically benign intestinal illness of unknown origin is manifested by multiple, adjacent, intramural, generally separate, gas-filled colonic cysts, ovoid to spherical in shape. The number of hypotheses about their development may one day approach the number of reported cases. Clearly benign, pneumatosis cystoides intestinalis is often discovered on a routine, plain abdominal film, which is sometimes performed in evaluation of painless rectal bleeding, the illness's commonest symptom. On plain film, the lesions appear as multiple radiolucencies, spherical or egg-shaped, resembling the bubbles in plastic sheet wrapping (Fig. 5–28).

A relatively frequent association with pulmonary disease (e.g., asthma, emphysema, and use of respirators) raises the possibility that some thoracic-gas access into the bowel wall is etiologic. While no intestinal infestation by gas-forming bacteria is reported, increased breath hydrogen in pneumatosis patients is noted. Secondary recurrent but low-grade pneumomediastinum and pneumoperitoneum have been described; these are generally benign and do not mandate exploratory or resection surgery, instead requiring only careful observation.

Physical examination may reveal pliable masses over the involved areas, and sigmoidoscopy or colonoscopy demonstrates a mucosa disrupted by reddened friable elevations of translucent mucosa. Since the condition is so clearly quiescent, it is clinically distinguishable from the bowel wall gas of necrotizing enterocolitis that may occur in chronically ill, immunosuppressed patients and in very young children.

Pneumatosis developing during nebulization or inhalation therapy, endotracheal intubation, or acute asthma often resolves after cessation of the specific treatment. Inhalation of 40% oxygen or use of oral broad-spectrum antibiotics effective against anaerobic bacteria (e.g., metronidazole or clindamycin) have been followed by reports of diminution or disappearance of cysts. Resection of the involved area is usually curative. An unrelated true cystic disorder of the distal bowel (colitis cystic profunda) involves entrapped mucus, not gas.

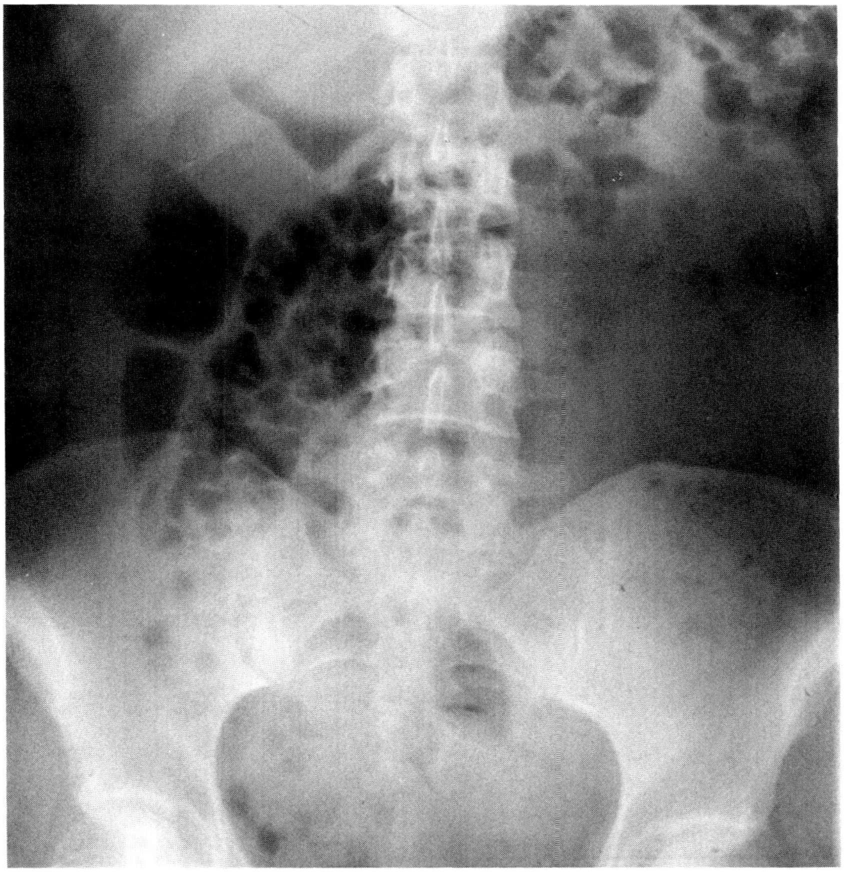

FIG. 5–28. Plain film, revealing innumerable bubble-like gas collections in wall of the ascending colon.

CHAPTER 6

A FEW FINAL THOUGHTS

1. Try to provide your radiologist with as many clues as possible regarding your (and now his) patient's history, particularly what you are looking for and where. Viewing his examination as a form of "exploratory," the serious radiologist should be armed with at least as much information as you would give your surgeon.
2. Never refrain from repeating an incomplete or inadequate x-ray study. Patients may grumble, but most will appreciate the diligence implied. Your radiologist cannot help but notice and should respond by providing you with examinations he only has to do once.
3. Limit your referrals to as few radiologists or radiology groups as possible. Learning of your insistence on quality, they will come to depend on and strive to retain your consultations, providing you and your patients with a quality "product."
4. Distrust radiologists whose reports are one- or two-line "rubber stamps," including those who employ identical computerized printout interpretations. Doctors who think they can complete a task by pressing a button will be tempted to try, and will miss diagnoses or omit important ancillary information. They are cutting intellectual and economic corners. No x ray should be thought of as routine, and no two normal x rays are identical.
5. Insist that the radiologist deliver or mail all your patient's films to you. Knowing that the examinations will be reviewed by the referring physician encourages their special first scrutiny.
6. Develop the habit of reviewing your patient's films. Accordingly, your personal office should have a bank of at least four x-ray viewboxes, preferably above a flat-topped table or cabinet. A single viewbox teetering on a windowsill or bookcase makes film reading a hardship.
7. Distrust radiologists who take too few films at fluoroscopy. A proper barium enema, for example, must contain a minimum of 8 to 10 different exposures, taken in various positions, with and without added air.
8. For patients with chronic illness, identify those films that may require comparison with future studies, and consider giving the patient custody of the films. The misfiled, lost earlier x ray, now perhaps critical to decision-making, is a tragically frequent, avoidable occurrence.
9. When an x ray reveals a clinical problem for which special surgery is required, the world is your oyster. Choose surgeons on the basis of proven excellence, and know or learn of the leaders in a field, particularly if you have reason to doubt the competence of those in your immediate area. Tourist-class airfare anywhere costs far less than a day in the average intensive care unit.

INDEX

Page numbers in *italics* refer to illustrations.